Music Therapy Research
and Practice in Medicine

T0385096

of related interest

Case Study Designs in Music Therapy
Edited by David Aldridge
ISBN 184310 140 8

Health, the Individual, and Integrated Medicine
Revisiting an Aesthetic of Health Care
David Aldridge
ISBN 1 84310 232 3

Music Therapy in Dementia Care
Edited by David Aldridge
ISBN 1 85302 776 6

Music Therapy in Palliative Care
New Voices
Edited by David Aldridge
ISBN 1 85302 739 1

Music Therapy with Children
David Aldridge
ISBN 1 85302 757 X (CD Rom)

Spirituality, Healing and Medicine
Return to the Silence
David Aldridge
ISBN 1 85302 554 2

Suicide
The Tragedy of Hopelessness
David Aldridge
ISBN 1 85302 444 9

Music Therapy Research
and Practice in Medicine
From Out of the Silence

David Aldridge

Jessica Kingsley Publishers
London and New York

First published in the United Kingdom in 1996 by
Jessica Kingsley Publishers Ltd
116 Pentonville Road
London N1 9JB, England
and
29 West 35th Street, 10th fl.
New York, NY 10001-2299, USA

www.jkp.com

Copyright ©1996 David Aldridge

Second impression 1998
Printed digitally since 2004

Library of Congress Cataloging in Publication Data
Aldridge, David
Music therapy research and practice in medicine: from out of the
silence / David Aldridge.
p. cm.
Includes bibliographical references and index.
ISBN 1-85302-296-9- (pbk.)
1. Music therapy. I Title.
[DNLM: 1. Music Therapy. WB 550 A361m 1996]
ML3920.A33 1996
615.8'5154--dc20
DNLM/DLC
for library of Congress   96-11249
CIP

British Library Cataloguing in Publication Data
Aldridge, David
Music therapy research and practice in medicine : from out
of the silence
1. Music therapy
I. Title
615.8'51'54

ISBN 1-85302-296-9

This book is dedicated to Gudrun

Acknowledgements

I would like to acknowledge the help of the numerous therapists who have contributed their time and patience in letting me into their therapeutic world. In particular I would like to thank my colleagues whose work is presented here in this book: Gudrun Aldridge, Dagmar Gustorff, and Lutz Neugebauer. My introduction to music therapy was through Rachel Verney, to whom I am forever indebted. Konrad Schily, in his understanding of the need for art as well as science in modern medicine, made it possible for me to work in Germany and thereby to develop the work to where it is today. Finally, my thanks go to the Stiftung zur Förderung der Nordoff Robbins Musiktherapie in their continuing support of both research and practice in this field.

Contents

List of Figures

List of Tables

CHAPTER ONE

Getting Started

One Tuesday morning in the spring of 1986, I set out with a colleague to visit a clinic where she was working as a music therapist. My job at the time was to assess various complementary therapies for the benefits that they would bring in general medical practice. On arriving at the clinical unit for mentally and physically handicapped adults, the unit psychologist soon made it clear to me that really I was on a fool's errand. While music therapy, he said, was an entertaining diversion, there was little that it could bring in the way of real change for the patients in his care. Being multipally handicapped, nothing further could be done for them. These people could barely communicate it seemed. However, he did say that with the appropriate techniques, their 'communication behaviour' could be modified in terms of compliance with the rules of the unit. That they should want to express themselves, or that we should wish to understand those expressions, were concepts seemingly alien to his understanding of those within his care. It was enough simply to get through the day. For those of us who have worked in such establishments, such a sentiment can be readily understood. However, I suspect that most of us at some time really would like to do more than contain those charged to our care, that our lives as custodians could be enlivened as creators.

Amongst the impulsive flights of various individuals across the room, and amidst the cacophony of moans, shrieks and whistles, it seemed almost impossible to hear oneself think, let alone sing. The psychologist could have been right in his behavioural assessment. Yet, from out of this chaos, a group of people formed, instruments were distributed, and songs were sung. Music was fun and a diversion. There was nothing wrong in that. Far from it. To laugh and sing are activities that no one should be denied, and that many of us would be pleased to achieve. But as an academic researcher in a modern medical school, what was I going to make of all this other than to echo a platitude, no matter how profound? How was I going to convince my other colleagues that this was a therapy in which we should invest our time and expertise? So far, my optimism was simply a mirror-image of the psychologist's pessimism.

Following this group activity, a young woman was selected for an individual music therapy session. Her dress hung limply on her thin body. A body that, because of her physical and mental handicaps, had aged prematurely. Although in her early twenties, she appeared to be in her forties. She could not speak, and her only utterances were high-pitched shrieks and wails. Yet, while outwardly nervous, she came to sit directly by the music therapist at the piano. The music began and her therapist improvised a song. What happened next gave the impetus to the rest of my professional working life, and is the basis of this book. The young woman began to wail in answer to the music therapist. But her wailing was in the tonality of the music being played on the piano and matched roughly the melodic form that the music therapist had sung. A dialogue had begun. Phrase for phrase, both women sang together improvising a duet. The quality of the woman's voice lost its wail. As she began to sing more freely, the timbre of her voice changed. With these changes, it became clear to me that I was witnessing an intense form of human communication, such that this person before me, who had seemed hopelessly handicapped, emerged from out of her handicap to display the person that was trapped within that body. How was I going to explain this to my colleagues? How was I going to be able to tell other practitioners, 'Let your patients sing and play; there is healing in making music'?

This book is an attempt to do just that. It is the biography of a researcher attempting to explain to himself and his colleagues the importance of music in our culture of healing. In some ways too this is the story of a scientist reconciling the artist within himself. Perhaps this act of reconciliation reflects that schism within our society whereby the rationality of science and technology threaten to run out of balance and we forget the necessity of art, dream and mythology. In the following pages, then, I shall attempt to present various grounds for using music therapy in medical practice. The book describes a journey both through the territory of music therapy practice as it is used in medical settings, but also the development of a research programme. All too often it appears that we can simply take one form of research practice and apply it to any matter that interests us as scientists. In the case of music therapy this was not so. Music therapists were quick to point out that they did not want their way of working explained away as a series of psychological responses, as a set of behavioural repertoires, as a range of physiological reactions. Yet what did they want? My question about how to inform others of the importance of this therapy, and their question about how to talk about their work with other professionals, became similar. We were searching for a way to talk about therapy that made sense to others but maintained some authenticity to the art of music itself.

Fortunately, this search for an appropriate way of doing research was not an isolated activity. In the mid-1980s there was a hot argument raging about the validity of complementary therapies in medicine. One criticism aimed at such therapies was that they were inadequately researched. My job at the time was to find, or formulate, ways of doing research that would adequately describe in a systematic way what the clinical benefits of such therapies would be. One way of finding out is to ask an expert. Although my colleagues and I were convinced that our new 'holistic' medical project at Marylebone in the centre of London was indeed a project that the world would follow, and would be held as the model for health care delivery in the twenty-first century, it was pointed out that a hospital in Germany had been working in this way for at least ten years and had the expertise we needed. It seemed to be a good idea to ask these pioneers about their research. So off I went to Germany, to the Gemeinschaftskrankenhaus Herdecke, where the practice of medicine includes various art therapies as part of the integrated treatment package.

I knew that in various other hospitals patients were referred to art therapy or music therapy or occupational therapy. But in Herdecke, clinical treatment decisions were made involving information from medical practitioners, nursing staff and the various creative arts therapists. An arts diagnosis, and an arts assessment of progress, played a significant role in treatment decisions. The creative arts therapies were truly complementary.

Such therapies must be seen in the light of a different attitude to health care in mainland Europe. In Germany, and some neighbouring countries, there has been a long tradition of 'Kur'. The 'Kur' is a time that one takes, usually on medical recommendation, at a spa town. While there is medical supervision, the treatment plan also includes eating healthily, outdoor and indoor exercise, plenty of walks in fresh air, various water activities in thermal spas, and often mud packs combined with physiotherapy. There are special 'Kur', or spa, hotels that include medical treatments. Health care is seen as an enjoyable activity, and the boundaries between hospital and hotel treatment and recreation are subtly eroded. While Herdecke is a general hospital, not a 'Kur' resort, there is an acceptance amongst people in Germany of a wide range of possible therapeutic activities and particularly amongst the patients attending this hospital. Being creative is seen as an important step on the road to recovery.

While my initial experience in Germany showed that music therapy played a significant role in general medicine, the ability to research adequately such practice was lacking still. Here too, there was no accepted research method for music therapy, and no tradition of such research. The following chapters tell the tale of this research development, the search for appropriate models and some of the findings that are pertinent to practice. Hopefully, those interested in research will see that it is not necessary to spring immediately into a full-blown research project, with a vast research budget and an active staff of scientists. It is possible to start small with our selves as the primary resources.

When I first moved to Germany, the university, to which the hospital at Herdecke was attached as a co-operating clinic, offered me a post as research consultant. While sounding rather grand, what this post really amounted to was a substantial salary, a desk with a chair, a room to work in and the freedom to write. Above all there was no pressure to produce results, for there was enough trust on the part of my employers to know that the results would come. Having arrived from a project were results were urgent, and having been hampered by a steering committee, each member of which believed he could do my job better himself, such an atmosphere of leisurely trust meant that results did indeed come quickly. Indeed trust and respect for expertise are crucial dimensions for fostering a productive research atmosphere.

The material circumstances were somewhat restricted. Five years after beginning work in Germany, I had a telephone. My office was in the corner of the former architect's hut, next to the horse stables. In winter, the heating failed regularly and the initially interestingly textured grey-green patterned walls proved to be mildew in various exotic forms. In summer, the moist darkness of the slowly rotting wood floors were an irresistible enticement for the flies from the stables. There was no research budget; being a private university we had to find our own funding. After a year, I had a computer, and three months later enough money for a printer. I could begin to write and, I hoped, to publish. The following chapters are examples of that developing work, and are presented approximately in the sequence in which they were written. In some ways I hope to present a picture of how, even within financial limitations, theoretical and clinical research can be achieved.

First comes the paper and pencil work that can be done by going out and asking questions. Second comes the basic thinking and theoretical work related to reading the material that is available, and trying to bring ideas and questions together. Third is an investigation of putting ideas into practice and seeing what happens in the clinical situation. There is no guaranteed way of success. If our idea of success is to produce a world-shattering document that will prove what we are doing is better than any other clinical approach, and infallible to criticism, then we are in all probability doomed to failure. What emerges from my experience, and particularly in the light of what my former academic colleagues said in terms of my 'throwing my career away', is that a deep commitment to finding out the truth, combined with clear presentation and a respect for both clinicians and patients, taking small steps at a time, brings success of a different nature. What is presented here, then, is a series of partial truths, glimpses of a reality that at times may be contradictory. But what remains, I hope, is the impression that I have tried to remain authentic to that impulse heard in the musical duet mentioned at the start of this chapter, to discover what it is in music that heals, and when it is pertinent to use music as therapy.

I believe that it is important also to bear in mind that invigorating feeling which many of us encounter when we first set out upon the research trail. Finding out is exciting. 'Re-searching', 'looking again', 'getting to know' are challenges to our intellectual capacities that enliven us. While our computers get faster and bigger promising an information super-highway, and we have world literature at our fingertips, such aids do not bring us knowledge. Time to think and write, access to a good library, sympathetic colleagues and supportive management are the primary resources for such work. Above all, a desire for research – to discover, not necessarily to prove – enriches a working atmosphere. There is that necessary balance between the excitement and enthusiasm of questions based on a belief in the work we are doing, and the scepticism of intellectual activity that challenges us to reveal our biases.

In 1995, we moved into the new campus building at the University of Witten Herdecke where the computer has indeed grown bigger, the printer quieter and our list of publications longer. Our students have begun to think in terms of research, and their dissertations reflect the influence of grounding ideas on empirical data collected from practice. Two colleagues have completed, and been awarded, doctoral dissertations, and a third has begun her doctoral work. Other colleagues are beginning to formulate questions that they could translate into research activities. A colleague from England who came to study with us, and then worked for a while in our team, has himself gone on to a doctoral study and produced a pioneering book about creative music therapy with adult patients (Ansdell 1995). We have developed a research service to allow other music therapists working without university or academic support access to literature and research supervision.

When no research tradition exists, it is possible to encourage a research culture that encourages practitioners to take part. However, if practitioners are to take part they must feel that research has relevance for them; either professionally in terms of qualification leading to status or promotion, or in terms of enhanced practice. What I have tried to do is not to promote research that is done by me, the researcher. My aim is that the research methodologist supports the practitioner to research his or her idea in clinical practice, such that the results are valid primarily for the practitioner, and his or her colleagues, and then to see what wider relevance such studies can have. Research that remains as a dissertation, or even a report, standing on a shelf gathering dust is a waste of time and money. Such research can be dusted off now and again to rebuff questions about academic validity; but if that research remains unpublished, the work has little chance of being considered for use in practice. What I have tried to do is to foster a climate of clinical research that produces material pertinent to the daily practice of the music therapist as clinician. That this practice must be focused on the patient is a central tenet of our music therapy approach.

Not all research is inward-looking. It is necessary to establish a publishing career, either as an individual or as an institute for music therapy. In our institute, we have to generate our own funds and articles that are published, in terms of peer-reviewed professional journals, help us to establish our credibility when we ask funding organizations for money.

A further positive benefit of written publications is that when we work with new referring clinicians we can often give them a written account of what we do in practice. While case studies presented on audio- or videotape are initially convincing, it is the combination of personally presented case-material and published material that convinces potential sponsors, referring clinicians and, in terms of health insurance, the third-party funding agencies. If such work is published in a peer-reviewed journal, then we have gone some way to establishing our credibility with a wider group of professionals. In some ways this is a form of external validation where the research work we are doing is examined as being of a standard acceptable to the profession in which we work, and with whom we work. One of the strategies of our publishing has been to submit papers to music therapy journals and medical journals. I knew that if we could build bridges between our work and the practice of medicine, by developing a language that could be understood by other clinicians, then we had gone some way to promoting the wider practice of music therapy. By publishing in established peer-reviewed journals we have ensured also that the contents of our work appear in electronic databases and are thereby available to a broader readership. This means that our hypotheses regarding the work with Alzheimer's disease, for example, are being investigated by colleagues worldwide from other disciplines.

Research has a benefit for teaching too. We educate young musicians to become music therapists. Our research feeds into the practical and theoretical work of our postgraduate study-course. Not only are we preparing future music therapists, some of whom I hope will want to do research, but we are refining the practice of music therapy itself to understand what works and why. This understanding is a process of unfolding. It take place over time, for the individuals involved, but also for us as a group working together. In recent years, various national and international groups have come together to share their research experiences, and it appears that a new era is beginning where music therapists are beginning to co-operate by bringing their various research skills and expertise together (Bunt 1994; Wheeler 1995).

In the coming chapters, the reader will find an emphasis on music therapy research as it appears in medical settings such as hospitals or clinics. While music therapy is also practised in other educational and social settings, this book concentrates on my limited perspective. The reason for this decision is that the group I was working with had a need to communicate within the context of the hospital in which they worked. While we now work in several hospitals and rehabilitation clinics, those settings are still predominantly medical.

A Research Strategy for a Small Institute

In January 1987 the research work began in earnest. The aim of the initial part of the project was to establish specific research strategies for music therapists in the hospital where they were working. Such an approach is a practical reflection of the method recommended by McNiff (1987), which suggests that we must pursue research and scholarship to serve both clinical practice and higher education. In this case the practice was in the music therapy clinics, and the higher education was the training of our students.

My intention was to devise a way of researching into the phenomena of a *particular creative arts therapeutic* approach (music therapy) in a way that generated exciting ideas pertinent to the *practitioners* (in this case music therapists) and their colleagues, and that was applicable to the *institutional* context (the hospital). This way of working, while meeting specific needs, also considers the ecological niche in which those needs reside. Particular research interventions are designed to 'fit' into the broader setting of the hospital community in which they are applied. Such a fit is made not only on the practical grounds of clinical practice and patient access, but also in terms of philosophy.

I want to propose here that there is such a phenomenon as an *ecology* of ideas. When we consider the healing process we must incorporate the many activities that contribute to our health. Orthodox and complementary medical practitioners are currently seeking ways of carrying out research that addresses the needs of clinicians and considers the whole person. This project keeps such clinical and holistic perspectives in mind. This work was also happening at a time when other research commentators in the creative arts were advocating broad research perspectives that included qualitative and quantitative data. An ecology of ideas, then, will contain ideas from colleagues both near and distant, from patients, from students and hospital practitioners. What the doctor thinks, what the patient believes, what the therapist plays, what the spouse expects and what the hospital promotes have ramifications for each other. Researching such a milieu will be more likely to resemble clinical anthropology than laboratory experimentation (Aldridge and Pietroni 1987).

The setting

The general hospital at Herdecke is a large district general hospital serving the immediate community. It has inpatient and outpatient facilities. The underlying philosophy of the hospital is anthroposophical and based on the teachings of Rudolf Steiner (Steiner 1970). While our music therapy approach is not anthroposophical, in that it is not based on Steiner's teaching, we had to take into account the ethos of the institution in which we were working.

Anthroposophical medicine is an extension of orthodox medical practice. Its basic tenets are:

○ Each person is a unique individual and treatment decisions must recognize this individuality.

○ Scientific, artistic and spiritual insights, which recognize the whole person, need to be applied together in our therapeutic endeavours.

○ Life has meaning and purpose. If these qualities are lost then there is a deterioration of health.

○ Illness may provide opportunities for positive change and new balance in a person's life.

Creative music therapy had been an important part of therapeutic approaches since the hospital began. As a discipline it had always been part of the medical faculty of the University of Witten Herdecke, of which Herdecke hospital is a co-operating clinic, and enjoyed the co-operation of medical practitioners. For a researcher it was an ideal virgin environment to formulate research strategies. There was no established way of researching. The only stipulation was that the methodology maintained the integrity of music therapy and did not attempt to impose a restrictive methodology on the practice.

Our approach is based upon, and an extension of, Nordoff–Robbins' *Creative Music Therapy* (Nordoff and Robbins 1977). It is an approach, as the name suggests, that actively involves the patient in making music creatively. The therapist encourages the patient to improvise music using percussion and tuned percussion instruments, by singing with the patient, and by encouraging the patient to play with the therapist at the piano. No attempt is made to interpret the music psychotherapeutically. The process of creatively improvising music, and the development of a musical relationship between therapist and patient, are seen as the vehicles of therapy. Visual arts and eurhythmy are also practised within this hospital. Health is seen as an activity that occurs within an environment of creativity.

A strategy for research was gradually developed with music therapy colleagues. Strategy indicates a general approach to the research campaign in the hospital setting and was a statement of intent. More detailed and particular research designs were to be developed in later years, as we will see in the following chapters. In these later designs it is possible to state particular research criteria of patient selection, variable definition, experimental control, instrumental measures, and methods of analysis.

In the preliminary stages I met the five hospital music therapy staff collectively, and then singly each month for six months. I also went out into the hospital and interviewed those senior medical practitioners who worked in teams with music therapists. These interviews were then written up as an internal paper and submitted departmentally as well as to those previously interviewed. All practitioners involved were then invited to a common meeting and asked for their comments about the work so far. This meant that the work stayed close to the comments of the practitioners directly or peripherally involved.

From these early discussions it was possible to see what common areas of interest were available to build on as foundations for the future development of the institute for music therapy.

Areas of research

Three main themes, centred around physiological work, clinical application studies and theoretical work, were recommended for the research in the music therapy department (see Table 1.1). These emerged from the discussions with the doctors and therapists in the hospital who were asked directly what they wanted to see from the music therapy department and how much they were willing to co-operate, and from extensive talks with the music therapists. A fourth theme relating to publication was added as the expectation of the university that we would forge an academic reputation within Europe.

A significant feature in developing the research ideas was to get music therapists to present their taped work to the researcher, and to say what questions were raised by that work. All the discussions focused on clinical practice, not idealized abstractions about research. One of the difficulties of research until then – and this was reflected in the field of complementary medicine in general – was knowing where to start. Some practitioners wanted to debate the very concept of research itself, an activity that repeated unproductively what they had been doing for the last ten years. While this debate may be necessary sometimes, my position was that until any research had actually been realized, the arguments surrounding the nature of research would be so far removed from reality as to be useless. Furthermore, of the clinicians involved, whether music therapist or medical practitioners, none had had a training in research methodology. There was a strange situation where music therapists would insist that only musicians with a specialist training in music therapy could do clinical work, yet the same therapists would assume anyone could do research regardless of their expertise and academic preparation. However, by taking a pragmatic stance of 'doing research' and questioning that research as part of the cycle of inquiry, practitioners were involved in the research agenda and saw it as being relevant to their daily work.

One of the difficulties facing music therapists is that although they have no established research tradition, they often know what kind of research they do not want to do. This rebuttal of formal clinical research is based on a rejection of methodologies psychologists or medical practitioners have previously attempted to impose on music therapy practice. However, what some therapists appear to have learned is a litany of rejection towards structured studies, some of which appear to be based on the argument stemming from qualitative researchers in their rejection of quantitative work. This argument has historically a political base where professional music therapy organizations have struggled to establish their credibility. In establishing their credibility, it has been necessary to discredit the work of others as being too deterministic or, contrarily, too vague. What few therapists have done is actually to complete any research themselves.

What we sometimes forget in the high-mindedness of theoretical discussion is that our theories are probably more extreme than the practice. What I was trying to do was first to establish a culture of systematic clinical observation that mirrored the systematic observations found in the music therapy practice. It must be mentioned here that all the music therapists audiotape their therapy sessions, and make an index of the sessions afterwards, so there was already an established basis of 'good practice' regarding documentation.

The general intent of this work was to develop a common structure for single case designs such that individual analysis and comparative analysis could be made. Music therapists in the hospital were working with individuals, and were referred a series of individuals with similar problems by physicians. For example, particular therapists were referred patients who had chronic bowel disease, AIDS, cancer, anorexia nervosa, and neurological problems, as we shall read in later chapters. The initial session for therapy was one of assessment, and we had hoped that a common format for assessment could be negotiated between music therapists to allow comparison between single case studies. These therapists could have then compared their assessments and notes of the therapeutic process with notes made by other therapists of patients having the same problem. This proved to be unrealistic as the patients themselves were so varied, even though they had a similar disease in common. Indeed, the classification of patients by disease, while maybe necessary for the practice of conventional medicine, seems unbelievably crude in terms of the creative therapies. What emerged was the idea that in music therapy, being creative may not have anything to do with the illness, but it may have something very important to do with regaining health. Categories of illness were going to tell us little about becoming healthy.

Three themes for future research were identified.

PHYSIOLOGICAL
The aim of this area was to discover the physiological implications of improvising music with a therapist. As the music therapy department shared its accommodation with the department of physiology, and the professor of physiology was himself a musician, it made sense to co-operate, bringing together mutual interests and expertise.

The questions to be asked were:

1. What changes occur during the process of playing music together – (a) in the individuals concerned, and (b) in the interaction between patient and therapist?

2. What are the implications of those changes – (a) for the patient, and (b) for the course of the therapy?

Table 1.1 Phases of the research plan

	Physiological work	Clinical applications	Theoretical work	Publications
Phase One	establish physiological criteria of change in therapist/patient interaction	single case studies, develop working methods appropriate to a hospital setting	literature reviews, theory development	case studies and position papers
Phase Two	refine hypotheses and test out methods, establish experimental method	develop working relationships with the hospital staff, attempt feasibility study of co-operative work	collect case examples from recorded work	case studies and clinical outcome material
Phase Three	continue work, identify clinical problems and refine hypotheses	look for larger scale clinical trials, establish contacts with other clinical groups	develop theory and refine techniques assessment	develop database, research methods and literature service, produce collected works and CD-ROMs for teaching and research

Note: None of these areas of work was exclusive, and each part informed the other. For the sake of practicality and to avoid confusion, it may help to think of three areas: physiological working, teaching/theory work and the clinical case studies. Not all therapists wanted to concentrate on all three areas. The clinical case study work and the physiological work provided a framework for more refined and formal research studies. These studies informed, and were informed by, the developing theory. This approach gave the work both conceptual and practical coherence. Knowledge gained in this way had meaning for the practitioners and retained the integrity of therapeutic practice, which was enlivened by the rigour of systematic observation.

There has been a considerable amount of research work on the influence of receptive music on physiological parameters (see Chapter 3). However, there had been little work on the interaction between the physiological parameters of therapist and patient when playing music together. This investigation of mutual influence in therapy was potentially of great benefit in understanding therapist–patient interaction in contexts other than music therapy.

The initial part of this programme monitored the heart rate of the patient and the heart rate of the therapist, and the recorded playing of the therapist on the piano and the playing of the patient on a drum. These parameters were recorded in real time onto a videotape. Each interaction was structured as a series of episodes: rest, playing a composed work, and creative improvised playing. In some ways this was an attempt to monitor *the physiology of creative dialogues*, a feature many wanted to include in our clinical practice, and which a colleague, Lutz Neugebauer (1992), was later to write up as his doctoral thesis.

The reasons for choosing heart rate were that:

(1) It was a relatively easy parameter to measure and observe.

(2) It indicated important aspects of listening and the activity of communication.

(3) It was a parameter acceptable to medical scientists in the wider community with whom we were attempting to promote a dialogue, and

(4) There was also an immediate relevance for patients suffering with heart disease.

THEORETICAL

This work focused on the audiotaped work of the therapy sessions. Careful systematic observation based on recorded data, which can be made accessible to another clinician/researcher, is a significant feature of any research approach and emphasizes the rigour of music therapists.

The questions to be asked were:

(1) How do music therapists talk about their work?

(2) What are the questions music therapists ask of their own therapeutic endeavour?

(3) How can music therapy with adult patients be documented in an acceptable way for the music therapists to exchange and compare clinical understandings as a group?

(4) Can some terms be defined in a way to form a common vocabulary for talking about music therapy with peers and colleagues – a music therapy lexicon, for example?

(5) How does therapy work?

(6) What happens during the course of therapy?

(7) What is the relationship between the music and the patient as a whole person?

(8) Can a patient's state of health or illness be heard in the way in which he or she improvises music; and if so, how could this be demonstrated?

These questions were concerned with *internal* validity, that is, what was valid within the thinking of the music therapists.

CLINICAL

The clinical work concentrated on understanding outcomes of practice and questions about the nature of therapeutic change. It was carried out within the context of the hospital wards and in co-operation with interested doctors and therapists.

The questions to be asked were:

(1) What changes during the process of therapy in terms of the patient's problem?

(2) How is this change recognized by the music therapist?

(3) How can this change be communicated to other professional practitioners?

(4) What is evidence of therapeutic change for the patient?

(5) What are the clinical criteria of the referring practitioners in terms of patient referral, therapeutic change, and clinical prognosis?

(6) How can observed changes be documented and correlated with those of other practitioners and family members?

These questions were concerned with *external* validity, that is, what is valid to those practitioners with whom the therapists were working.

It is important to note that in this approach the process of therapy and outcome are not separate activities. It is convenient to consider them as separate but this does not happen in clinical practice. Similarly, clinician and researcher work together, not separately.

The biased researcher

Perhaps before the book really begins it remains necessary for me to declare my interest in music. That the researcher reveals a bias by the selection of his topic is a truism reflected here. Whether this bias is a strength or a weakness, the reader must decide. As a child I was brought up by my grandparents. My grandmother sang all day long. My grandfather was a professional musician and employed by the local colliery to conduct their brass band and teach budding musicians. I was a readily available, if singular, audience for his theories and speculations, and he spared me, even as an infant, no respite from my birthright to the world of music. Music was blown into me from an early age. Hearing the orchestral works of French impressionistic composer transposed live for brass instruments was an experience that perhaps many parents would shrink away from inflicting upon their children. However, for a child about to start school, the imperatives of timbre and its ramification for melody, and the architecture of harmony, were a world of wonders achieved not through books but through listening.

I began this introduction by declaring that hearing a seemingly hopelessly handicapped young woman communicate gave me the impulse to research further in this field. Apart from the indignity that all of us feel in the face of our own inarticulacy, I was annoyed by the pessimism of the psychologist that day who could not face the simple fact before his eyes. His own frustration about being unable to achieve clinical change had deafened him to the potentials of this woman locked within her body. We can handicap others further within their own handicap by the way in which we respond to them. Yet what was apparent for me was that this woman's singing, despite her handicap, was a communication. This communication reminded me that the possibility is always there for us to realize a hidden potential. Our inarticulacy is only in particular realms. We too can find a way of realizing our potential in the world such that it can find a form of expression.

In these pages, I argue that music is the end and means of such expression. That this musical expression has a benefit for our health I hope to demonstrate through the use of the written word that, like written music, always has an element missing. For a man in a post-modern society, it is also pertinent to mention that I too was struggling to accept and express the feminine within myself, and to reconcile my own inner feelings of inarticulacy and handicap as the shadow of an outer, worldly display of success and achievement. That inarticulacy should assume such a role in my own research interests betrays the so-called neutrality of my approach. However, I would argue that this element is always present in our choice of research topics, and the attempted neutrality of many research endeavours is an actual denial of a potent force of knowing inherent in the endeavour.

While science represents an important force of rationality within our culture, where ideas are contained within given bounds and gain their validity when they assume an accepted form, the activity of research proposed here resembles the form of improvised music, where something new is sought, where new forms can emerge. Research from this perspective is not science, it is jazz. Just as we have classical music in our culture, which is formed and beautiful, there is also the notion of jazz, which is also beautiful but demands the new.

The Politics of Self and the Language of Therapy

There is, however, a basic dilemma in researching the clinical practice of a music therapist. Some therapists will say that they are not to be judged. They are artists, and what they do should be heard as a mutual musical activity without concern for the impact on the problem that the patient has. Such a view seems to me to be as blind, or perhaps as deaf, as those researchers who want to reduce the music to a series of responses. People when they are suffering, when they are indeed patients in the context of a clinic, expect that what is done with them under the label of 'therapy' will have some estimated benefit for them. When treated, or after undergoing therapy, we expect something to change, and this should be evaluated. This is not to say that the evaluation of change should solely be in medical or psychological terms. However, once we embark upon a clinical practice, or call ourselves in some way a therapist, then we must open ourselves up in some way to an assessment of what we do. Such evaluation can incorporate the view of the person with whom we have worked in the therapist–patient relationship. Change can be described in music therapy terms, and there lies the rub. While music therapists have an established language of musical terms, the language used for describing therapy is rarely debated and seldom accepted.

When we come to interpret what takes place in therapy we can rely, in part, upon artistic terms. Creativity is a process which exists within a framework of the aesthetic. The status of health is the striving for creative realization. Within the individual the ability for self-regulation is based upon a repertoire of improvisational possibilities. While it is essential to have a standard repertoire of responses for everyday life, it is also necessary to improvise solutions when necessary. This is true of the biological, as it is of the musical, as it is of the existential. There exists a balance between stability and change; both the conventional and unconventional lie in a healthy tension. For example, the music therapist talks about the patient's ability to maintain the logic of a sustained melodic line alone. For the patient, as we will read in Chapter Ten, this is her melody according to her inner logic. We can assume that this is a part of therapeutic change in that the patient finds and expresses her own inner logic. Yet this individual expression is contained within the context of a relationship. The personal and the social are balanced. Health is a statement about an ecology.

The European tradition influenced Western post-war culture both in the arts and psychotherapy. Such a culture has emphasized the individual as self and recognized a need for personal expression. What we are attempting to address in our work is the existential quality of the arts where the self finds expression. This stands in contrast to the scientific movement which seeks to understand the individual according to the group. However, as we know from twentieth-century history, the cultural tradition that enlivens self-expression can be used for both good and evil. The expression of the self unfettered by social concerns can lead to tyranny. So too, the music therapist who says listen to my work as a work of art alone, without concern for its clinical relevance, imposes an individual tyranny apart from indulging in solipsism.

The classification of activities is a political act: it is a way of saying 'See this activity in this way'. The feminist movement has alerted us to the right to call our own activities by the names we give them. When we come together to establish a united voice in the healing arts we must be aware that we are making a political status within the field of healing. We are saying that what we do is not psychology and not science but artistic, and that the terms which we use have their own legitimacy. Our task then is to negotiate those terms among ourselves. While we may differentially express creativity, improvisation, form, structure, dynamic, time and space within our own therapeutic modalities, we do need to learn a language based on these concepts such that we can maintain a unified discourse about what we do. This is not a new endeavour within the tradition of Western art, particularly European art, and it should be possible to extend this discourse into the realm of therapy. At the same time, we have to locate that discourse within the realm of health care delivery if we are working as therapists in medical settings. In the following chapters I hope to show that music therapists can maintain a dialogue with practitioners from other persuasions while maintaining their identities as creative arts therapists. What makes this process difficult is that music therapists are indeed artists and therapists, and it is this duality that lies at the root of the dilemma.

The role of the aesthetic in healing

At the centre of this therapeutic work is the creative art in performance or composition. The creative expression is not the same as cathartic expression. Whereas personal emotive expression may be the first step in the process of healing, the continuing therapeutic process is to give articulation to a broad range of human feelings. While passionately playing music can lead to an emotional catharsis it lacks the intensity of form which articulates the whole range of personal aspiration. When we introduce form and order into the creative act then we promote a higher form of human articulation. This is the process of healing; the escape from emotive fragmentation to the creative act of becoming whole. Our inner lives in all their depth and richness are given coherence and presented externally as created form. In this way we help our patients to articulate their inner realities as beautiful; this is the manifestation of the aesthetic.

We have a cultural tradition within twentieth-century modern art where music, poetry, art, drama and dance are considered together. This was prefigured by the late nineteenth-century movement in German culture which also expressed the role of the healing arts as a necessary antidote to the rigorous soulless advance of technological medicine. The international movement known as Expressionism, which began in the early part of this century and was based on those nineteenth-century Romantic ideas, embraced concepts of personal liberation and placed a passionate emphasis on heart and spirit. It stood against the disintegration of communities and the personal isolation caused by increasing urbanization and industrialization (Kellner 1988).

These ideas are still available to us today. The art of healing is a practice in which we can participate as creative arts therapists from our own cultural foundations. Perhaps the time, like the idea, has come when we can articulate our own healing purposes for those with whom we work in a common language.

Round and round, the cycle of research

The central message of this book is that in music therapy, research has to be done. Research is a performed act. Research is jazz. Research is not the Cartesian 'I think, therefore I am', but 'I do, therefore I am'. We have to try it out, rather than sit around for ever discussing what will be the best way. We can only find the best way by trying it out to see what works, and then comparing our best way with others with common purposes. This is not to advocate blind undirected activity. We have to go to theory and the previous writings of practitioners and researchers. This guides our practice. We produce a strategy and then try it out. From this trial, we have results that modify, either supporting or contradicting our original thoughts. From these results, and the ideas of others, we can begin the research cycle anew by submitting our renewed ideas to scrutiny. This is the process of re-search, 'looking again'. In the following pages, the reader will see how thoughts have been tried out in practice, based on the experiences and practices of music therapists (Chapter Two), relating this work to a broader field in the published literature (Chapter Three), and then going further by suggesting a schema for the next stage in the cycle.

CHAPTER TWO

Health as Performance

This chapter is an effort to make a connection between the perception and the performance of music, and the implications that this may have for health when music is used as a form of therapy. What I will propose is that becoming healthy is itself a creative performance. Rather than accept the Cartesian statement 'I think, therefore I am', what I am proposing is 'I do, therefore I am', thus shifting the emphasis from a separation of cognition and behaviour to a unified notion of creative performance. Performance is pertinent when the arts are considered as therapies. We already have within our Western culture an acceptance of the dramaturgical concept of human behaviour. The world is really a stage upon which we play. If the arts are to do with the successful creation of a performed reality, then such creative activity can enable the analogous activity of successfully performed health.

In modern times, health is no longer a state of not being sick. Individuals are choosing to become healthy and, in some cases, declare themselves as pursuing the activity of being well. This change, from attributing the status 'being sick' to engaging in the activity of 'becoming well', is a reflection of a modern trend whereby individuals are taking the definition of themselves into their own hands rather than relying upon an identity being imposed by another. Being recognized as a 'healthy' person is, for some, an important feature of a modern identity. While personal active involvement has always been present in health care maintenance and prevention, in that people have strategies of distress management (Aldridge 1994), a new development appears to be that 'being healthy', being a 'creative' person, being a 'musical' person and being a 'spiritual' person are significant factors in the composition of an individual's 'lifestyle'. Rather than strategies of personal health management in response to sickness, we see an *assemblage* of activities like dietary practices, exercise practices, aesthetic practices, psychological practices, spiritual practices designed to promote health and prevent sickness. These activities are incorporated under the rubric of 'lifestyle' and sometimes refer to the pursuit of 'emotional well-being', as well as concerns for the work–home environment (Furnham 1994). Furthermore, such a lifestyle is intimately bound up with how a person chooses to define him or herself. Thus I am arguing here that modern identities are constructed. Although such identities are bound up with cultural values, they focus primarily on the body. What we need to take heed of as health care professionals is that this 'body work', this embodiment of culture, this corporeality of expression, is a pleasurable activity, often recreational and not simply medical.

The definition of health, who is to define what health is and who is to be involved in healing is not a new activity. Such issues are raised at times of transformation when the old order is being challenged (Aldridge 1991c). In post-modern society, orthodoxies are challenged, and as truth is regarded as relative with few fixed authorities to turn to, identities can be composed from a palette of cultural alternatives.

Health is also appearing in modern society as a commodity. Far from being a simple object, health is concerned with social relationships representing personal worth, market values, existential principles and theological niceties. However, the location of health in modern terms is often within the body, albeit paying lip-service to the mind. People are demanding recognition that they play an active role in their own health care, and that some can act as lay health-care practitioners. Indeed, before we ask a doctor or any licensed practitioner we have been through varying cycles of self-care, asking family and friends or just hoping that the problem will go away. This shift away from authority and orthodoxy towards democratization and choice reflects a change from a belief in the certainties of science and religion to a relativist position where people literally 'make up' their own minds and work on their bodies; that is, we construct our own identities.

By concentrating on the modern sense of self, there is a continuing focus on the body. Our corporeality is both objectified and subjectified, in that the body has become the major site of subjectivity and agency (Waterhouse 1993). 'Bodywork', a term that occurs in numerous complementary medical approaches, locates cultural disciplines within a particular site – the body.

While body size and shape are aspects of personal identity, it is how the body is interpreted, the aesthetics of health beliefs that play an important role in forming identity. Such beliefs play an active part in how we recognize illness and what therapy form we choose (Aldridge 1992). Meaning provides a bridge between cultural and physiological phenomena. The diagnosis of a medical complaint is also a statement about personal identity (van der Geest 1994) and the stigma that may be attached to such an identity (Crossley 1995), as we saw in the introduction. Symbolic meanings are the loci of power whereby illness is explained and controlled. Definition of health occurs in a cultural context.

It is clear that in our modern cultures several belief systems operate in parallel, and can co-exist. Patients have begun to demand that their understandings about health play a role in their care, and practitioners too are seeking complementary understandings. Health itself is a state subject to social and individual definition. What counts as healthy is dependent upon cultural norms. Health and disease are not fixed entities but concepts used to characterize a process of adaptation to meet the changing demands of life and the changing *meanings* given to living. Negotiating what counts as healthy is a process we are all involved in, as are the forms of treatment, welfare and care which we choose to accept as adequate or satisfactory (Aldridge 1990).

Spickard (1994) reminds us that modern people do not merely accept the identities passed down by authorities. Instead, they construct their identities from various sources. Modern identity is eclectic. As in the age of Romanticism, when revolution demanded a new way of being, the primacy of the perceiver is once more being emphasized. Subjectivity becomes paramount, on the one hand reifying the individual, but on the other hand running the risk that the individual will become isolated. Indeed, while post-modernism is perhaps itself characterized by a revolt against authority and tends towards self-referentiality, its very eclecticism leaves the individual valued but exhausted of significance – what Gergen (1991) refers to as 'the saturated self'. Brewster-Smith (1994) suggests that the inflated potential for self-hood dislocated from traditional values increases the potential for despair.

The notion of 'lifestyle' also appears to be important in describing modern approaches to health care use and its delivery. The self is not an assemblage of functional components, but a unified style of behaviour (Dreyfus 1987). Rather than there being a human nature, the self-interpreting practice of being human enables us to have varying natures or various repertoires. In this way our lives have the potential to become a work of art in that our identities are constructed and maintained each day (Aldridge 1989). The activity of healing is concerned not with restricting us to a one-dimensional sense of being according to an accepted and orthodox world-view, but a possibility of interpretation of the self as new.

Individuals, however, make claims about their personal identity to someone else to whom they matter; that is, in interaction. Claiming to be a well, fulfilled, empowered, artistic or spiritual person, is a way of presenting self that will elicit a response from others. Schwalbe (1993) interprets this action of deciding which identity to present, and of how we present ourselves, as one of moral agency. In modern descriptions of alternative healing, it is the body that is the stage for the interaction of the self and its interaction with culture.

The Expressive Body: Music as Identity

I want to introduce here the idea that the dynamic interplay of maintaining our personal identity is an expressive activity akin to improvising music. Indeed some young people do regard themselves against a background that is musical, and some people refer to themselves as being 'musical' (Ruud 1995). An extension of the understanding is the notion of *being* as it is characterized by the tradition of phenomenological philosophy, which looks towards 'being in the world' as a unified experience. This phenomenological approach sees a correlation between musical form and biological form. By regarding the identity of a person as a musical form that is continually being composed in the world, a surface appears on which to project our understanding of a person as a physiological and cultural being. The thrust of this endeavour is to view people as 'symphonic' rather than 'mechanical'. By considering how persons come into the world as whole creative beings one can speculate on their potential for health and well-being.

The perception of music

As Dennis Fry (1971) wrote:

> In the case of music there is also continuously interaction between the physical character of the musical stimulus and its physiological and psychological effects so that a more thorough study of music would demand at least the combining of a physical, physiological and psychological approach. Modern science has relatively little information about the links between physics, physiology and psychology and is certainly not in a position to specify how the effects are related in music, but most scientists would recognize here a gap in scientific knowledge and would not want to deny the fact of a connection. (p. 1)

The problem in understanding the perception of music is inherent too in understanding personal health. Health is complex, yet how is one to make a unified sense of the complexity that avoids fragmentation and reduction? Furthermore, how can one begin to understand qualitative aspects of personal life as they are expressed in terms of hope, joy, and beauty, which complement increasingly sophisticated quantitative knowledge of the human body?

Although there have been many attempts to describe the process underlying the perception of music there has been little success in presenting any satisfactory explanation. The perception is not limited solely by the acuity of the ear (Longuet-Higgins 1979) and all that impinges on the listener, but is achieved in combination with the conceptual structure imposed by the listener. In this way the knowledge of the phenomenon is intimately linked with the phenomenon itself. Both the knower and the known are part of the same process. Perception in this sense is a holistic strategy.

Much scientific research into the perception of music has concentrated on those aspects that can be measured quantitatively. In this way nature is organized according to the concepts that are imposed on it. This is the analytic mode of consciousness that is predominantly a product of the verbal intellectual mind (Bortoft 1986) where phenomena are represented by number, and variables in equations are represented by quantities.

This chapter attempts to demonstrate the need for a phenomenological understanding that is isomorphic with the medium of music itself; a holistic consciousness that is qualitative, non-verbal, and participatory appears in the very phenomenon of music. What is more, the element of participation by the knower speaks directly to the aspect of music as performance, an aspect that is sadly neglected by many researchers who reduce research into the perception of music to a restricted range of received sounds.

Heidegger (1962) emphasized the intuitive element in the comprehension of phenomena. When music is heard, the phenomenon becomes its own explanation. It is that which shows itself – in itself. Perhaps one can begin to understand people, as they come into the world, as music, that is, composed as a whole.

The explanatory idea of a 'frame of reference' is a common theme among a number of writers referring to musical perception and brain function (Longuet-Higgins 1979, 1982; Safranek, Koshland and Raymond 1982; Steedman 1977; Walker and Sandman 1979). Walker (1979) suggests an 'Ursatz' (the essential underlying principle) to music that is an all-embracing thought unifying the music and giving a musical structure accessible to analysis. However, he also states that this musical structure is ultimately unknowable, that is, beyond analysis. In this explanation lies the perennial difficulty of seeking a unifying explanation by an analysis into parts. Somehow that which is intuitively sought is lost in the process of description.

What results is a statement that what is sought is unknowable, rather than a questioning of the analytic method of knowing. This situation also prevails in the understanding of personal health.

According to the philosophy of empiricism, knowledge of the world is gleaned through experience. This knowledge comes through the senses. However, there is more to this sensory knowledge than meets the ear. There is always a non-sensory factor involved, that of cognitive perception, the dimension of the mind. This cognitive perception is a process of organization where meaning is imposed upon what is heard. In this way a seemingly meaningless ground of sound is given meaning. To perceive then is to give meaning to what is heard, an act of identity. However, the non-sensory process of cognition is transparent, or rather silent, and appears as if hearing were solely a sensory experience. The process of discovery in science is also one of the perception of meaning. What appears to be empirical is indeed cognitive.

If the phenomenon of music is considered as a unified whole the question arises whether this unity is imposed on the senses by the mind, or whether it is the phenomenon itself that is a whole. To a great extent organizational frameworks are imposed on experience; hence there are descriptions that call for a framework of reference in the perception of rhythm and of melody. However, there is a danger of being blinded to this imposed organization and thus to believe that this is the way the phenomenon really is.

Once an attempt is made to synthetically reproduce the act of musical perception, the framework analogy is seen as limited. Longuet-Higgins' (1979, 1982) careful and inspiring work demonstrates the utility of a frame of reference approach using tempo and metre for the perception of rhythm. This approach fails, as he remarks, when it is understood how a particular choice of phrasing affects the rhythm. Furthermore, the perception of atonal and arrhythmic music is still a mystery to analytical methods. Yet one can hear and play arrhythmically and atonally.

However, there is an approach to understanding phenomena as unified wholes. The roots of this approach are in the work of Goethe's scientific consciousness and the work of Franz Brentano (Bortoft 1986). Both of these men were to be influential in the development of phenomenology. Goethe perceived the wholeness of the phenomena not as imposed by the mind but by a conscious act of experience. This experience could not be reduced to an intellectual construction in terms of the way the phenomena are organized. Bortoft (1986) uses the following example to explain this change of consciousness:

> if we watch a bird flying across the sky and put our attention into seeing flying, instead of seeing a bird which flies (implying a separation between an entity 'bird' and an action 'flying' which it performs), we can experience this in the mode of dynamical simultaneity as one whole event. By plunging into seeing flying we find that our attention expands to experience this moment as one whole which is its own present moment. (p.31)

In this phenomenological approach sounds are heard as sensory information and as a unified experience, which is music as consciousness. How then can personal health be perceived as a unified experience?

Language as music

> Thus feelings lose nothing by not being expressed. Perhaps they even gain in sincerity and intensity the less they are verbalized...there is a fundamental communication which embraces all forms of existence and which, because of its immediacy, must abandon the medium of words. (Herrigel 1988, p.26)

Whether or not music is a language is a running debate through the literature relating to the perception of music. Morley (1981) insists that music is a form of communication analogous to speech in that it has cadences and punctuation. Perhaps the restructuring of the primacy of language over music to suggest that language is a form of music may be more enlightening. It could be that speech is analogous to music and that the musical components of speech are abdicated in favour of the literal content.

Many of us in academic life rarely question the primacy of the word. As a form of communication the word appears to be central to endeavour whether written or spoken. Underlying this concern with language is an analytical consciousness. A subject–predicate grammar is used that gives a structure to language. This very structure, in turn, structures consciousness. It is a feature common to Western culture; in the beginning was 'the word'. To write that creation began with the 'word' hides the fact that the author is a writer whose consciousness is structured by the medium used.

It might profitably be asked, 'How would a musician communicate this primal understanding of consciousness? What is "in the beginning" for a musician?' In communicating in a different way perhaps communication with a different consciousness may take place. This understanding may also explain the difficulty of writing and talking about health using a verbal analytic language when there is concern with a realm of behaviour necessitating another, perhaps musical, mode of consciousness. From this perspective, an expression of health is something that could better be sung or played than spoken. When we consider symptoms as an unconscious form of expression, then we may better understand that expression when it occurs in another non-verbal form. It is not to deny the value of speech and the consciousness associated with speech, rather that we can perhaps attempt to bring into consciousness, by a premature emphasis on verbalization, that which is better left unsaid until it has a form suitable for expression. Mutuality of expression, whether it be in making music, making love or talking is primarily a performed activity that requires the temporal structural fluidity of music.

To move from a position that advocates the primacy of the word in speech, and to understand speech in terms of phrasing, rhythm, pitch, and melody, a different consciousness emerges. A consciousness that reflects a different range of logic from the predicatory logic of language. Here are dynamic, movement, interval, and time – the very essences of music and of biological function.

If consideration is given to what constitutes people as identity, attention may be better directed to how they are composed not only in quantitative terms of bones and blood, but how they are composed as musical beings in regard to relationship patterns, rhythms, and melodic contours. This may reflect the original biblical notion that in the beginning was 'logos', that is, order. In music lies the phenomenon of a person coming into order. It may perhaps be that when a sense of that order is lost a person experiences a loss of health.

HEMISPHERIC PROCESSING

In support of the above argument, the realm of cerebral processing and music perception may also be examined. Although language processing may be dominant in one hemisphere of the brain, music processing involves a holistic understanding of the interaction of both cerebral hemispheres (Altenmüller 1986; Brust 1980; Gates and Bradshaw 1977).

In attempting to understand the perception of music there have been a number of investigations into the hemispheric strategies involved. Much of the literature considering musical perception concentrates on the significance of hemispheric dominance. Gates and Bradshaw (1977) conclude that cerebral hemispheres are concerned with music perception and that no laterality differences are apparent. Other authors (Wagner and Hannon

1981) suggest that two processing functions develop with training. Left and right hemispheres are simultaneously involved and musical stimuli are capable of eliciting both right and left ear superiority (Kellar and Bever 1980). Similarly, when people listen to and perform music they utilize differing hemispheric processing strategies.

APHASIA

Evidence of the global strategy of music processing in the brain is found in the clinical literature. In two cases of aphasia (Morgan and Tilluckdharry 1982) singing was seen as a welcome release from the helplessness of being a patient. The authors hypothesized that singing was a means to communicate thoughts externally. Although the 'newer aspect' of speech was lost, the older function of music was retained possibly because music is a function distributed over both hemispheres.

Berman (1981) suggests that recovery from aphasia is not a matter of new learning by the non-dominant hemisphere but a taking over of responsibility for language by that hemisphere. The non-dominant hemisphere may be a reserve of functions in case of regional failure. A less defensive alternative explanation is that the strategies underlying musical process are those same strategies underlying biological process and the maintenance of the identity of the organism.

RHYTHM

Defining rhythm is not an easy matter; there are multivarious definitions in the Western world alone (You 1994). Yet a common underlying feature is the anticipatory nature of the phenomenon. While located in time, and simultaneously structuring time, there is in the present a tension that anticipates the future. In a current rhythmical event, there is an expectation of what is to come. This has led some authors to speak of rhythm, in a Platonic sense, as order in movement or as temporal patterning. Parncutt (1994) defines a musical rhythm as an acoustic sequence evoking a sensation of pulse, where pulse is a form of expectancy. Once a pulse sensation is established, events are 'expected' at equal time intervals (p.453). It is this establishment of pulse, of expected events, that will be later be argued as the fundamental property of communication, and the essential factor lying at the heart of music therapy practice. The anticipatory factor inherent in rhythm is perhaps that which lies in the intentional actions present in movement.

Rhythm is the key to the integrative process underlying both musical perception and physiological coherence. Barfield's (1978) approach suggests that when musical form as tonal shape meets the rhythm of breathing there is the musical experience. External auditory activity is mediated by internal perceptual shaping in the context of a personal rhythm. It is interesting to speculate here on the meaning of context, not as a container but as *con textere*, which is a weaving together. One pattern is then woven against another to produce an interference pattern, the basis for matter. Sound is woven together with rhythm.

When considering communication, rhythm is fundamental to the organization of that communication. Before any consideration of content we must connect rhythmically with another person and establish some commonality. This connection of rhythms is seen as the phenomenon of entrainment, which occurs in the circadian rhythms of temperature and sleep. Should those rhythms lose entrainment, then jetlag takes place. Scientists observing such phenomena often attempt to find an underlying mechanism for entrainment (Johnson and Woodland-Hastings 1986), a master clock, as it were. However, if we move from a mechanical clockwork perspective, a dynamic musical analogy for co-ordinating rhythm is more appropriate for describing human activity. The metaphor of man as machine is prevalent in our Western culture and influences health care thinking in terms of a mind and body with faults that need repair or replacement. I am arguing here for another metaphor to guide our thinking regarding health; that is, man as musical composition.

The pulses that entrain the rhythmic patterns of the human body are non-material. The senses – hearing, smell, taste, sight, touch in addition to balancing and moving are integrated as a musical form. It is rhythm that provides the ground of being, and a rhythm of which being is generally unaware. Rhythm is the matrix of identity.

Dossey (1982) writes of disorders of time being particularly prevalent in modern society. This may be rephrased as disorders of disrupted rhythm as we shall see in the next chapter. The work of Safranek, Koshland and Raymond (1982) demonstrates the use subjects make of a preferred personal tempo in the performance of a motor task. This personal tempo is reflected as a functional reflex in the muscle. However, by introducing a musical rhythm while a musical task is being performed, which is different from that of the personal tempo of the subject, a different response is invoked in the subject. The authors see this as a 'volitional response'. Control over seemingly involuntary movements can be achieved by meeting the personal tempo of a subject and then changing to a slower, even beat.

The existence and role of a personal tempo are refined even further in creative music therapy (Nordoff and Robbins 1977). It may be inferred then that people become aware of the ground of their being not in verbal logic, but in a logic analogous to the ground of their own functioning, that is, music. In this sense insight is made, not in a restricted verbal intellectual sense, but achieved as being in composition.

The frame of reference approach mentioned earlier is used indirectly by Povel (1984) to understand rhythm. Tones in sequence are seen as having a dual function. They are characterized by pitch, volume, timbre, and duration. They also mark points in time. These tones then produce both structure in time and *of* time. When tones are used in sequence as temporal concepts, they can be thought of as providing a temporal grid; a grid that is a time scale on which the tone sequences can be mapped for duration and location. It might profitably be asked what the isomorphic events in terms of physiology are that would meet such a dual function. There may be regular sequential pulses of metabolic, cardiac, or respiratory activity within the body that also have qualities of pitch, timbre, and duration. What is important in these descriptions of musical perception is the emphasis on context where there are different levels of attention occurring simultaneously against a background temporal structure (Jones, Kidd and Wetzel 1981; Kidd, Boltz and Jones 1984).

You (1994) takes this point further, defining rhythm 'functionally in terms of a temporal order that anticipates, suspends and fulfils on the level of the visceral, physical, ecological, institutional as well as the moral' (p.361). It is the anticipatory property of rhythm that shifts our awareness away from an objective definition to a qualitative definition of rhythm that categorizes temporal experiences at different conceptual levels but always with the element of expectancy.

MELODY

Rhythm too plays a role in the perception of melody. The perceptions of speech and music are formidable tasks of pattern perception. The listener has to extract meaning from lengthy sequences of rapidly changing elements distributed in time (Morrongiello *et al.* 1985).

Temporal predictability is important for tracking melody lines (Jones, Kidd and Wetzel 1981; Kidd, Boltz and Jones 1984). Melody has a structure in time and a regular rhythm facilitates the detection of a musical interval and its subsequent integration into a cognitive representation of the serial structure of the musical pattern. Adults identify familiar melodies on the basis of relational information about intervals between tones rather than the absolute information of particular tones. In the recognition of unfamiliar melodies, less precise information is gathered about the tone itself. The primary concern is with successive frequency changes or *melodic contour*. The rhythmical context prepares the listener in advance for the onset of certain musical intervals and therefore a structure from which to discern, or predict, change.

The implication of this work is that change, whether it be melody or rhythm, is dependent on a global rhythmic strategy. To extend this understanding to biological processes, it can be hypothesized that differences in contour (melody) (as in the release of hormones, fluctuations in temperature) and changes in rhythm are detected in reference to a global rhythmic context of the body. This global context may be regulated by the heart or breathing patterns, or may be an emergent property of the varying rhythmic patterns of the body. Disruption in this overall global strategy will influence a person's ability to detect new or changed non-temporal information (Cuddy, Cohen and Miner 1979; Jones, Kidd and Wetzel 1981; Kidd, Boltz and Jones 1984). We may not be aware of certain changes and become either out of tune or out of time.

The composed self as improvised order

The perception of music requires a holistic strategy where the play of patterned frequencies is recognized within a matrix of time. People may be described in similar terms as beings in the world who are patterned frequencies in time.

A phenomenological approach presses the scientist to understand phenomena as direct experiences before being translated into thoughts and feelings. The practice of creative music therapy adopts such a position. A person is invited to improvise music creatively with a therapist. It may be inferred from this playing that one is hearing a person directly in the world as a direct expression of those patterned frequencies in a matrix of time. Rather than subject a person to measurement, to be reduced to what is quantifiable, he or she may be experienced directly. This experience requires no verbal translation as in psychotherapy. What can be heard is the person being in the world. An extension of such improvised playing as an expression of the whole person is that tendencies to play in differing ways may be heard. There may be limitations in rhythm, melody, or musical structure. By challenging personal tempo one may hear the extent of his or her intent.

If musical form and biological form are isomorphic, improvised music may also provide a holistic strategy for the assessment of health and well-being. Feinstein (1966) stressed the importance of clinical logic in the diagnosis of cancer, and the importance of allowing the patient to speak: 'The complexity of man increases the difficulty of studying human disease, but also enables a diseased man to talk. His description of symptoms gives crucial information about the diseased structures under investigation' (p.245).

Speech itself is limiting both in content and in form. The creative playing of improvised music offers a holistic form of assessment that is relational, non-invasive, and non-verbal, and that allows the identity of the patient to be revealed and experienced in the world. This context allows the expression of tendencies that have potentials for those states called health and illness.

If music is an earlier form of communication than language, and the processing strategies for the perception of music are distributed over both hemispheres, it is possible to infer that this holistic strategy is closer in developmental terms to physiological processes and autonomic activity than language. There is an emerging tolerance and even acceptance of the influence of language on physiology. However, there is a more subtle and more precise medium with potentials for representation and influence, that is, the playing of music. What links the performance of music and the performance of health is the element of participation. The semiologist Nattiez (1990) refers to the aspect of performance as 'poietic process' and the aspect of listening, and making sense, as 'esthesic process', with the reality of the work itself as a material object, 'the trace'. In health terms we can also see the process of becoming healthy, and what we do to become healthy, the understanding of our own health and the material traces that those activities leave in our bodies. Indeed the body, like the musical work, is the trace of our health activity.

It may perhaps be that when a sense of that order is lost a person experiences a loss of health. When we seek to establish order, the flexible, kairotic, performed order of music, song or dance, then perhaps we are moving towards health. In the same way, we could argue from traditions of Indian and Oriental medicine that the pursuit of changes in breathing and posture, or the rhythmical changes from herbal medications, is establishing an order of the same dynamic dimension.

The problem of causal thinking is that although the influence of nature on the individual is explained, there is no allowance for the spontaneity of the living being (Tsouyopoulos 1984). Therefore any change, whether it be described as developmental or therapeutic, must include an element that is dynamic. What is being argued here is that our struggle to maintain our identity – that we see reflected in the integration of immunology and psychology – is a dynamic process of equilibrium and self-regulation that demands spontaneity (Tauber 1994). Achieving the new becomes an intentional act, promoting sustaining activities by creating the optimal conditions – physical, psychic and cultural – that some may call an ecology (Bateson 1978, 1991), and others may refer to as a milieu (Tsouyopoulos 1994).

Music is the ideal medium to discover how people are composed and how they come into the world as whole beings both to create and sustain identity. Not only can such personal expression be recorded for analysis, it can be heard and experienced directly as a whole. As beings in the world we are composed in the moment. Our health is improvised to meet the challenges and contingencies of life, whether these be internal or external. The structures of that improvisation are analogous to the dynamics of music. The means by which we then achieve health are performed improvisations and therefore susceptible to a creative music therapy. If we move from a mechanical materialistic concept of what it is to be human, and consider how we are organized as living beings emerging into the drama of daily life, then our focus shifts from a technological solution to an aesthetic expectancy.

CHAPTER THREE

Communication and the Playing
of Improvised Music

Arms, hands, or legs do not behave; it is the total person who behaves.
(Condon 1975, p.45)

It is important in explaining to others the benefit of music therapy, to know
what happens when people improvise music together. My intention is to be
able to demonstrate the influence music therapy has on the body of the
patient – that is, not only to accept the ramifications music has for mental
well-being, but the physical effect that music therapy has on the body of the
patient too. As I have argued in the previous chapter, both mind and body
are considered inseparable when we come to consider the condition of
human suffering. As we shall read later in the chapter, while music can be
demonstrated to have a direct physical effect on the body, it is organization,
the non-material aspect, that is vital to communication both within the
person and between persons. However, the ground from which I will argue
is that music has the ability to bring about physical changes in the human
body, an understanding that has been in our culture since antiquity (Khan
Inayat 1983).

In trying to demonstrate the change brought about by music therapy I
have looked for a simple physiological indicator. From a preliminary review
of the literature about communication, suitable indicators emerged from the
studies of cardiovascular change. The principal measures in such work were
those concerned with changes in blood pressure and heart rate. Heart rate
was chosen because it was a relatively easy parameter to observe and measure.
Perhaps more significantly, it was a parameter acceptable to medical science,
with which we, as a therapeutic discipline, are attempting to promote a
dialogue.

The previous chapter mentioned the important factors associated with
both biological form and musical form – time, phrasing, pitch, rhythm, and

34

melodic contour (Aldridge 1989a). Similar considerations apply for studies of communication. The basic pre-verbal fundamentals of human communication are called suprasegmentals – these are time, phrasing, rhythm, pitch, and voice tone (which would more accurately be called timbre). It is these qualities that are considered by music therapists when they assess tape-recorded sessions of improvised music therapy.

The literature that first alerted me to these factors concerned chronic heart disease and Type A behaviour (Aldridge 1989a; Dielman *et al.* 1987; Dimsdale and Stern 1988; Friedmann *et al.* 1982; Linden 1987; Lynch *et al.* 1981; Smith and Rhodewalt 1986). Heart disease patients were described in terms that owed as much to a musical basis as they did to a physiological process. Loud, fast speech using a limited range of voice timbre, and speech patterns that interrupted the responses of a partner, appeared to reflect qualities music therapists heard in their descriptions of patients when they creatively improvised music (see Table 3.1). Although these qualitative descriptions may only be regarded as noise in the formal terms of grammar, they provide the essential expressive context for communication.

Table 3.1 Speech characteristics, physiological changes and musical components

Type A behaviour	Type B behaviour	Musical and music therapy components
increased voice volume	voice quieter	volume
fast speech rate	slower speech rate	tempo
short response latency	longer response latency	phrasing
emphatic voice	less emphasis	expression
hard metallic voice	melodic voice	timbre
less mutuality	increased mutuality	musical relationship
trying to keep control	less need for control	musical relationship
increased reactivity		responsiveness
increased heart rate	decreased heart rate	tempo
higher cardiovascular arousal maintained	cardiovascular arousal returns to lower level quickly	dynamic

It seemed important to compare apparently similar statements from two different theoretical backgrounds to see if there was any commonality between them. As heart disease is such an important problem in both mortality and morbidity throughout the Western world, it made sense to propose how a discipline like improvised music therapy could offer a tool for both assessment and treatment.

The medium of improvised music offers possibilities for extremely varied communication and has a subtlety beyond that of interview techniques that are confounded by verbal content. In addition, in improvised playing there is both the possibility of hearing what may be pathological in terms of restriction and inflexibility under challenge, and that which indicates positive possibilities for growth and change. This is accomplished by an essential feature of the therapy of performance. The patient is an active participant, not a passive recipient, in the process of assessment or therapy.

Furthermore, what we are concerned with in music therapy is the mutual construction by partners in dialogue. The same situation exists in conversation. While most communication theorists apply themselves to the understanding of meaning in conversation, what we are primarily concerned with is a deeper and primary understanding of how dialogue is constructed. While meaning is important, the establishment of dialogic structure, that in itself enables meaning to be negotiated, is the first important step in communication. As Fais (1994) writes, conversation involves the simultaneous co-production by the participants involved, not merely the construction of meaning through alternating discrete contributions. We will see in a later chapter how encouraging improvised musical playing in children – that is, the simultaneous co-production of musical sounds or utterances – is an important stage in the development of improved communication.

Time

A central, albeit contentious, area of coronary heart disease research has been that of the Type A behaviour pattern, which is characterized by the way in which an individual responds to, and provokes, environmental demands. Helman (1987) refers to this view of the cause of heart disease as a cultural construction that involves the 'unique social and symbolic characteristics of Western time' (p.969). In this view we are 'the embodiment (both literally and figuratively) of the values of that society' (p.971). The individual is caught in the contradictions of self-demand and societal demand, which for some people may become pathogenic.

At the centre of this cultural construction (Helman 1985) is the notion of time. The predominant form of Western time is monochronic. This form is conceived as an external order imposed on the individual. It developed from the need of a modern industrialized society to have a universal public order by which the means of production could be co-ordinated and the actions of many individuals regulated. In this form, deadlines have to be met, the passage of time is linear, and its measurement is quantitative. This is time as *chronos*.

However, there is an alternative conceptualization of time that is personal rather than public. This is time as *kairos*. It is polychronic, and closer to the emerging biological understanding of physiological times that are rhythmically entrained (Johnson and Woodland-Hastings 1986), not to an external clock, but to the person as a whole organism. In this conceptualization, time is in a state of flux; it is concerned with flexibility and the convergence of multiple tasks. Time is seen as springing from the self.

Apart from these notions, there is also the qualitatively different time encountered in ritual, in prayer, and contemplation, during sex, or while dancing. Most are aware of the difference between an hour spent in the company of a lover, which seems like minutes, and an hour spent in an administrative meeting, which can seem like days.

Some authors (Dossey 1982; Helman 1987) suggest that when we try to impose a fusion between external clock time and personal physiological time our physiology is affected.

> Western society is unique in trying to impose a fusion between clock time and individual physiology – between rates of bodily movement, speech, gestures, heartbeat and respiration – and the small machine strapped to the wrist or hung on the wall. 'Rush hour', deadlines, diaries, appointments and timetables all affect the physiology of modem man, and help construct his world view and sense of identity. (Helman 1987, p.974)

There may then be a tension between private and public time resulting in stress and anxiety.

In music there are possibilities of experiencing these varying aspects of time as they converge in their seamless reality. The tension between personal and public time may be heard in improvised music and, apart from promoting experiences that differentiate and develop those conceptualizations, an experience of a timeless qualitative reality can also be promoted.

When illness is categorized in Western medicine the time concepts of acute and chronic are used. The presence of chronic illness is causing many problems for the delivery of health services throughout modern society and promoting a debate about the way in which such illness can be tackled in the latter part of the twentieth century. However, it may be that conceptualizations of illness on the acute and chronic dimensions of a linear reality are limiting, and it may be necessary to consider a concept of *kairotic* illness.

This illness may entail a personal attempt to maintain identity in the face of imposed environmental constraints and would be similar to the way in which family therapists talk about personal solutions to a problem located within an ecology of family members, cultural constraint, and individual development (Aldridge 1984, 1988; Aldridge and Rossiter 1985; Bloch 1987). These concepts of time (development) and space (relationship) are fundamental to our culture whether it be in terms of science or art.

Cardiovascular Change and Communication

Lynch (Friedmann *et al.* 1982; Lynch 1977; Lynch *et al.* 1981) carefully explored the relationship between human communication, principally talking, and elevations in blood pressure and heart rate. Reading out loud or talking to another person produced rapid and significant rises in heart rate. From this work he suggested that certain hypertensive individuals experience difficulties with communication, and that individual elevations in blood pressure may be manifested symptoms of difficulties with communication.

These communicational difficulties were then related to the personality traits attributed, albeit contentiously, to Type A individuals with coronary heart disease. Patients classified as Type A had been observed to speak fast, loud, have a tendency to interrupt, and use emphatic gestures. Friedman *et al.* (1982) proposed that tempo and volume were important characteristics of communication. Although tempo and volume were correlated with cardiovascular change, this correlation was not dependent on the affective content of conversation and, therefore, independent of cognitive processes. This finding is important for music therapists in the Nordoff–Robbins (1977) tradition who state that there is physical change during the process of music therapy and that it is not necessary to use only a psychotherapeutic model for change in music therapy.

The recommendations of this early research for patients with hypertension were to modify speech rate and volume using breathing techniques, and to control communication style. If cardiovascular response is a process out of the range of conscious awareness, then presumably cognitive approaches are likely to be only partial. Music therapy, with its intrinsic factors of tempo and volume as direct performance, may be better suited to changing communicational style than the so-called talking therapies.

A feature of assessing Type A behaviour and physiological reactivity has been some form of assessment using an interview (Dimsdale and Stern 1988). Unfortunately, these interviews have presented a rather negative picture of the Type A person as competitive, hard driving, ambitious, impatient, and often hostile. Yet, within these descriptions there are other categories of classification that are concerned with elements of speech stylistics. These speech stylistics are easier to objectify and are less like personal value judgements. For our research purposes they are also translatable into musical terms of tempo, phrasing and dynamic.

Some researchers (Dielman *et al.* 1987; Linden 1987; Siegman *et al.* 1987) recognize the following characteristics for assessing global Type A behaviour:

- voice volume
- speed of speaking
- accelerated speech at the end of statements
- duration of silent pauses
- duration of subjects responses
- interruptive and non-interruptive simultaneous speech
- response latency (the amount of time between the time the question is asked and the subject's answer), and
- voice timbre.

These researchers also go on to assess interaction patterns with the interviewer that they see as hostility and verbal competitiveness. Verbal competitiveness is a tendency to take control of the interview away from the interviewer by interrupting, asking for unnecessary qualifications, or raising the voice to drown out the interviewer's interruptions (Dielman *et al.* 1987).

These stylistic qualities and interactions can be observed in musical improvisation, and without the need for negative connotations of hostility. In the context of a spoken interview it is important to remember that the content of some of the questions may indeed be hostile or challenging. A further difficulty is that although speech rate and volume can be measured, hostility, impatience, and competition can only be assessed subjectively with poor interrater reliability.

In this approach there appeared to be two general categories of attentional styles. One, field-independent subjects appear to use bodily information more readily than others and make accurate perceptual judgements about the environment even though presented with distracting perceptual information. Such subjects appear to have a broad and differentiated range of physiological responses to various stimuli. For these subjects there is a concordance between how they say they feel and how they respond physiologically.

The other style is that of field-dependent subjects, who tend to base their perceptual judgements on distracting external information and use this external information to assess their own state. When reacting to stimuli they are less emotionally complex.

The implications for music therapy from these preliminary findings are that we may also hear such field-dependent or field-independent characteristics in the musical playing of the patient. For example, some patients may have an extensive repertoire of playing styles and be able to play both rhythmically and melodically while listening to themselves and to the therapist in the overall context of the music. Yet others may have a limited range of playing styles and, in response to changes in the music, may only change particular musical parameters (i.e., play louder or faster).

We speculate that repertoires of coping responses can be heard musically, and these reflect quantitative, differentiated physiological responses. It is this link that we wish to demonstrate in our physiological experiments. Note that these observed patterns are considered either musically or physiologically. We are not necessarily invoking any descriptions of psychological state.

Sandman was to develop his work further. He was interested in the pronounced, and paradoxical, decrease in heart rate of field-independent subjects in response to stressful information. He began to demonstrate that a learned heart rate deceleration could bring about an improved attention to the environment. Thus, he argued, by controlling heart rate, attention could also be influenced.

Awareness of the environment was partially regulated by interactions of the brain and the heart. When heart rate was low, subjects perceived stimuli significantly better than when heart rate was high. This view was also supported by indications that when heart rate decelerated, there was an increased blood flow to the brain. There appeared to be 'a fortuitous or purposeful synchronization between physiological systems' (Sandman 1984, p.118), and it appeared that the hemispheres of the brain were 'tuned' (Sandman 1984a; Walker and Sandman 1979, 1982) by the cardiovascular system.

These findings challenged the classical view that intellectual abilities were the sole province of the brain and promoted further investigations of links between both mind and body where the cardiovascular system influences the brain and behaviour. In some patients an inviolable relationship exists between the brain and the cardiovascular system that may be a biological marker for psychiatric state (Safranek, Koshland and Raymond 1982).

These researchers speculate that the heart has an influence on consciousness or awareness. The impact of heart rate is dynamic and fluctuates between suppressing and liberating the left and right sides of the brain. When heart rate increases, it is indicative of cognitive processing and a rejection of the environment; when heart rate decreases, there is a switch to environmental attention. The cardiovascular system reflects a person's intention to receive information. If this is so, music therapy is a sensitive tool for discerning the physiological state of a person as a whole. This tool is not fragmented by introducing a measuring instrument between researcher and subject that limits responses to a narrow mechanical range.

We anticipate that we can hear how changes in the improvised musical playing are reflected in changes in the heart rate of the patient. Hypotheses about a patient listening only to him or herself and not listening to another may be heard in their fast, or accelerating, heart rate.

If, as is also inferred in this literature, intellectual abilities are not solely begun and terminated in the brain but are whole body phenomena, then the active playing of the patient in music therapy is most important. The patient is involved physically in this therapy, is not expected to sit still and answer a questionnaire, or remain stationary while being monitored. He or she is asked to play. This improvised playing encourages the use of soma and psyche. To play rhythmically is a whole-person activity. To play rhythmically with another person is an extension of this activity that includes vital components of relationship.

As mentioned earlier, speech variables have been significantly correlated with coronary difficulties in terms of Type A behaviour. These variables need not be discovered in a provocative or challenging manner (Siegman *et al.* 1987). Short response latency and accelerated speech are also expressions of anxiety.

Music therapy can also offer a context for communication. It is not provocative in a hostile sense, and has the possibility to promote all the elements inherent in speech stylistics without the confounding aspect of affective components. These variables can be heard in a way that is not solely voice-dependent. Communication is not only concerned with the use of the voice; it also includes those gestures and movements that accompany vocal behaviour. Condon (1975) calls these co-ordinated sounds and movements the quanta of behaviour or 'linguistics-kinesics'.

In the playing of improvised music it may be observed how the person moves and also hear how the patient communicates non-verbally. It is this musico-kinesic behaviour that contributes to the assessment of how a person plays and as we shall see later is vital for the cognitive development of young children. A central feature of this assessment is the elusive quality of intentionality. The movement of the body provides an indicator of whether the patient is playing with the therapist and intends to play the instrument or whether the patient is just going along with the music. These kinesic considerations are also an important indicator of self-synchrony within the person – either as bilateral synchrony (right and left hand playing together), or at the level of hearing and responding to what is heard.

Music therapy, in the improvised sense used here, is also dependent on the relationship between the patient and the therapist – an interactional synchrony. It may be that a vital aspect of communication, which is missed by some researchers, is not the ability to produce sound but the ability to listen and respond appropriately to sound. Smith and Rhodewalt (1986) consider this circular process of listening and responding. They suggest an interactional understanding where people with Type A behaviour not only respond in a certain way but also provoke situations that will allow them to respond in a characteristic fashion.

Heart rate and attention

While some researchers were studying the implications of heart rate and communication, others were studying the relationship between a process like attention, which is classically attributed to the brain, and emotion, which is related to the body. This mind–body unity debate heralded an era of interest in holistic medicine.

Sandman (1984, 1984a) began investigating the relationship between physiological responses and stressful, neutral, or pleasant stimuli. In particular he was interested in the apparent relationship between attention and emotion where attentional style could influence physiological responses to affective stimuli. His work was based on the premise that the viscera, the muscles, the heart, and the endocrine system provided peripheral information to the brain and provided a context wherein perceptions gained meaning.

Sandman was to develop his work further. He was interested in the pronounced, and paradoxical, decrease in heart rate of field-independent subjects in response to stressful information. He began to demonstrate that a learned heart rate deceleration could bring about an improved attention to the environment. Thus, he argued, by controlling heart rate, attention could also be influenced.

Awareness of the environment was partially regulated by interactions of the brain and the heart. When heart rate was low, subjects perceived stimuli significantly better than when heart rate was high. This view was also supported by indications that when heart rate decelerated, there was an increased blood flow to the brain. There appeared to be 'a fortuitous or purposeful synchronization between physiological systems' Sandman

(1984a, p.118), and it appeared that the hemispheres of the brain were 'tuned' by the cardiovascular system.

These findings challenged the classical view that intellectual abilities were the sole province of the brain and promoted further investigations of links between both mind and body where the cardiovascular system influences the brain and behaviour. In some patients there appears to exist an inviolable relationship between the brain and the cardiovascular system that may be a biological marker for psychiatric state. Meehan (1986) has also emphasized the interaction of the two main stress response systems involving depression and relaxation, and their importance in coronary care.

These researchers speculate that the heart has an influence on conscious-ness or awareness. The impact of heart rate is dynamic and fluctuates between suppressing and liberating the left and right sides of the brain. When heart rate increases, it is indicative of cognitive processing and a rejection of the environment; when heart rate decreases, there is a switch to environmental attention. The cardiovascular system reflects a person's intention to receive information. If this is so, music therapy is a sensitive tool for discerning the physiological state of a person as a whole. This tool is not fragmented by introducing a measuring instrument between researcher and subject that limits responses to a narrow mechanical range.

We anticipate that we can hear how changes in the improvised musical playing are reflected in changes in the heart rate of the patient. Hypotheses about a patient listening only to him or herself and not listening to another may be heard in their fast, or accelerating, heart rate.

If, as is also inferred in this literature, intellectual abilities are not solely begun and terminated in the brain but are whole body phenomena, then the active playing of the patient in music therapy is most important. The patient is involved physically in this therapy, is not expected to sit still and answer a questionnaire, or remain stationary while being monitored. He or she is asked to play. This improvised playing encourages the use of soma and psyche. To play rhythmically is a whole-person activity. To play rhythmically with another person is an extension of this activity that includes vital components of relationship.

Given that in a study by Bason and Celler (1972) it was possible to influence the heart rate of a patient by externally matching the pulse of their heart rate, then we must conclude that studies of the influence of music on heart rate must match the music to the individual patient. This also makes psychological sense as different people have varied reactions to the same music. Furthermore, improvised music playing which takes meeting the tempo of the patient as one of its main principles, may have an impact other than the passive listening to music. In addition, the work of Haas (1986) showed that listening, coupled with tapping, synchronizes respiration pattern with musical rhythm, further emphasizing that active music playing can be used to influence physiological parameters and that this synchronization can be learned. Thaut (1985) also found that children with gross motor dysfunction performed with significantly better motor rhythm accuracy when aided by auditory rhythm and rhythmic speech. We may infer that musical rhythms can be used for their therapeutic influence on physiological parameters.

Breathing

The relationship between listening to music and physiological change, notably respiration, has also been investigated in situations other than coronary care (Brody 1988; Fried 1990; Gross and Swartz 1982). Breathing training itself is believed to have a physical benefit in increasing tidal volume without excessive loss of CO_2 (hypocapnia) (Fried 1990). Typically anxious patients have relatively rapid shallow chest breathing and may hyperventilate. However, music appears to have a paradoxical effect; while subjects report music to be highly relaxing, soothing and sedative, their physiological reactions indicate otherwise. Nursing approaches have also utilized the anxiolytic effect of music in combination with massage and breathing exercises to relax patients, as we will read in the next chapter.

In recent work, two distinct components of psychosomatic symptoms are reported; one that is primarily psychological, and another that reflects physiological functioning (Wienties and Grossman 1994). It is these relationships between heart rate, attention and breathing that we will see in the next section as they are applied in clinical practice.

Music Therapy and Intensive Care

> however great the organic damage…there remains the undiminished possibility of re-integration by art, by communion, by unlocking the human spirit; and this can be presented in what at first seems at first a hopeless state of neurological devastation. (Sacks 1986, p.37)

The neurologist Oliver Sacks reminds us of the necessary balance we must bring to our work with patients in the field of medicine. All too often we are concerned with testing the patient for deficits, for measuring and for assessing problem-solving capacities. As a balance to testing and measuring, he urges us to consider the narrative and symbolic organization of the patient, such that we consider their possibilities and abilities. What seems to be damaged, ill organized and chaotic becomes composed and fluent. This is the function of the creative arts. Through art and play we realize other selves elusive to measurement and fugitive to assessment. Furthermore, there is a quality of time apparent in arts activities that is 'intentional' and involves the will of the patient. Her spirit is set free. When we consider the situation of intensive care, where patients are often damaged, disorganized, intubated, machine-regulated, often unconscious, and unable to communicate; then we must consider a way of introducing activities which will stimulate communion with those patients.

The ground of consciousness exists in time, a subjective present that organizes the various pulses of the body. When this organization fails then communication fails. Yet we know from patients who have recovered that there is a continuing awareness. Although brain activity is negligible, the person endures. This enduring identity raises questions about the location of the self in patients who are comatose and about the nature of communication with patients who are unconscious. In the following pages modern medicine will be challenged to realize the human body itself as an instrument of knowledge more precise, and infinitely more flexible, than its technological inventions. The ramifications are that the clinician, whether doctor or music therapist, has at her disposal the essential means of communication even when the awareness of the patient is apparently absent.

Some aspects of modern medicine have become increasingly technological. Such is the case of intensive care treatment. Even in what may appear to be hopeless cases, it can save lives (Hannich 1988) through the application of this modern technology. However, albeit in the context of undoubted success, intensive care treatment has fallen into disrepute. Patients are seen to suffer from a wide range of problems resulting from insufficient communication, sleep and sensory deprivation (Hannich 1988; Ulrich 1984) and lack of empathy between patient and medical staff. Many activities in an intensive care situation appear to be between the unit staff and the essential machines, that is, subjects and objects. To a certain extent patients become a part of this object world. Improvised music therapy can be a useful adjunctive therapy in such situations both for the patient and the staff.

The music therapy sessions
At the suggestion of a hospital neurologist, a music therapy colleague began working with patients in intensive care (Gustorff 1990). To investigate this approach further, the work was monitored in the intensive treatment unit of a large university clinic. Five patients, between the ages of 15 and 40 years and with severe coma (a Glasgow Coma Scale score between 4 and 7), were

treated. All the patients had been involved in some sort of accident, had sustained brain damage, and most had undergone neurosurgery.

The form of music therapy used here was based on the principle in Chapter Two that we are organized as human beings not in a mechanical way but in a musical form; i.e. a harmonic complex of interacting rhythms and melodic contours. To maintain our coherence as beings in the world then we must creatively improvise our identity. Rather than search for a master clock which co-ordinates us chronobiologically, we are better served by the non-mechanistic concept of musical organization. Music therapy is the medium by which a coherent organization is regained, i.e. linking brain, body and mind. In this perspective the self is more than a corporeal being. As Sacks (1986) writes, 'the power of music or narrative form is to organize' (p.177). What music and narrative structure organizes is the recognition of relationships between elements, not in an intellectual way, but direct and unmediated. With coma patients we see signs of activity, albeit often machine-supported, but totally disorganized. The person exists, sometimes in what is described as a vegetative state, but hardly 'lives'.

Each music therapy contact lasted between eight and twelve minutes. The therapist improvised her wordless singing based upon the tempo of the patient's pulse, and more importantly, the patient's breathing pattern. She pitched her singing to a tuning fork. The character of the patient's breathing determined the nature of the singing. The singing was clearly phrased so that when any reaction was seen then the phrase could be repeated.

Before the first session the music therapist met the family to gain some idea of what the patient was like as a person. On contacting the comatose patient she said who she was, that she would sing for the patient in the tempo of his or her pulse and the rhythm of his or her breathing. The unit staff were asked to be quiet during this period and not to carry out any invasive procedures for ten minutes after the contact.

There was a range of reactions from a change in breathing (it became slower and deeper), fine motor movements, grabbing movements of the hand and turning of the head, eyes opening to the regaining of consciousness. When the therapist first began to sing there was a slowing down of the heart rate. Then the heart rate rose rapidly and sustained an elevated level until the end of the contact. This may have indicated an attempt at orientation and cognitive processing within the communicational context. EEG measurement of brain activity showed a desynchronization from theta rhythm, to alpha rhythm or beta rhythm in former synchronized areas. This effect, indicating arousal and perceptual activity, faded out after the music therapy stopped.

If we consider that cells firing with a cardiac rhythm have been recorded in the medullary area of the brain, and that there is a synchronous relationship between the contraction of the heart and the 'ascending' wave of alpha rhythm (Sandman 1984) of brain activity, then it is possible to hypothesize that the rhythmic co-ordination of the cardiovascular system with cortical rhythmic firings is of primary importance for cognition. What we have is a weaving together of basic primitive human rhythms, which produce an interference pattern which itself may be that of cognition. It is proposed here that the rhythmic co-ordination of basic functions in the human body is a fundamental healing activity.

Parncutt (1987) refers to the sounds associated with heartbeat and walking movements of a mother as being the most important for conditioning the perception of rhythm. It is the perception of such pulses as events that forms the basis for establishing a rhythmic pattern. This, he argues, is not a structural characteristic of the brain, but a feature of how we interact with the environment. A pulse is best described by two factors. One is called the period and is the time interval between successive events. The other factor is the phase and is the actual time at which any event occurs relative to some reference time.

Periodicity is an important key to understanding the problem of patients who are in coma. For a musical pulse to be perceived it must fall within a certain time limit before a feeling of pulse can be evoked. The duration of short-term memory as the psychological present is restricted to several seconds. Gerstner and Goldberg (1994) have demonstrated in several mammalian species, other than human beings, that the time span required to integrate successive events into a 'subjective present' requires a duration of about three seconds. Complex human motor behaviours and movement patterns require a co-ordinating activity that is based upon pulse as its establishes a rhythmic pattern. For patients in coma, the regaining of complex movements patterns demands the establishment of a rhythmic pattern. This is essentially a musical activity, and as we have seen earlier is not solely a brain activity but is an interaction between person and their environment. Furthermore, for pulse events to be perceived as a rhythmic sequence they need to be uneven in chronological time, time as 'chronos'. Thus machine noises will not provide a rhythmical context in which human beings can experience themselves as being present and so co-ordinate their movements. Singing with a patient, or making music that has another time structure, can provide such a context. We then have a basic context of time for co-ordinating human movement patterns, and it is such patterns we observe as the first signs of awakening in coma patients when they are sung with, time as 'kairos'.

The ward situation

Sleep disturbance is a major problem in intensive care units and the effect of a disturbed waking/sleeping rhythm upon other metabolic cycles is critical (Johnson and Woodland-Hastings 1986; Reinberg and Halberg 1971). The rhythmic entrainment of cardiovascular and somatic activities may be the key ground for recovery. This means that we must consider the total 'behavioural' (Engel 1977) activity of the patient such that seemingly independent systems are integrated. The context (Latin *con textere* = weaving together) of this integration is rhythmical, involving the co-ordination of the major tidal rhythms of the body and timing mechanisms within the hypothalamus in the brain.

As an organizational problem we must look to the way in which staff are employed in work shifts. It can occur during a 24-hour period that patients are constantly in contact with nursing staff, no matter what time of day or night. These nursing staff have their own cycles of activity separate from the patients' night–day rhythm. For rhythmically disoriented patients, this constant activity is a problem. No wonder that there are sleep problems when patients must respond to carers who are in a phase of their own activity cycle and, thereby, unsynchronized with the patient. Nursing staff, while synchronized with management needs and hospital routine, may need to attend to the sleep/activity rhythm of the patient to communicate effectively.

In response to music therapy, some ward staff are astonished that patients can respond to quiet singing. This highlights a difficulty of noisy, busy, often brightly lit units. All communication is made above a high level of machine noise. Furthermore commands to an 'unconscious' patient are made by shouting formal injunctions, such as 'Show me your tongue', 'Tell me your name', 'Open your eyes'. Few attempts are made at normal human communication with a patient who cannot speak, or with whom staff can have little if any psychological contact. It is as if these patients were isolated in a landscape of noise, and deprived of human contact.

A benefit of music therapy is that the staff are made aware of the quality and intensity of the human contact. In the intensive care unit environment of seemingly non-responding patients, dependent upon machines to maintain vital functions and anxiety-provoking in terms of possible patient death, then it is a human reaction to withdraw personal contact and interact with the machines. While the machines themselves are of vital importance, they present data which are independent one from another, and which are often considered in isolation whereas the integration of the systems being measured is the clue to recovery. This is further exacerbated by a scientific epistemology which emphasizes the person only as a material being and which equates mind with brain.

At yet another level, we must consider the fixed chronological pulses of machines as opposed to the kairotic time of organisms. If human activity is based on pulse, the nature of those pulses is that they are variable within a range of reactivity. Those pulses are lively and accommodate other pulses to form interacting rhythms. This is not so with machines; they are fixed in their range. Therefore, what is a variable in human activity (the tempo of varying pulses) becomes a constant in coma patients. The task then is to introduce co-ordinated variety with the intention to heal, something which as yet machines cannot do. Perhaps the key lies in the fact that it is the consciousness of the therapist which stimulates the consciousness of the patient, and this consciousness is not divorced from the living rhythmic reality of our physiology.

A period of calm is also recognized as having potential benefit for the patient. What some staff fail to realize is that communication is dependent upon rhythm, not upon volume. We might argue that such unconscious patients, struggling to orient themselves in time and space, are further confused by an atmosphere of continuing loud, disorienting random noise and bright light. For patients seeking to orient themselves then the basic rhythmic context of their own breathing may provide the focus for that orientation. This raises the problem of intentionality in human behaviour even when consciousness appears to be absent. Reflexes do not occur in a vacuum; they are conditional, occurring in a context of other behavioural activity. If bodily systems are proactive, as well as reactive, then purposive behaviour and consciousness may require the context of human communication to function. It is also vital that staff in such situations do not confuse 'not acting' on behalf of the patient with 'not perceiving'.

We can further speculate that the various body rhythms have become disassociated in comatose states and following major surgery. The question then remains of how those behaviours can be integrated and where is the seat of such integration. It is quite clear that integration then is an organizational property of the whole organization in relationship with the environment and not located materially in any cell or any one organ. The environment of the patient includes the vital component of human contact and there is reason to believe that the essential ground of this social contact, too, is rhythmical.

Communication, contact and consciousness

Improvised singing appears to offer a number of possible benefits for working in intensive care both in terms of human contact and promoting perceptual responses. Human contact as communication is a creative art form. Although what we know from machines is valuable, there are other important subtle forms of knowledge that are best gleaned through personal contact with the patient. Mindell (1989) took the courageous step of attempting process oriented psychology with comatose patients accompanying them on their great symbolic journey. The drama of our contact with such patients at a time of existential crisis points to a fundamental aesthetic of living systems creatively realized such that we, as artist therapists, can go beyond the confines of a soulless technology. This is not to deny technology and its benefits, simply to remind us of our human intention as it is realized in art, play, drama, music.

What we may also need to consider in future is not how to observe more, but how to question the quality of what we are observing and the premises on which this observation is based. In such situations of intensive monitoring and machine support, particularly in the case of comatose patients, we may ask of ourselves, 'Where is the self of the patient?' Needleman (1988) reminds us that the power of scientific thought has been to organize our perceptions in such a manner that we can survive in the world. Hence the value of scientific medicine and instrumentation. However, he goes on to say that science has also neglected the human body as an instrument of knowledge and as a vehicle for sensations as direct as ordinary sensory experience, but as subtle as consciousness. He writes, 'it is not simply the intellect which science underestimates, it is the human body as an instrument of knowledge – the human body as a vehicle for sensations as direct as ordinary sensory experience, but far more subtle and requiring for their reception a specific degree of collected attention and self-sincerity' (p.169).

The question still remains for us as clinicians and scientists when faced with a patient in coma, or a persistent vegetative state, 'Where is the person and how can I reach her?', and then for ourselves as fellow human beings, 'Where am I?' What part of the therapist is contacting the unconscious patient? Could it be that if the musical form of our communication touches the patient, as singing, then we can also attend to how we speak with the patient in their breathing patterns, and attend to them with the very form of our own bodies?

This ability to communicate with unconscious patients raises further the ethical issues of decisions about terminating life support when the brain and the person are no longer seen as one and the same entity (Mindell 1989).

When patients do not respond it may be that we are not providing them with the human conditions in which, and with which, they can respond. We as therapists are those conditions that are the context for healing to take place.

Music, Communication and Medicine

> The body of the speaker dances in time with his speech. Further, the body of the listener dances in rhythm with that of the speaker! (Condon and Ogston 1966, p.338)

The main argument of this book so far, then, is that musical components are the fundamentals of communication; and that rhythm, in particular, is the primary aspect of communication in which we relate to ourselves and to others. Communication in this sense is not solely restricted to the transmission of information, but is also concerned with the establishment and management of relationships (Penn 1983).

If this argument is true then music is a powerful and subtle medium of communication which is, as suggested in Chapter Two, isomorphic with the process of living (Aldridge 1989, 1989a, 1991a). As we have seen in the previous section, even with patients who are regarded as unconscious, music therapy is a powerful therapeutic medium for promoting communication.

The focus for understanding communication is how the human being can maintain a coherent identity in a personal and interpersonal milieu. This continually maintained coherence is a creative act. None of us as human beings is an island isolated in the universe. We are organisms which act and interact with the environment. We experience the world and attempt to influence it. Communication is the process by which we interact with our environment which includes the interpersonal milieux of our friends, colleagues and lovers. It is the medium by which we negotiate our self-image in those relationships and integrate ourselves with others.

Dialogue and exchange of information, the regulation of interpersonal distance and personal boundary, the mutual expression of human emotion and the sharing of ideas are based upon communication. These are located within a matrix of time which is not static. Sequence, order and phrasing, the fundamentals of musical form are vital elements in maintaining coherence whether in physiological systems, personal development or interpersonal relationships. In conversations, as well as in musical dialogues, a mutual structure is improvised between the communicators. Such a structure is co-produced, and is maintained not only by the speaker, or performer, but also by the listener. Jeannerod (1994) argues that even for the observer of another's action there is a concomitant kinaesthetic activity.

Physiology and communication

At the molecular level the immune system and nervous system communicate with each other. Psychological stress and social stress influences the immune system, sometimes adversely. The relationship between neuroendocrine and immune systems is one of mutual communication (Tee 1987). Our bodies are engaged in a continuing communicative process out of the range of conscious awareness. These communications are vital for life. We can, as Rossi (1987) says,

> conceptualize a fairly complete channel of information transduction between mind as it is experientially encoded in the limbic-hypothalamic system filter, and the autonomic endocrine, immune, and neuropeptide systems that transmit their 'messenger' molecules to the organs and tissues and to the cellular, genetic, and ultimately molecular levels. (p.52)

In this approach mind and body are united within a rhythmic context of communication which enables healing to take place. At the core of this work is the idea that the suprachiasmatic nucleus of the hypothalamus is a regulator of the ultradian (within a day) rhythms (Moore-Ede, Czeisler and Richardson 1983) responsible for autonomic system regulation and cerebral dominance. When the normal periodicity of these rhythms is disturbed by stress then psychosomatic reactions may occur. The restoration of an integrated rhythmic hypothalamic response should be an important factor in the process of healing. It is feasible then that music therapy is an ideal medium for promoting such integration and regulation through rhythm.

SYNCHRONY, RHYTHM AND COMMUNICATION

> Curative chronobiotics may be visualized for disease such as certain emotional disorders or rheumatoid arthritis – if, and only if, rhythm alternation can be recognized to be etiologically significant. (Reinberg and Halberg 1971, p.487)

For communication to occur, as we have seen with comatose patients, there has to be an element of predictability by which events are structured. This communication occurs within a matrix of time and is manifested as particular rhythms. These may be the circadian rhythms (literally about a day) of temperature and sleep in humans, the shorter ultradian (within a day) rhythms of autonomic system regulation and metabolic processes, or the shorter periodicities of respiration, peristalsis and heart rate (Johnson and Woodland-Hastings 1986; Moore-Ede *et al.* 1983; Reinberg and Halberg 1971). These are the regulatory mechanisms by which self-synchrony is maintained as a process of internal communication.

The work of Condon (1975, 1980, Condon and Ogston 1966) clearly shows the integration in terms of verbal behaviour, including silence, and bodily gestures. There is a self-synchronous organization to speech and movement which is essentially rhythmic. Rhythm provides the means by which behaviour is organized.

However, Condon (1980) goes on to write that as human beings we also communicate with other people. This he calls 'interactional' synchrony. We are active participants in communication. When we listen we move synchronously with the articulatory structure of the speaker's speech. As the speaker moves with his own speech, then so does the listener too. What is 'sent' and 'received' are inseparable in the ordered context of communication. This gives additional support to the idea, to which some music therapists refer, that therapist and patient are 'united in the music'. In Condon's words (1980):

> But what flows through them is a similar order; so that what is sent and what is received are understood and shared by both speaker and listener. What all aspects of this process have in common is the propagation and reception of order. There is no 'between' in the continuum of order. (p.56)

As rhythms are entrained, or synchronized, within the individual, then the listener will entrain with the emergent rhythmic structure of the speaker, singer or player. By watching the movement of the listener's body as well as by observing the way in which the listener plays it is possible to glean some ideas about their perceptual involvement.

PHRASING

A central feature of both musical and biological form is phrasing. When we speak in dialogues then we must know when a phrase is ending, and how to begin another. This occurs in speech by accented differences in a rhythmic context. When we listen we give a continuous feedback by small motions and gestures of our heads and bodies, and vocalizations. When a phrase is coming to an end there is an increase or change in such activity (Kempton 1980).

Interactional synchrony between people, and the co-ordination of phrasing in communication, cannot be explained as reaction or as a reflex response to sound or movement. Synchronization is achieved by a shared interaction in a rhythmic context known to both participants. The basis of such mutual knowledge is both physiological, in that we share common physiologies, and cultural (Key 1980). The forces which bind us together, which are the essence of our mutuality, are musical.

Child Development and Rhythmic Interaction

The development of language and socialization in the infant depends upon learning the rhythmic structure of synchronization (Kempton 1980). From birth the infant has the genetic basis of an individually entrained physiology, i.e. a self-synchronicity. The infant has its own time as 'kairos'. Yet the process of socialization and the use of language depend upon entraining those rhythms with those of another. This interactional synchrony reflects those neural timing mechanisms which form the ground of communication. Interactional cycles of attention and affect are entrained with homeostatic mechanisms in the nervous system (Linden 1987).

Lester, Hoffman and Brazelton (1985) investigated the synchronization of neonatal movement and the speech sounds of the adult talking to the baby and argued that the ability of the infant to attend to social stimuli was related to the infant's capacity for self regulation. Cycles of rhythmic interaction between infants and mothers reflected an increasing ability by the infant to organize cognitive and affective experience within the rhythmic structure provided by the parent.

However, this was not a one-sided phenomenon. Infants produce forms of expression and gesture that are not imitations of maternal behaviour (Murray and Trevarthen 1986; Trevarthen 1985). Both baby and mother learn each other's rhythmic structure and modify their own behaviour to fit that structure. Arousal, affect and attention are learned within the rhythm of a relationship.

This is the method employed in music therapy. The rhythmic structure of the patient is discovered by the therapist, and the patient is then met within that rhythmic structure.

Stern *et al.* (1975) studied the non-verbal behaviour of mothers and infants. They found two parallel modes of communication. One form of communication was that of *co-action*. In this form both mother and infant vocalize together. These authors suggest that co-actional vocalizing is an early pattern of behaviour which is structurally and functionally similar to mutual gaze, posture sharing and rhythm sharing. It occurs during the highest levels of arousal and is indicative of emotional tone. In adults co-actional vocalizing occurs in situations of interpersonal arousal such as intense anger, sadness, joy or lovemaking.

The contrasting form of communication is that of *alternation* and is found in conversation where speaker and listener alternately exchange roles. It is a dialogic pattern valuable for the exchange of symbolic information. This alternative mode is valuable for the acquisition of language. It allows information to be sent by one person while being processed by the other. However, it is a different pattern from that of co-action.

Co-action emphasizes the event of communication itself rather than the content of the communication. Simultaneous vocalization promotes mutual experience and may be essential to the process of bonding and feeling of relatedness. These two structurally different forms are present in the playing of improvised music with a partner.

Communication and Pathology

If musical elements are essential to communication, then the improvised musical playing of people may make manifest both underlying pathology and possibilities for growth and change.

Condon and Ogston (1966) compared normal and pathological behaviour between patients and therapists using the medium of film. Human interaction was filmed. The films were then viewed repeatedly one frame at a time, and analyzed. Each frame was numbered and sequences of frames analyzed according to speech and vocalization correlated with body movements. The authors call this the study of 'linguistics-kinesics' (p.38).

When the same authors studied a chronic schizophrenic patient they found that there was a noticeable lack of head movements and rigidity of posture in the patient compared to the relatively free head movement of normal speakers. The expressive qualities of speech and movement were severely restricted. A self-dyssynchrony also appeared in the schizophrenic patient where body movements appeared to be laterally separate.

In the micro-analysis of films of depressed patients by Condon (Condon and Ogston 1966) prosodic features of pitch, stress, phrasing and timbre were found which seemed indicative of underlying pathology:

> A marked laxity of articulatory movements characterized the speech of these patients. With its sparing use of pitch and accent, their voice had a dead listless quality: changes of pitch covered a narrow tonal range and were predominantly stepwise rather than gliding; hovering tones appeared at the end of sentences…intonations tended to occur in the same stereotyped patterns; and emphatic accents were either rare or absent entirely. Their speech gave an impression of being slow

and halting because of the frequent appearance of hesitation pauses interrupting the flow of their phrases. (p.344)

It is evident from this description that these are also musical qualities, and if we listened to the improvised playing of a depressed patient then a music therapist would be making similar comments to those in the passage above (as Pavlicevic and Trevarthen 1989 have).

Fraser *et al.* (1986) showed similar discriminating linguistic profiles of schizophrenic and manic patients. There was a continuum of linguistic degeneration across the psychotic spectrum. In an experimental control group 'normal' subjects produced fluent, complex and error-free utterances. Schizophrenic patients produced dysfluent, simple and error-ridden speech. Interestingly, when these patients improved clinically sentences became more tightly constructed and pitch widened in range and became more melodically varied. Again clinical improvement can be heard in the musical (prosodic or suprasegmental) aspects of speech style.

Condon (1975) continued to develop this diagnostic work, further studying the integration of body motion and speech across many dimensions, particularly in the field of autistic-like behaviour. His frame-by-frame filmed micro-analysis of patients with various syndromes like petit mal, Huntington's chorea, autism, stuttering, Parkinsonism and aphasia led him to believe that there may be some relationship between their problems and an underlying dysfunction in sound processing. Many of the behavioural mannerisms he observed in children appeared to be related to a multiple response to sound; there was both an immediate response and a delayed response to a sound event, or 'dyssynchrony'.

This work resulted in Condon postulating a continuum of degrees of delayed response to sound with autistic-like behaviour at the severe end and learning disabilities at the milder end. (While not evident as a motor abnormality during conversation, these children had difficulty with reading and mathematics.) The observed children responded to an immediate actual sound but also appeared to respond again to that same sound with a delay 'by as much as a quarter to a full second' (Condon 1975, p.47).

He gives the example of a two-and-a-half-year-old child throwing a block on a table. The block lands on the table and the child picks up another such block. Some microseconds later, the child's hands suddenly move in a jerky and seemingly bizarre manner. These hand movements were isomorphic with the sound and movements which occurred 16 film frames earlier. (There were 24 film frames per second.) By delaying the film sound to coincide with the movement the child was seen to move in precise synchrony with the sound of the brick hitting the table. It was possible to see and hear the occurrence of a sound on film and predict the occurrence of a bodily movement 16 frames later, although no sound occurred at the time of the hand movement.

In children with a delayed response to sound their behaviour appeared to be dominated by that delay. Furthermore, these children often lacked a co-ordination between hearing a sound and visually locating that sound. These children were literally out of time with the sensory structure of their world.

The entrainment of vision and sound gives an important spatial location in the world. To communicate we need to be entrained both within ourselves and with our environment. A delay in sound processing can lead to estrangement from the world and personal incoherence. We will see the ramifications of this early work of Condon in a later chapter regarding the role of focused listening and hand co-ordination in facilitating the development of young children.

A Musical Being

The basic elements of human communication are musical. Physiological, psychological and social activity occur in a context of time which is dynamic and the structure of which is musical. At a fundamental level human activity is organized as a hierarchy of rhythmic entrainment; within the individual as self-synchrony, and within relationships as interactional synchrony.

As we have seen regarding patients in a coma, and we shall see later regarding patients suffering with dementia, it is the co-ordination of pulses into a musical gestalt that underlies recovery, and it is speculated that it is the ground for higher cognition. Where a physicalist medical approach looks for a material time-giver (Zeitgeber), or a site where such co-ordination takes place, we may be better served by a musical metaphor that looks for a stability of process. Such stability of process is non-substantive. Stability of process, that is, organization, happens. We can see the products of organization, but 'organization' itself cannot be located. Such an understanding of phenomena as process and organization as a pattern in time is demanded if we are to grasp the healing powers of music.

When the breakdown of this synchronous behaviour occurs then pathology is evident. The restriction of musical aspects of communication, pitch, stress, articulation, timbre and fluency, appear to be indicative of psychopathology. An improvement in these qualities appears to be evident in a return to health and the maintenance of a coherent identity.

It is possible to hypothesize that improvised music therapy (Nordoff and Robbins 1977) is a powerful tool for promoting communication in terms of personal and interpersonal integration. Alternative creative dialogues may be encouraged within the person such that they are not out of synchrony with themselves, or estranged from others. Furthermore, clinicians, no matter in which discipline they have their origins, may be advised to attend to the musical components of communication. In this way the arts, as well as science, may inform the practice of medicine.

In creative music therapy lies the possibility of hearing, in a dynamic way, the individual as a whole self as well as in relationship with another person. We can hear the person coming into being as he or she creates a relationship in time. In addition music therapy offers the individual a chance to experience the self in time concretely, to hear his or her own self literally coming into being. If human survival is concerned with a repertoire of flexible coping responses to both external and internal demands, then we may hear in the playing of improvised music the creative way in which a person meets those demands. It could be that illness is a state where there is (a) a restriction in the ability of the person as a whole to improvise creatively (i.e., develop new solutions to problems), or (b) a limited repertoire of coping responses. By promoting creative coping responses we may be establishing the possibilities for renewed health. These are based on the creative qualities of the whole person that promote autonomy.

The next chapter compares our speculations and experiences from clinical practice with those of other researchers within medical settings.

CHAPTER FOUR

Music Therapy Research in the Medical Literature

I have suggested in earlier chapters that it is necessary to negotiate a common language between those of us involved in the creative arts therapies and those with whom we work in clinical practice. While we are trying to find a suitable language for music therapy, and must not necessarily translate what we know into a language of psychological science or medical terminology that is inappropriate, it is necessary to build bridges between understandings. One step forward in negotiating those understandings is to establish procedures and methods of research. An aspect of this research is to find out what has gone before, what is needed in the future and how current research fits into a broader perspective of clinical practices as they are presented in the health care literature. This chapter presents a general overview of music therapy research as it has been published in medical journals for the years 1983 to 1994. As this material is rather fragmentary, other related articles have been included to put the material into a broader music therapy context.

There have been a series of overviews about music therapy in the medical and nursing press ranging from letters through to full-scale articles. The principal emphasis is on the soothing ability of music and the necessity of music as an antidote to an overly technological medical approach (Aldridge 1993). Most of these articles are concerned with passive music therapy and the playing of pre-recorded music to patients emphasizing the necessity of healthy pleasures like music, fragrance and beautiful sights for the reduction of stress and the enhancement of well-being.

Hospital-based overviews

After the Second World War music therapy was intensively developed in American hospitals (Schullian and Schoen 1948). Since then some hospitals, particularly in mainland Europe, have incorporated music therapy within their practice (Goloff 1981), carrying on a tradition of European hospital-based research and practice (Leonidas 1981).

The nursing profession has seen the value of music therapy, particularly in the United States of America, and championed its use as an important nursing intervention (Cook 1986; Fletcher 1986; Frandsen 1989; Frank 1985; Glynn 1986; Grimm and Pefley 1990; Kolkmeier 1989; Marchette, Main and Redick 1989; Moss 1987; Mullooly, Levin and Feldman 1988; Prinsley 1986; Sammons 1984; Updike 1990; Walter 1983), even when music therapists are not available (Cook 1981). Although there is little work published about the benefits of music therapy in general medicine, the overall expectation is that the recreational, emotional and physical health of the patient is improved (Goloff 1981). This expectation of an overall improvement in health brought about by music therapy has not yet been substantiated by a broad base of research studies.

Psychiatry and Psychotherapy

The published work covering psychiatry has its basis in hospital treatment (Benjamin 1983; Courtright et al. 1990; Devisch and Vervaeck 1986; Engelmann 1995; Meschede, Bender and Pfeiffer 1983; Tang, Yao and Zheng 1994) and reflects the psychotherapeutic approach signalled by the psychiatrist Altshuler (1948).

In a study of chronic psychiatric patients who exhibited disruptive and violent behaviour at meal times, the playing of taped music as a background stimulus with the intention of providing a relaxed atmosphere reduced that disruptive behaviour (Courtright et al. 1990). Meschede and colleagues (Meschede et al. 1983) observed the behaviour of a group of chronic psychiatric patients over eight weeks of active music-making sessions and discovered that the subjective feelings of the patients had no correlation with the observations of the group leaders about the outward expression of those feelings.

Continental Europe has encouraged the use of music, particularly in terms of individual and group psychotherapy (Behrends 1983; Gross and Swartz 1982; Heyde and von Langsdorff 1983; Kaufmann 1983, 1985; Lengdobler and Kiessling 1989; Moreno 1988; Pfeiffer et al. 1987; Reinhardt, Rohrborn and Schwabe 1986; Schmuttermayer 1983) for the encouragement of awakening the emotions of the patient, and in helping them cope with unconscious intrapsychic conflicts. This situation is not surprising given that the roots of psychoanalysis are middle European.

Group psychotherapy has been used on an inpatient and outpatient basis by Kaufmann (1983, 1985), in what was formerly East Germany. He based his work on the psychodynamic music therapy methods of Schwabe (1978). Reinhardt (Reinhardt and Ficker 1983; Reinhardt *et al.* 1986) also developed Schwabe's method while working with depressed patients, the purpose of which was that patients would be led through listening to music to a confrontation with themselves and their surroundings, giving them a chance to overcome conflicts experienced in the past. Schmuttermayer (1983), also working in the East of Germany, utilized four types of music therapy (listening, singing, dancing, and playing instruments) which were combined to obtain a 'graduated group-centred music therapy' with a group of psychotic patients. Each of the therapy types acted in a different way on the variables 'anxiety' and 'activity'. Therapy influenced these variables during group-centred treatment and led the group towards modes of communication and behaviour that were more appropriate to reality, although the grounds for the author making such an observation are elusive.

Schizophrenia

Schizophrenia has been the subject of varying studies in applied music therapy (Pavlicevic and Trevarthen 1989; Pfeiffer *et al.* 1987; Schmutter-mayer 1983; Steinberg *et al.* 1985; Tang, Yao and Zheng 1994; Wengel, Burke and Holemon 1989). It is interesting to see, in the previously mentioned work of Altshuler, that 40 years ago psychotic patients were being treated with cold wet sheet packs in tubs of water as well as listening to music. The conclusion was that overall the presence of music in the hydro-therapy room was beneficial!

While modern music therapy techniques may seem less drastic in application, the difficulty of researching into the treatment of schizophrenic and psychotic patients remains. Pfeiffer's study (Pfeiffer *et al.* 1987) highlights such difficulties. First, it was difficult to find matching groups of acute psychotic patients using the parameters of age, syndrome, and diagnosis which were not complicated by other problems (for example, alcohol- or drug-related). Second, these patients were also being handled using particular psycho-medication which itself introduced variability. Third, the patients themselves were prone to crises which necessitated a change in their handling, which could also mean a change in medication. As the patients were being treated over a period of 27 weeks, it might have been foreseeable that by the nature of acute psychosis there would be predictable crises. Fourth, all the patients improved, including those on the control waiting list, as the psychotherapeutic support services in the area of Munich were favourable for helping such patients. With only 14 patients it was difficult to come to conclusions about the value of the music therapy, as the treated patients on follow-up had gradually deteriorated in functioning towards their original scores. It is clear that with psychotic patients, no matter how apparently effective the music therapy, their health does not survive the test of daily living and the temptations of normal life. One of the subjects who appeared to be improving received a letter from her divorced husband, thus precipitating a crisis. Another patient went on a weekend drinking spree.

Schmuttermayer's approach (1983) attempted through combined musical activities to reduce anxiety and improve communication in a group of schizophrenic patients. Overall communication, as measured by observed behaviour and self-reports using a checklist of adjectives, appeared to be improved by the development of a common rhythm within the group. Activity was enhanced by the instrumental playing, but reduced during the dancing and listening to music. While there was an increase in anxiety during the instrumental playing and dancing this could be handled within the therapeutic context of the group. Singing brought about a reduction in anxiety. It could well be in this study that the overall context of rhythm encouraged emotional control in terms of establishing predictability.

Within recent years researchers have attempted to understand the musical production of schizophrenic patients (Steinberg and Raith 1985, 1985a; Steinberg *et al.* 1985) in terms of emotional response. The underlying reasoning in this work is (a) that to produce music depends upon the mastery of underlying feelings, and (b) in psychiatric patients musical expression is negatively influenced by the disease. Steinberg and colleagues found that in the musical playing of endogenous-depressive patients there were weakened motoric qualities influencing stability and rhythmicity, while manic patients also exhibited difficulties in ending a phrase with falling intensity. Tempo appeared uninfluenced by depression, but was susceptible to the influence of medication. Schizophrenic patients exhibited changes in the dimensions of musical logic and order.

More recently Pavlicevic and Trevarthen (1989) have compared the musical playing of 15 schizophrenic patients, 15 depressed patients and 15 clinically normal controls. Significant differences in musical interaction between therapist and patient were found between the groups on a self-developed scale to test musical interaction. This musical interaction scale was developed to assess the emotional contact between therapist and partner according to musical criteria based upon six levels of interaction ranging from no contact (Level 1) to established mutual contact (Level 6). A critical element of the musical contact is the establishment of a common musical pulse which is defined as a series of regular beats.

In the above study, schizophrenic patients appeared musically unresponsive and idiosyncratic in their playing, which correlates with other studies of schizophrenia (Fraser *et al.* 1986; Lindsay 1980). The depressed patients appeared to take fewer initiatives in the music although it was possible for the therapist to make contact with them. Controls were able to enter into a musical partnership with the therapist and take musical initiatives. The lack of reciprocity from the schizophrenic patients seemed to be the factor which prevented contact and thereby disturbed communication. However, this finding with individual patients is in contrast to the previously mentioned group studies which refer to 'open' communication within the group. The strength of the Pavlicevic and Trevarthen paper is that it is firmly grounded in empirical data and, unlike many of the group therapy papers, gives clear evidence of how conclusions are reached.

The peculiarities of language which accompany some forms of schizophrenia has led to the inevitable link between speech disorders and musical components of language (Fraser *et al.* 1986) and the processing of language and musical information (Green 1986). Fraser's study suggested that the speech of schizophrenics had fewer well-formed sentences, often contained errors with many false starts and was simpler than the speech of controls which was fluent, error-free and complex. Lindsay (1980) argues that social behaviour is dependent upon social language skills of communication. Withdrawn patients speak with less spontaneous speech utterances, and their speech is improved by matching their utterances and building up dialogues from simple interactions to complex sequences; which is a feature of dialogic playing in improvised music therapy.

Tang *et al.* (1994) in a randomized controlled study of 76 inpatients found also found an increased ability to converse with others. Furthermore, negative symptoms were diminished, social isolation was reduced and those in the treatment group increased their interest in outside events. As we will read later in the work relating to patients suffering with dementia, music therapy makes a significant contribution to enhancing communication, reducing isolation and promoting interest in others. All three factors we could hypothesize are interlinked, and all three fostered by making music together.

Adolescent psychiatry

Group music therapy is the principal music therapy approach to the treatment of adolescent problems (Behrends 1983; Friedman and Glickman 1986; Mark 1986, 1988; Phillips 1988). Friedman (Friedman and Glickman 1986) recommends the use of creative therapies in general for the treatment of drug abuse in adolescents as it encourages spontaneous activity, motivates the client's response and fosters a culture of free expression.

Pop music is used by Behrends (1983) to provide a party atmosphere for adolescents with the intention of promoting 'communicative movement therapy'. This, the author claims, motivates deviant adolescents to take part in the necessary psychotherapy which they need to resolve their crises of identity, and this relates to other work which uses music as a precursor to psychotherapy itself. Mark (Behrends 1983; Mark 1986, 1988) also uses rock music, and in particular rock lyrics, as a bridge to reach 'highly resistant' adolescents enabling them to communicate their feelings about their roles in society, to express their opinions non-aggressively and to listen to others. In this sense music is an aid to articulacy, self-expression and communication in a context of psychotherapy. As one author (Saari 1986) says, adolescents are too old for play therapy.

Phillips (1988), as psychotherapist and jazz fan, provides an overview of improvisation in psychotherapy and the way in which it relates to adolescent patients. He identifies four important qualities as bases which enable the therapist to improvise in clinical practice: (a) to have access to his or her past, (b) to be able to focus attention solely on the present, (c) to be comfortable enough to give up control over the outcome of the task to experiment during the session, and (d) recognize the significance of accidental expression (p.184). He relates this ability to improvise to the therapeutic task of treating adolescents who call upon a wide range of responses which relate to the past experience of the therapist and which may require quite novel solutions.

Culture

Most of the references to the use of music therapy in medicine are predominantly Western, although the use of music as a therapeutic medium is found in most cultures. Two papers (Benjamin 1983; Devisch and Vervaeck 1986) describe the use of music in African hospitals, both locating the use of music within a cultural context, and combining this music with drama and dance. As in other group therapy methods, music is used as a vehicle to reach those who are isolated and withdrawn and reintegrate them into social relationships.

In South Africa (Benjamin 1983) the group consists of about 100 female patients sitting in a circle directed by a doctor. Music, through increasing tempo in singing and dancing, is used as an activator for the psychodrama techniques of Moreno (1946).

A Tunisian approach is far more radical in terms of psychiatry. Through 'art group therapy' (Devisch and Vervaeck 1986, p.541) utilizing dance, painting, therapy using clay, role play and singing, patients are encouraged to integrate personal experiences and emotions within a social context of relationships. The explanatory principle behind this work is that of 'the door' whereby fixed barriers between experiences are broken down, but the concept of threshold between experiences remains. In support of this integration family members of patients can be included in the singing and dancing to facilitate the patient returning to a family or wider social environment. For the individual patient it is argued that individual expression, when given the form of a work of art (to include singing and dancing), allows the person to experience themselves as something orderly and subjective; and, like a door, be able to be opened or closed to others and participate in interaction. This ability to discriminate between activities is called by the authors (who are social anthropologists) 'the liminal or threshold function of the body and the door' (p.543). Such an approach attempts to establish a meaningful relationship between the inner rhythms of the body, outer rhythms of personal interaction and broader patterns of cultural activity.

The Arab tradition, which regards the body as the meeting place of psyche and soma, and locates psychiatric illness within social relationships, gives cultural support to the ideas practised in such an institution. Culture is a source of meaning which does not only act through cognition, but also through personal interaction. The way in which people greet each other, listen to each other, and play with each other structures the meaning of that interaction and has a direct experience on the body. Similarly bodily experiences shape social contact. The act of kissing as a greeting, for example, has an external effect on relationship; and an internal effect on the emotional experiences of the body. This symbolic reality is not restricted solely to cognitive activity. We can further infer that the playing of music, and encouraging a person to express themselves in an articulate form within a relationship, promotes experiences which integrate the person inwardly within themselves and outwardly with others independent from cognition. Such relationships between emotions, relationships and body chemistry are being formally described as psychoneuroimmunology (Solomon *et al.* 1988; Stein, Keller and Schleifer 1985; Wiedermann and Wiedermann 1988).

Rehabilitation

Strategies for rehabilitating psychiatric patients using group and family approaches are not solely confined to African traditions (Ba 1988; Jochims 1990; Reinhardt and Ficker 1983), and music therapy has a broad base within the tradition of psychiatric and general rehabilitation (Bason and

Celler 1972; Gilbert 1977; Heyde and von Langsdorff 1983; Jochims 1990; Lengdobler and Kiessling 1989; Pfeiffer *et al.* 1987; Porchet-Munro 1988; Updike 1990).

Haag (Haag and Lucius 1984) discusses theories including psychosocial factors involved in the development of, and in coping with, disability. Psychological intervention approaches are set out, focusing on their particular relevance to rehabilitation. Music therapy is also recommended for the rehabilitation of patients who have difficulty in expressing their feelings and communicating with others. In an Italian psychiatric hospital, which includes family counselling (Ba 1988), regressed psychotic patients are referred to active music therapy; and patients who are less disturbed, and able to face their own emotional problems, are referred to passive music therapy.

Psychosomatics

Where both physical and mental processes overlap within medicine, i.e. the field of psychosomatics, then individual and group music therapy appears to play an important role (Lengdobler and Kiessling 1989).

Multiple sclerosis is a chronic neurological disease of unknown origin which can result in severe neuropsychological symptoms. Difficulties of anxiety, resignation, isolation and failing self-esteem seen in this disease are not easily relieved by symptom oriented medication or physiotherapy. Lengdobler and Kiessling (1989) set out to treat in a clinic, over a two-year period, 225 patients with multiple sclerosis with group music therapy. Each treatment period lasted for four to six weeks. A further part of their work was to discover the musical parameters of the playing of such patients using methods which were based on active improvisation; group instrumental playing, singing, listening, and free-painting to music. Unfortunately the size of the groups is not recorded, patient attendance at the groups was uncontrolled and the reports made by the patients were unstructured. Those reports which are published are vague and general, highlighting the need for rigorous research design with an underlying structure to display what may be valuable work at its best.

Music as therapy was used in the reduction of rheumatic pain in antiquity (Evers 1990), and latterly with the emphasis on emotional relief and rehabilitation. Sources citing the use of music specifically in rheumatism are rare. Terms like 'gout' or 'joint-pain', rather than rheumatism, are mentioned; which emphasizes the difficulty of making historical comparison in that terms change and have differing meanings. Recently Schorr (1993) has found a favourable response among women suffering from rheumatoid arthritis in relationship to the relief of chronic pain.

Elderly

The psychosocial rehabilitation of older persons is one of the main problems in health policy (Haag 1985). About one quarter of the over-65-year-olds face psychic problems without receiving adequate treatment and rehabilitative care. Substantial deficits exist above all in the outpatient and non-residential service sector, and the development of ambulatory, community-based services as well as intensive support for existing self-help efforts are necessary. Music therapy has been suggested as a valuable part of a combined treatment policy for the elderly (Dellmann-Jenkins, Papalia Finlay and Hennon 1984; Fenton and McRae 1989; Gilchrist and Kalucy 1983; Gross and Swartz 1982; Morris 1986; Prinsley 1986).

Music and dementia in the elderly

The responsiveness of patients with Alzheimer's disease to music is a remarkable phenomenon (Swartz *et al.* 1989). While language deterioration is a feature of cognitive deficit, musical abilities appear to be preserved. Beatty (Beatty *et al.* 1988) describes a woman who had severe impairments in terms of aphasia, memory dysfunction and apraxia yet was able to sight read an unfamiliar song and perform on the xylophone which to her was an unconventional instrument.

Certainly the anecdotal evidence suggests that quality of life of Alzheimer's patients is significantly improved with music therapy (Tyson 1989), accompanied by the overall social benefits of acceptance and sense of belonging gained by communicating with others (Morris 1986). Prinsley (1986) recommends music therapy for geriatric care in that it reduces the individual prescription of tranquillizing medication, reduces the use of hypnotics on the hospital ward and helps overall rehabilitation. He recommends that music therapy be based on treatment objectives; the social goals of interaction co-operation; psychological goals of mood improvement and self-expression; intellectual goals of the stimulation of speech and organization of mental processes; and the physical goals of sensory stimulation and motor integration. Such approaches also emphasize the benefit of music programmes for the professional carers (Kartman 1984) and families (Tyson 1989) of elderly patients.

Musical hallucinations

Hallucinations may occur in any of our senses, and auditory hallucinations take various forms; as voices, cries, noises, or, rarely, music. However, the appearance of musical hallucinations, often in elderly patients, has generated interest in the medical literature (Aizenberg, Schwartz and Modai 1986; Berrios 1990; Fenton and McRae 1989; Gilchrist and Kalucy 1983; Hammeke, McQuillen and Cohen 1983; Keshavan, Kahn and Brar 1988; McLoughlin 1990; Patel, Keshavan and Martin 1987; Wengel, Burke and Holemon 1989). When such hallucinations do occur they are described as highly organized vocal or instrumental music. In contrast, tinnitus is characterized by unformed sounds or noises that may possess musical qualities (Wengel, Burke and Holemon 1989).

The case histories of patients with musical hallucinations suggest an underlying psychiatric disorder (Aizenberg, Schwartz and Modai 1986; Wengel, Burke and Holemon 1989), which may be exacerbated by dementing illness occurring with brain deterioration (Gilchrist and Kalucy 1983); or that patients with musical hallucinations and hearing loss become anxious and depressed (Fenton and McRae 1989). Fenton challenges the association of psychosis and previous mental illness, preferring an explanation that relies upon the degeneration of the aural end-organ whereby sensory input, which suppresses much non-essential information, fails to inhibit information from other perception-bearing circuits. Other investigators (Gilchrist and Kalucy 1983) argue for a central brain dysfunction as evidenced by measures of brain function. In a sample of 46 subjects experiencing musical hallucinations musical hallucinations were far more common in females; age, deafness, and brain disease affecting the non-dominant hemisphere played an important role in the development of hallucinations; and psychiatric illness and personality factors were found to be unimportant (Berrios 1990).

For these patients the application of music therapy to raise the ambient noise level, to organize aural sensory input by giving it a musical sense and counter sensory deprivation, and to stimulate and motivate the patient seems a reasonable approach.

Music Therapy, Heart Rate and Respiration

The effect of music on the heart and blood pressure has been a favourite theme throughout history. In an early edition of the medical journal *Lancet* (Vincent and Thompson 1929) an attempt was made to discover the influence of listening to gramophone, and radio, music on blood pressure. The effects of music were influenced by how much the subjects appreciated music. Differing groups of musical competence responded in relation to volume, melody, rhythm, pitch, and type of music. Interest in the music was an important factor influencing response. Melody produced the most marked effect in the musical group. Volume produced the most apparent effect in the moderately musical group. In general, listening to music was accompanied by a slight rise in blood pressure in the listener.

If music produces physiological and psychological effects in healthy persons as listeners, then it may be assumed that persons with various diseases respond to music in specific ways. A particular hypothesis, which is yet to be substantiated empirically, is that people with known diseases respond to music in a way which is mediated by that disease. Also, in terms of music therapy, if music is known to influence a physiological parameter such as heart rate or blood pressure then, as argued in the previous chapter, music can be used therapeutically for patients who have problems with heart disease or hypertension.

Bason (Bason and Celler 1972) found that the human heart rate could be varied over a certain range by entrainment of the sinus rhythm with external auditory stimulus, which presumably acted through the nervous control mechanisms, and resulted from a neural coupling into the cardiac centres of the brain. An audible click was played to the subject at a precise time in the cardiac cycle. When it came within a critical range then the heart rate could be increased or decreased up to 12 per cent over a period of time up to three minutes. Fluctuations caused by breathing remained, but these tended to be less when the heart was entrained with the audible stimulus. When the click was not within the time range of the cardiac cycle then no influence could be made. Bason and Celler's paper is important for supporting the proposition often made by music therapists that meeting the tempo of the patient influences their musical playing and is the initial key to therapeutic change.

An extension of this premise, that musical rhythm is a pacemaker, was investigated by Haas and her colleagues (Haas, Distenfeld and Axen 1986) in terms of the effects of perceived rhythm on respiratory pattern, a pattern which serves both metabolic and behavioural functions. Metabolic respiratory pathways are located in the reticular formation of the lower pons and medulla, whereas the behavioural respiratory pathways are located mainly in the limbic forebrain structures which lead to vocalization and complex behaviour. There appear to be both hypothalamic and spinal pattern generators capable of synchronizing this respiratory and locomotor activity. Therefore, Haas hypothesized that an external rhythmical musical activity, in this case listening to taped music, would have an influence on respiratory pattern while keeping metabolic changes and afferent stimuli (i.e. no gross motor movements) to a minimum.

Twenty subjects were involved in this experiment, four of whom were experienced musicians and practising musicians, six had formal musical training but no longer played a musical instrument, and the remaining ten had no musical training. Respiratory data including respiration frequency and airflow volume was collected alongside heart rate and end-tidal CO_2. Subjects listened to a metronome set at 60 b.p.m. and tapped to that beat on a microphone after a baseline period. The subjects were then randomly presented with four musical excerpts and a period of silence which they tapped along to. There were no appreciable changes in heart rate during the experiment, but there was an appreciable change in respiratory frequency and a significant decrease in the coefficient of variation for all respiratory parameters during the finger tapping. For non-musically trained subjects there was little co-ordination between breathing and musical rhythm, while for trained musicians there was a coupling of breathing and rhythm. That singers have more efficient pulmonary strategies than non-trained musicians, even when talking, is supported elsewhere in the literature (Formby *et al.* 1987).

Auditory cues, then, appear to be important in the synchronization of respiration and other motor activity. This finding supports other evidence linking a decrease in muscle activity while performing a motor task accompanied by a musical rhythm (Safranek *et al.* 1982); that respiratory rhythm follows that of music within certain limits of variability (Diserens 1920); and that there is a relationship between disturbed functional cardiac arrythmias and musical rhythmic ability (Richter and Kayser 1991).

Richter and Kayser (1991) hypothesized that patients with cardiac arrhythmias perform worse in rhythm perception and production than healthy controls. Thirty-one patients with functional cardiac arrythmias were compared with 31 control subjects. Subjects were required to mark on a sheet of paper rhythmic patterns which were played to them by a tape-recorder, and tap synchronously with repeating patterns from a tape-recorder. Patients with dysrhythmias have significantly poorer abilities in musical perception and rhythmic anticipation than healthy controls. Patients with tachycardia show a particularly poor sense of rhythm perception and synchronization.

Coronary care

Several authors have investigated this relationship in the setting of hospital care (Bolwerk 1990; Bonny 1983; Davis-Rollans and Cunningham 1987; Gross and Swartz 1982; Guzzetta 1989; Philip 1989; Wein 1987; Zimmerman, Pierson and Marker 1988) and in dentistry (Lehnen 1988), often with the intent of reducing anxiety in chronically ill patients or treating anxiety in general (Chetta 1981; Daub and Kirschner-Hermanns 1988; Elliott 1994; Fagen 1982; Gross and Swartz 1982; Heyde and von Langsdorff 1983;

Lengdobler and Kiessling 1989; Schmuttermayer 1983; Standley 1986; Zimmerman *et al.* 1989).

A hospital situation which is fraught with anxiety for the patient is the intensive care unit. For patients after a heart attack, where heart rhythms are potentially unstable, the setting of coronary care is itself anxiety-provoking, which recursively influences the physiological and psychological reactions of the patient. In these situations several authors, in varying hospital intensive care or coronary care clinics, have assessed the use of tape-recorded music delivered through headphones as an anxiolytic with the intention of reducing stress (Updike 1990). Bonny (Bonny 1975, 1983; Bonny and McCarron 1984) has suggested a series of musical selections for tape-recordings which can be chosen for their sedative effects and according to other mood criteria, associative imagery and relaxation potential (Bonny 1978); none of which has been empirically confirmed; although Updike (Updike 1990), in an observational study, confirms Bonny's impression that there is a decreased systolic blood pressure, and a beneficial mood change from anxiety to relaxed calm, when sedative music is played.

Rider (1985, 1985a) proposed that disease related stress was caused by the desynchronization of circadian oscillators and that listening to sedative music, with a guided imagery induction, would promote the entrainment of circadian rhythms as expressed in temperature and corticosteroid levels of nursing staff. This study found no conclusive results, mainly because there was no control group and the study design was confused, highlighting the essential difference between music when applied as a music therapy discipline, and music as an adjunct to psychotherapy or biofeedback.

Davis-Rollans (Davis-Rollans and Cunningham 1987) describes the use of a 37-minute tape-recording of selected classical music[1] on the heart rate and rhythm of coronary care unit patients. Twelve of the patients had had heart attacks and another 12 had a chronic heart condition. Patients were exposed to two randomly varied 42-minute periods of continuous monitoring; one period with music delivered through headphones, the other control period without music and containing background noise of the unit as heard through silent headphones. Eight patients reported a significant change to a happier emotional state after listening to the music (a result replicated by Updike (1990)), although there were no significant changes in specific physiological variables during the music periods. A change in mood, how-

---

1   Beethoven's Symphony No.6 (first movement), Mozart, *Eine kleine Nachtmusik* (first and fourth movements), and Smetana, 'The Moldau'.

ever, which relieves depression is believed to be beneficial to the overall status of coronary care patients (Cassem and Hackett 1971).

Bolwerk (1990) set out to relieve the state anxiety of patients in a myocardial infarction ward using recorded classical music.[2] Forty adults were randomly assigned to two equal groups; one of which listened to relaxing music during the first four days of hospitalization, the other received no music. There was no controlled 'silent condition'. While there was a significant reduction in state anxiety in the treatment group, state anxiety was also reduced in the control group. The reasons for this overall reduction in anxiety may have been that after four days the situation had become less acute, the situation was not so strange for the patient, and by then a diagnosis had been confirmed.

State anxiety is an individual's anxiety at a particular state in time, as opposed to trait anxiety which is an overall prevailing condition of anxiety unbounded by time and determined by personality. The relationship between stress and anxiety is that stimulus conditions, or stressors, produce anxiety reactions; i.e. the state of anxiety. Anxiety as a state is characterized by subjective feelings of tension, worry and nervousness which are accompanied by physiological changes of heart rate, blood pressure, myocardial oxygen consumption, lethal cardiac dysrhythmias and reductions in peripheral and renal perfusion (Guzzetta 1989). Admission to the coronary care unit is itself a stressor, and the environment produces further stress, therefore the importance of managing state anxiety.

The purpose of a study by Guzzetta (1989) was to determine whether relaxation and music therapy were effective in reducing stress in patients admitted to a coronary care unit with the presumptive diagnosis of acute myocardial infarction. In this experimental study, 80 patients were randomly assigned to a relaxation, music therapy, or control group. The relaxation and music therapy groups participated in three sessions over a two-day period. Music therapy comprised a relaxation induction and listening to a 20-minute musical cassette tape selected from three alternative musical styles: soothing classical music, soothing popular music and non-traditional music (defined as 'compositions having no vocalization or metre, periods of silence and an asymmetric rhythm' (Guzzetta 1989, p.611)). Stress was evaluated by apical heart rates, peripheral temperatures, cardiac complications, and qualitative patient evaluative data. Data analysis revealed that lowering apical heart rates and raising peripheral temperatures were more successful in the relaxation

---

2   Bach, 'Largo', Beethoven, 'Largo', Debussy, 'Prelude to the Afternoon of a Faun'.

and music therapy groups than in the control group. The incidence of cardiac complications was found to be lower in the intervention groups, and most intervention subjects believed that such therapy was helpful. Both relaxation and music therapy were found to be effective modalities of reducing stress in these patients, and music listening was more effective than relaxation alone. Furthermore, apical heart rates were lowered in response to music over a series of sessions, thus supporting the argument that the assessment of music therapy on physiological parameters is dependent upon adaptation over time. Further research strategies may wish to make longitudinal studies of the influence of music on physiological parameters.

This positive finding above was in contrast to Zimmerman (Zimmerman, Pierson and Marker 1988) who failed to find an influence of music on heart rate, peripheral temperature, blood pressure or anxiety score. However, Zimmerman's study only allowed for one intervention of music. In this experimental study the authors examined the effects of listening to relaxation-type music on self-reported anxiety and on selected physiologic indices of relaxation in patients with suspected myocardial infarction. Seventy-five patients were randomly assigned to one of two experimental groups, one listening to taped music and the other to 'white noise'[3] through headphones, or to a control group. The Spielberger State Anxiety Inventory (Spielberger 1983) was administered before and after each testing session, and blood pressure, heart rate, and digital skin temperature were measured at baseline and at 10-minute intervals for the 30-minute session. There was no significant difference among the three groups for state anxiety scores or physiologic parameters. Because no differences were found, analyses of the groups combined were conducted. Significant improvement in all of the physiologic parameters was found to have occurred (a finding that was to be replicated in 1995 (Barnason, Zimmerman and Nieveen 1995)). This finding reinforces the benefit of rest and careful monitoring of patients in the coronary care unit, but adds little to the understanding of music interventions. Time to listen, separated from the surrounding influence of the hospital unit by the use of headphones, may itself be an important intervention. Although Rider (1985a) did not reach this preceding conclusion (he found that perceived pain was reduced in a hospital situation in response to classical music delivered through headphones) it could be concluded from his work that isolation from environmental sounds, cancelling out external noise, has a

---

3   'White noise' or 'synthetic silence' is an attempt to block out environmental noise. In this case it was a tape-recording of sea sounds, which themselves were rhythmic (Philip 1989; Zimmerman 1989).

positive benefit for the patient regardless of inner content, i.e. music, relaxation induction or silence.

Given that Bason's study (Bason and Celler 1972) could influence heart rate by matching the heart rate of the patient, we must conclude that studies of the influence of music on heart rate must match the music to the individual patient. This also makes psychological sense as different people have varied reactions to the same music. Furthermore, improvised music playing which takes meeting the tempo of the patient as one of its main principles, may have an impact other than the passive listening to music. In addition, the work of Haas (Haas, Distenfeld and Axen 1986) mentioned above showed that listening, coupled with tapping, synchronizes respiration pattern with musical rhythm, further emphasizing that active music playing can be used to influence physiological parameters and that this synchronization can be learned. Thaut (1985) also found that children with gross motor dysfunction performed significantly better motor rhythm accuracy when aided by auditory rhythm and rhythmic speech.

Breathing

The relationship between listening to music and changes in respiration has also been investigated in situations other than coronary care (Brody 1988; Formby *et al.* 1987; Fried 1990; Gross and Swartz 1982; Lehmann, Horrichs and Hoeckle 1985; Tiep *et al.* 1986).

Fried (1990) presents a general overview of music as it is integrated in breathing training and relaxation. Breathing training itself is believed to have a physical benefit in increasing tidal volume without excessive loss of CO_2 (hypocapnia). Typically anxious patients have relatively rapid shallow chest breathing and may hyperventilate. However, music appears to have a paradoxical effect; while subjects report music to be highly relaxing, soothing and sedative, their physiological reactions indicate otherwise.

Music and breathing have been used to induce alternative states of consciousness and Fried's paper correlates the characteristics of consciousness and the role of music in altering those states, and the qualities of music which can be used to invoke calm and inner peace (McLellan 1988).

Nursing approaches have also utilized the anxiolytic effect of music in combination with massage and breathing exercises to relax patients (Lehrer *et al.* 1994).

Anaesthesia

The ability of music to induce calm and well-being has been used in general anaesthesia. Patients express their pleasure at awakening to music in the operating suite (Bonny and McCarron 1984) where music was played openly at first, and then through earphones during the operation. In a study by Lehmann (Lehmann, Horrichs and Hoeckle 1985) patients undergoing elective orthopaedic or lower abdominal surgery were given either placebo infusion (0.9% NaCl) instead of Tramadol in a randomized and double-blind manner in order to evaluate Tramadol efficacy as one component of balanced anaesthesia. Post-operative analgesic requirement and awareness of intra-operative events (tape-recorded music offered via earphones) were further used to assess Tramadol effects. Although anaesthesia proved to be quite comparable in both groups, striking differences between the two groups were shown with respect to intra-operative awareness: while patients receiving placebo proved to be amnesic, 65 per cent of Tramadol patients were aware of intra-operative music. The ability to hear music during an operation is also reported by Bonny (Bonny and McCarron 1984).

Cancer Therapy, Pain Management and Hospice Care

Cancer and chronic pain care require complex co-ordinated resources which are not only medical but psychological, social and communal (Aldridge 1987a, 1987b, 1987c; Coyle 1987; Fagen 1982; Frampton 1986, 1989; Gilbert 1977; Heyde and von Langsdorff 1983; Walter 1983). Hospice care in the United States and England has attempted to meet this need for palliative and supportive services which provide physical, psychological and spiritual care for dying persons and their families (Aldridge 1987a; Coyle 1987; Frampton 1986, 1989; Heyde and von Langsdorff 1983; Jacob 1986; Lindsay 1993). Such a service is based upon an interdisciplinary team of health care professionals and volunteers which often involves outpatient and inpatient care.

In the Supportive Care Program of the Pain Service to the Neurology Department of Sloan-Kettering Cancer Center, New York, a music therapist is part of that supportive team along with a psychiatrist, nurse-clinician, neuro-oncologist, chaplain and social worker (Bailey 1983; Coyle 1987). Music therapy is used to promote relaxation, to reduce anxiety, to supplement other pain control methods and to enhance communication between patient and family (Bailey 1984, 1985, 1983). As depression is a common feature of the patients dealt within this programme, then music therapy is hypothetically an influence on this parameter and in enhancing quality of life.

Although quality of life has assumed a position of importance in cancer care in recent years (Aaronson 1989; Clark and Fallowfield 1986; Gilbert 1977; Gold 1986; Heyde and von Langsdorff 1983; Oleske, Heinze and Otte 1990; Spitzer 1987); and music therapy, along with other art therapies, is thought to be important, the evidence for this belief is largely anecdotal and unstructured. Bailey (1983) discovered a significant improvement in mood for the better when playing live music to cancer patients as opposed to playing taped music which she attributes to the human element being involved.

A better researched phenomenon is the use of music in the control of chronic cancer pain, although such studies abdicate the human element of live performance in favour of tape-recorded interventions. Combinations of pharmacological and non-pharmacological pain management are acceptable in modern medicine (McCaffery 1990), with non-pharmacological interventions offering a form of distraction.

Such diversion from attention to pain was the subject of a study by Zimmerman who investigated the influence of playing preferred taped music, combined with suggestion, on a controlled sample of patients suffering with chronic pain. The objective of the study was to determine the self-reported relief obtained by patients receiving pain-medication where the blood level of analgesic was controlled. Music was found to decrease the overall level of the pain experience as reported by patients randomly assigned to the music treatment group. Furthermore, the sensory component, as well as the affective component, of the pain as measured by the McGill Pain Questionnaire (Melzack 1975) was significantly reduced for patients who listened to music. Not only was suffering as an emotional experience reduced, the actual *sensation* of pain was experienced as reduced. This would appear to confound the common belief that music therapy is primarily an intervention based upon qualitative emotional experiences, and support the contention that music therapy also has a direct influence upon sensory parameters.

In addition to reducing pain, particularly in pain clinics (Foley 1986; Godley 1987; Locsin 1988; Wolfe 1978); music as relaxation and distraction has been tried during chemotherapy (Kammrath 1989) to bring overall relief and to reduce nausea and vomiting (Frank 1985). Using taped music and guided imagery in combination with pharmacological antiemetics, Frank (1985) found that state anxiety was significantly reduced, resulting in a perceived degree of reduced vomiting, although the nausea remained the same. As this study was not controlled the reduced anxiety may have been a result of the natural fall in anxiety levels when chemotherapy treatment ended. However, the study consisted of patients who had previously experienced chemotherapy and were conditioned to experience nausea or vomiting in conjunction with it. That the subjects of the study felt relief was seen as an encouraging sign in the use of music therapy as a treatment modality.

Neurological Problems

In many cases neurological diseases become traumatic because of their abrupt appearance, resulting in physical and/or mental impairment (Jochims 1990). Music appears to be a key in the recovery of former capabilities in the light of what at first can seem like hopeless neurological devastation (Aldridge 1991b; Jones 1990; Sacks 1986).

For some patients with brain damage following head trauma, the problem may be temporary, resulting in the loss of speech (aphasia). Music therapy can play a valuable role in aphasia rehabilitation (Lucia 1987). Melodic Intonation Therapy (Naeser and Helm-Estabrooks 1985; O'Boyle and Sanford 1988) has been developed to fulfil such a rehabilitative role and involves embedding short propositional phrases into simple, often repeated, melody patterns accompanied by finger tapping. The inflection patterns, of pitch changes and rhythms of speech, are selected to parallel the natural speech prosody of the sentence. The singing of previously familiar songs is also encouraged as it encourages articulation, fluency and the shaping procedures of language which are akin to musical phrasing. In addition the stimulation of singing within a context of communication motivates the patient to communicate and, it is hypothesized, promotes the activation of intentional verbal behaviour. In infants the ability to reciprocate or compensate a partner's communicative response is an important element of communicative competence (Murray and Trevarthen 1986; Street and Cappella 1989) and vital in speech acquisition (Glenn and Cunningham 1984). Music therapy strategies in adults may be used in a similar way with the expectation that they will stimulate those brain functions which support, precede and extend functional speech recovery, functions which are essentially musical and rely upon brain plasticity. Combined with the ability to enhance word retrieval, music can also be used to improve breath capacity, encourage respiration–phonation patterns, correct articulation errors caused by inappropriate rhythm or speed and prepare the patient for articulatory movements. In this sense music offers a sense of time which is not chronological, which is fugitive to measurement and vital for the co-ordination of human communication (Aldridge 1989a, 1991d).

Jacome (1984) tells of a stroke patient who was dysfluent and had difficulty finding words. Yet, he frequently whistled instead of attempting to answer with phonemes...he spontaneously sang Spanish songs without prompting with excellent pitch, melody, rhythm, lyrics and emotional intonation. He could tap, hum, whistle and sing along... Emotional intonation of speech (prosody), spontaneous facial emotional expression, gesturing and pantomimia were exaggerated. (p.309)

From this case study Jacome goes on to recommend that singing and musicality in aphasics be tested by clinicians, a point also recommended by Morgan and Tilluckdharry (1982) in terms of aphasia following stroke.

Evidence of the global strategy of music processing in the brain is found in the clinical literature. In two cases of aphasia (Morgan and Tilluckdharry 1982) singing was seen as a welcome release from the helplessness of being a patient. The authors hypothesized that singing was a means to communicate thoughts externally. Although the 'newer aspect' of speech was lost, the older function of music was retained, possibly because music is a function distributed over both hemispheres. Berman (1981) suggests that recovery from aphasia is not a matter of new learning by the non-dominant hemisphere but a taking over of responsibility for language by that hemisphere. The non-dominant hemisphere may be a reserve of functions in case of regional failure indicating an overall brain plasticity (Naeser and Helm-Estabrooks 1985), and language functions may shift with multilinguals as compared with monolinguals (Karanth and Rangamani 1988), or as a result of learning and cultural exposure where music and language share common properties (Tsunoda 1983).

That singing is an activity correlated with certain creative productive aspects of language is shown in the case of a two-year-old boy of above-average intelligence who experienced seizures, manifested by tic-like turning movements of the head, which were induced consistently by his own singing, but not by listening to or imagining music. His seizures were also induced by his recitation and by his use of silly or witty language such as punning. Seizure activity on an EEG was present in both temporocentral regions, especially on the right side, and was correlated with clinical attacks (Herskowitz, Rosman and Geschwind 1984).

Aphasia is also found in elderly stroke patients and music therapy, as reported in case studies, has been used effectively in combination with speech therapy.

Gustorff (Aldridge, Gustorff and Hannich 1990) has successfully applied creative music therapy to coma patients who were otherwise unresponsive. Matching her singing, as music therapist, with the breathing patterns of the patient she has stimulated changes in consciousness which are both measurable on a coma rating scale and apparent to the eye of the clinician.

Mental Handicap

Adults

Music appears to be an effective way of engaging profoundly mentally handicapped adults in activity (Bolton and Adams 1983; Colletti *et al.* 1988; Knill 1983; Oldfield and Adams 1990). The functional properties of music have implications for the treatment of the mentally handicapped in that (a) exposure to sound arouses sensory processes, (b) a musical event is an organized temporal auditory structure with a beginning and an end, (c) music facilitates memory recall and expectation ('the signature tune effect'), and (d) a sequence of musical themes can enhance memory recall and the organization of a sequence of cognitive activities (Knill 1983).

For a group of profoundly mentally handicapped adults, music therapy was used to encourage those adults to attempt movements and actions, and achieve non-musical aims within the music therapy sessions (Oldfield and Adams 1990). Music therapy was compared with play activity using two groups of subjects. Each group received either music therapy or play activity for six months, at which time the groups were reversed to receive the comparison treatment. As the handicaps were so profound and varied between individuals then a separate behavioural index was formulated for each subject. It was hypothesized that each objective would be achieved to a greater extent in the music therapy group than in play activity. While the study was restricted in terms of numbers, and the behavioural indexes were varied, there was a significant difference in the performance in music therapy than in play therapy. This improved performance was not attributable to greater attention in the music therapy group. The type of input was noticeably different in the two groups; in the music therapy group improvisations were based on the subjects' own musical productions. However, for one subject there was greater improvement in the play activity which came before the music therapy treatment.

Children

Much of modern music therapy was developed in working with children (Nordoff and Robbins 1977; Probst 1976), and the diversity and richness of this work are reflected in several papers (Froehlich 1984; Grimm and Pefley 1990; Marley 1984; Sharon 1985).

Stern *et al.* (1975) emphasize the importance of the creative arts in general to child development as they involve the child's natural curiosity. However, she also proposes that in terms of child development then therapies must involve the family of the child particularly in the case of child disability. For children with multiple disabilities there is need for stimulation and this can be achieved using music, which also provides a sense of fun and enjoyment. Stern's approach suggests that songs stimulate a bond between therapist and patient, and that for one particular disabled patient, 'The music entered Susan's frame of reference' (p.649). An alternative explanation could be that music *was* Susan's frame of reference by which she co-ordinated her own activities, and those activities with another person. It may well be that families of handicapped children need to learn the rudiments of music therapy, as organized rhythmic communication, such that they can provide a structure for their mutual communications (Aldridge 1989, 1989a). In this sense it makes sense for therapists to work with both parents and children.

Songs, both composed and improvised, provide the vehicle for working with hospitalized children. Grimm and Pefley (1990) and her colleagues commissioned specially composed songs recorded on a cassette to cover important issues of hospitalization for children (see Table 4.1). In this case it was the symbolic content of the songs which was effective, rather than the pure musical effect.

Table 4.1 Issues of hospitalization for children

Issues
Separation from parents, family, school and friends
Misunderstanding the nature of the illness and the cause of the disease
Facing the reality of physical disability
Promotion of self-esteem and sensitivity to others
Stimulate motivation and reinforce strengths
Control over loss of privacy, loss of control, powerlessness and embarrassment
Use of imagery to help the healing process
Hospital fears and fantasies, fear of anaesthesia
Prepare for pain management
Coping with loss and disappointment
Integration of child and family

Songs were also used in the pre-operative preparation of children in an attempt to relieve fear and anxiety by transmitting surgery-related information. To ascertain the efficacy of using information alone, or information with songs, three groups of children were prepared on the day before surgery; one group with information alone, one group with information followed by specially prepared songs which were based on that information; and a third group which also had information followed by songs, with an additional session of songs immediately in the pre-operative phase on the day of the operation. The group receiving music therapy on the morning prior to the induction of pre-operative medication exhibited significantly less anxiety based on a number of observed variables. Lessons to be learned from this research may be that although information is made available it does not mean to say that the child will be able to use this information when it is needed. No amount of information will make a procedure less painful, and a cognitive understanding of pain made during a therapy session is not necessarily translated into physical or emotional relief during the context of surgical preparation. Music therapy in its immediacy may have been a critical factor in reducing anxiety, as anecdotal reports suggest, but in this study no group received music therapy alone.

In a general study of music therapy as applied to newborns and infants in hospital (Marley 1984), music appeared beneficial as a calming effect inducing sleep and relaxation. The methods ranged from simple tapping on the back to simulate a heartbeat, through rocking of children in time to played music, to receptive music therapy. It is difficult to understand the nature of this work as music therapy. The researcher reports that in 13 of the rooms the television was off, and in 14 rooms the television was on. When the television was on in most cases the sound was either too low or too loud. It must be added that the children were between the ages of 5 weeks and 36 months old. With continuous sound stimulation, it is little wonder the children responded to the television being switched off and guitar music being played to them.

Fagen (1982), working with terminally ill paediatric patients, also emphasizes the psychosocial setting of the family and the hospital as important. Music therapy in this setting was used to improve the quality of life of the patients in an attempt to broaden and deepen their range of living. However, no quality of life scale was used, nor are the criteria for assessing the quality of life in dying children made clear. This is not surprising as no quality of life scales for children with terminal illness exist at present. In her music therapy practice Fagen was eclectic, borrowing from various music therapy schools but concentrating on songs to confront the issues of hospitalization and dying. These songs often had improvised lyrics according to the needs of the situation, or songs which had given meanings and were appropriate to the patient. No attempt was made to force patients to confront their own dying.

Creative expression, as reported in the work with children, is generally accepted as a means of coping whereby pain and anxiety are channelled into activities (Lavigne, Schulein and Hahn 1986). In an attempt to encourage children to cope with the trauma of hospitalization by verbalizing their experiences, Froehlich (1984) compared the use of play therapy and music therapy as facilitators of verbalization. When specifically structured questions about hospitalization were asked of the children after sessions of music therapy or play therapy, music therapy elicited more 'answers' than 'no answers', and a more involved type of verbalization involving elaborated answers, than play therapy.

Autism

Music therapy allows children without language to communicate (Barison, Pradetto and Valer 1984), possibly to orient themselves within time and space, and has developed a significant place in the treatment of mental handicap in children (Knill 1983; Preza et al. 1990; Wesecky 1986; Zappella 1986) as it has with mental handicap in adults (Adams 1988; Bolton and Adams 1983; Oldfield and Adams 1990).

Children exhibiting autistic behaviour appeared to prefer a musical stimulus rather than a visual stimulus when compared with normal children (Thaut 1987). Although the significance of this finding was not statistically valid, the study does report that autistic children showed more motor reactions during periods of music than normal children, and that autistic children appeared to listen to music longer than their normal peers who preferred visual displays.

In a later study comparing autistic children and their normal peers (Thaut 1988), autistic children produced spontaneous tone sequences almost as well as normal children and significantly better than a control group of mentally retarded children. Each child sat at a xylophone with two beaters, after having had a short demonstration from the researcher, who then asked them to play spontaneously for as long as they liked until they came to a natural ending. The musical parameters, of the first 16 tones of these improvisations, which were assessed and used as the basis for group comparisons were: rhythm (representing the imposition and adherence to temporal order); restriction (representing the use of all available tonal elements); complexity (representing the generation of recurring melodic patterns; rule adherence

(representing the application of melodic patterns to the total sound sequence); and originality (representing the production of melodic patterns
that occurred only once but fulfilled criteria of melodic and rhythmic shape).
Autistic children perceived and explored the xylophone as normal children
did in terms of originality and restriction, but tended to play with short
recurring motives rather like the mentally handicapped children. Thaut
(1988) concludes that 'The low performances on complexity and rule
adherence of such children suggest an inability to organize and retain
complex temporal sequences' (p.567). This relationship between cognition
and motor behaviour as it is co-ordinated in rhythmical performance, as we
have read above in terms of heart rate, breathing, muscle performance and
speech rehabilitation, would appear to be worthy of investigation in a wide
variety of patients with communication difficulties regardless of the source
of those difficulties.

The Need for Method in Research

While there is a broad literature covering the application of music therapy
as reported in the medical press, there is an absence of valid clinical research
material from which substantive conclusions can be drawn. The obscure
observations in the realm of psychotherapy highlight a critical feature of
music therapy research; well intentioned, and often rigorous work, is spoiled
by a lack of research methodology. This is not to say that all clinical research
should conform to a common methodology (Aldridge 1991), or that it be
medical research, rather that standard research tools and methods of clinical
assessment be developed which can be replicated, which are appropriate to
music therapy, and develop a link with other forms of clinical practice. In
this way we develop working tools which allow us to inform ourselves and
others. While there is a lively debate in music therapy circles about appropriate methods, maybe a time has come when application may both prove
those methods better than continuing philosophizing and develop a base of
research expertise within the music therapy profession itself.

The research which has been produced is notably lacking in follow-up
data, without which it is impossible to make any valid statements about
clinical value. The assessment instruments are generally lacking by which
internal or external validity can be conferred. For example, as 'depression'
appears to feature in many chronic diseases then a clinical rating of depression, using a validated scale, would be appropriate to include in a research
design. If this assessment of depression could be combined with an overall
assessment of life quality then a significant step forward would be made in
establishing a minimal data set for assessing clinical change.

Much of the research work has been developed within the field of nursing, where the use of music is accepted as a useful therapeutic adjunct. Not surprisingly, the work from this field has concentrated on medical scientific perspectives. There is almost a complete absence of cross-cultural studies, or the use of anthropological methods which would bring other insights into music therapy. That music has been used therapeutically in other cultures cannot be denied, and other perspectives regarding the application of music therapeutically would highlight the limitations of modern Western scientific approaches when used as the sole means of research.

While the influence of music on heart rate and breathing is evident, it is difficult to find any work referring to the influence of music therapy on immunological parameters. Lee (1991) has written of the necessity for working with HIV and AIDS patients, emphasizing the value of music therapy while raising the question of clinical objectives. Apart from the significance of quality of life measures which could be used as criteria for such research, there remains the possibility that immunological parameters may be also be influenced by creatively improvising music. Such research would bring a parallel realm of clinical information to complement musical analyses such that therapeutic correlations can be attempted (Aldridge and Brandt 1991), and would provide a link with the current initiatives being made in psychoneuroimmunology.

CHAPTER FIVE

Aesthetics and the Individual
in the Practice of Research

While there is a demand made of music therapists by the wider community that they validate their work with clinical studies, this demand is often countered by music therapists with the argument that scientific methods are often inappropriate to the study of these forms of creative therapy. A similar cry is also heard in orthodox medicine that the strict methodology of science is often found wanting when applied to the study of human behaviour and has stimulated calls for innovation in clinical medical research (Hart 1984). A significant factor of that innovation is a growing awareness by the doctor of the patient's social and cultural milieu, and an understanding of health beliefs (Gregg 1985; Underwood, Gray and Winkler 1985; Wilkin 1986). What we need in clinical research is to facilitate the emergence of a discipline which seeks to discover what media are available for expressing clinical change. These media may be as much aesthetic as they are scientific thereby emphasizing the art of healing in parallel with the science of healing, as we read at the end of Chapter Three.

Both science and art are activities which attempt to bring certain contents of the world into cognition. The contention of this chapter is that when we study human behaviour, and in particular what it means to be sick, to become well again or the process of dying, then both forms of acquaintance, artistic and scientific, are necessary for the practice of research.

In medical research most of the modern initiatives for that research have come from the field of natural science. Such research when applied to the study of human behaviour is partial and neglects the important creative elements in the process and practice of healing. This is not to deny the scientific, rather to emphasize the aesthetic such that both may be considered together. Unfortunately the tension of understanding both elements of human understanding results in one or the other being denied. Such is the current situation in modern medicine. However, the continuing problems of chronic illness and human suffering urge us to go beyond our partisan beliefs and look again at how we know as well as what we know, literally the art of re-search.

The problem facing the clinician is that he must often mediate between the personal needs of the patient and the health needs of the community. These needs are informed by differing world-views. Similarly there is often a split in medical science between researchers and therapists: one group seeing themselves as rational and rigorous in their thinking and others as sentimental and biased, which in turn elicits comments about inhuman treatment and reductionist thinking. Neither of these stances is true; each perspective has something to offer. However, the predominant ideas in published medical research are those of natural science as informed by statistical data.

Historical context

The science of statistics developed in eighteenth-century France (Tröhler 1988) as part of the centralized apparatus of the State (Foucault 1989). 'Statistics' as the science of state was the empirical numerical representation of the resources available to the State and formed the components of a new power rationality. Health care became, as it is now, a political objective, as well as a personal objective. Health, from this perspective, is seen as the duty of each member of society and the objective of all. Individual needs are subsumed within the goals of the collective; the private ethic is informed by the public ethic; and objective empirical data are the means by which goals are assessed (see Table 5.1). These data are related to the economic regulation of health care delivery (health as commodity); public order (the regulation of deviance); and hygiene (the quality of food, water and the environment).

From this viewpoint we have the notion of health care, and knowledge about that health care, which is regulated by the State. The objects of that health care (patients), the practitioners of that health care (therapists), and the providers of that health care (health and State insurance) are informed by the same world-view. Such was the strength of modern science, it offered a replicable body of knowledge in the face of the ever-increasing solipsism of metaphysics in the eighteenth century.

From a modern scientific stance the body is to be manipulated as an object of the State whose ends it serves. Such manipulation is served by the processes of classification and normalization. People are observed, classified and analyzed as 'cases' according to their deviance from a given norm. Disease becomes a category like any other, rather than the unique experience which it is.

Table 5.1 Comparative and complementary perspectives on health research

scientific perspective	*individual perspective*
state regulation of health	personal regulation of health
constancy, predictability and control: *the future is based on past data*	creative irrationality: *being and becoming*
technology of the body: *observations, examinations and case reports*	techniques of the self: *music, art, personal narratives and poetry*
objective statistical reality based on instrumentally monitored data	subjective and symbolic reality based on the senses and human consciousness
the health of the body is an imperative of the State	self maintains own identity
scientific	aesthetic
time as *chronos*	time as *kairos*

The epistemology of this normative process is that of natural science which emphasizes reason, constancy and predictability. In the face of death and disruption the imperative of health is to maintain continuity and control. It is a philosophical assumption that the positive instance of an hypothesis will give ground for further instances. However, there is no logical necessity which will safeguard our passage from past to future experiences (Ayer 1982). Creative music therapy stands in complete opposition to this philosophy. The future is fashioned always as a new possibility, albeit maintaining a coherent identity.

A Critique of Scientific Methodology

Implicit in many criticisms of art therapy research is the notion that there are 'right' premises for doing science. The implication is that there is a common map of the territory of healing, with particular co-ordinates and given symbols for finding our way around, and that the orthodox map of scientific medicine is the only one. Any different map is seen as deviant, and any challenge to the construction of that map as heretical (Watzlawick 1984).

The implication of such heresy is that those who question the method of mapping human experience, or offer an alternative map, will be excommunicated from the scientific and therapeutic community. Alternative practices are implied to be 'cultish' and at best 'unscientific'. Bateson (1978), however, reminds us that although we think in terms of coconuts or pigs there are no coconuts or pigs in the brain. In clinical research that which we report on is a product of our own perceiving. This is not to put forward a purely nominalist argument (Gillon 1986) which would be to plunge us backwards into the darkness of metaphysical speculation and dogma, rather to emphasize the relativity of perspectives in thinking about healing.

Similarly, when we speak of scientific or experimental validity, that validity has to be conferred by a person or group of persons on the work or actions of another group. This is a 'political' process. With the obsession for 'objective truths' in the scientific community then other 'truths' are ignored. As therapists we have many ways of knowing; by intuition, through experience, and by observation. If we disregard these 'knowings' then we promote the idea that there is an objective, definitive external truth which exists as 'tablets of stone' to which only we, the initiated, have access.

Methodological issues
While clinical controlled trial methodology may appear to be scientifically sound a number of articles have questioned the scientific premises of such methods.

The first of these criticisms is that a random selection of trial subjects cannot be achieved because any group of patients comprises a highly selected non-random group. Any results concerning this trial group cannot be generalized to other trial groups. These inductive generalizations, it is argued, are no more respectable than those made from anecdotal experiences (Burkhardt and Kienle 1980, 1983).

Second, group generalizations from research findings raise problems for the clinician who is faced with the individual person in his or her consulting room. Individual variations are mocked by the group average (Barlow, Hersen and Jackson 1973; Barlow and Hersen 1984). If a group of 50 patients in a treatment group does statistically better than a control group of 50 patients, then such a difference could be due to a small number of patients in the treatment group showing a larger change while the majority of patients show no changes or deteriorate slightly. It is the patients who change significantly who are of interest to us as therapists and we would want to know the significant factors involved in that change. These, factors, however are lost within the group average.

Third, there are issues of reliability which are linked to the practice of scientific research. The reliability of our knowledge is only as good as the underpinning hypothesis (Dudley 1983). A hypothesis by definition is capable of being disproved. Inevitably the reliability of a trial when extended to a broader population is an act of induction (Burkhardt and Kienle 1983).

Not everything is measurable by numbers

At a fundamental level there is a major fault in much research thinking about human behaviour. This is the confusion of number with quantity. Numbers are the result of counting and can be accurate because there is a discontinuity with one integer and the next. We can count one boy, two boys, three boys and see the difference. When we come to the measurement of quantity then we have greater difficulty in being precise. Quantity is approximate.

It is easier to see three boys than it is to measure exactly three litres of water. When we come to 'measure emotion' or assess musicality then we encounter even greater difficulties. This problem has bedevilled clinical measurement. Although methods of measurement are continually being refined, the very process of measuring, when introduced into a clinical trial, influences the trial itself.

The people with whom we work in the therapist/patient relationship are not experimental units. Nor are the measurements made on these people isolated sets of data. While at times it may be necessary to make this split we must be aware that we are making the act of separating data from people.

When we come to measure particular personal variables then we face many complications. Consider a person who sits before a practitioner in a surgery who has been treated unsuccessfully for chronic leukaemia with a bone marrow transplant. The clinical measurements of blood status, weight and temperature are important. However, they belong to a different realm from those of anxiety about the future, the experience of pain, the anticipation of personal and social losses and the existential feeling of abandonment. These defy comparative measurement. Yet, if we are to investigate therapeutic approaches to chronic disease we need to investigate these subjective and qualitative realms (Aldridge 1991a, 1992).

In terms of outcomes measurement we face further difficulties. The people we see in or surgeries, or in our clinical trials, do not live in isolation. Life is rather a messy laboratory and continually influences the subjects of our therapeutic and research endeavours. Even more daunting is the fact that subjects influence themselves.

Finally, there is no such thing as a purely 'physical' treatment (Heron 1984). Treatment always occurs in a psychosocial context. Medicine is a social as well as a natural science (Kleinman 1973; Mechanic 1986). The way people respond in situations is sometimes determined by the way in which they have understood the meaning of that situation (Harré and Secord

1971). By studying the accounts people give of their symptoms in the context of their intimate relationships then we can glean valuable understandings of illness behaviour. The meaning of a headache in the context of a therapist–patient relationship may be a far cry from the meaning of a headache in a husband–wife relationship.

This reflects one of two fundamentally differing approaches to science. One is to develop precise and fixed procedures that yield a stable and definite empirical content. We have this in controlled trial methodology. The other approach to investigation depends upon careful and imaginative life studies which although lacking some of the precision of technical instruments have the virtue of continuing a close relationship with the natural social world of people.

Ethical and Political Issues

The subject matter of our research endeavours, and the way we carry out those endeavours, reflect our views of the society we wish to live in, how we wish to deal with our fellow human beings and how we want to be dealt with by them.

As therapists the concern for the subject prevails over the interest of society at large and scientific medicine as an institution. Individuals are not treated as a means to some collective end in clinical practice, although we may subscribe to a notion of community health. Furthermore, we discover a dilemma for research in that scientific standards of acceptability are juxtaposed with the ordinary therapeutic standards of the therapist. The standards of probability necessary for scientific statistical validity may be more exacting than the standards of probability acceptable to either the patient or the therapist. Such standards can vary according to the context in which they are applied. For the dying person the rigour of the clinical trial and the level of probability in terms of treatment efficacy may be quite different from that of the 'healthy' person, a woman in mid-term or an infant.

A further difficulty of accepting levels of probability is that trials of treatment are often scrutinized or judged by therapists and scientists who have a world-view which is different from that of those carrying out the trial. While it is necessary to have questions posed by 'outsiders' it is important that trials of art therapies are assessed by panels which have representatives of these therapeutic directions. By incorporating experts from differing disciplines it is then possible to design procedures whereby any prevailing dogma is not granted a monopoly status as a compulsory 'current status of scientific knowledge' and that minority groups representing other forms of therapeutic practice are not suppressed by the majority vote. This plurality of opinion will enliven research endeavours and offer a broad platform of therapeutic practice.

While trials may be set up to conform to an experimental methodology, those practising within the trial invariably approach their work from a clinical viewpoint. For the subjects of the trial their agenda is likely to be 'clinical' in so far as their expectations are of treatment. Similarly the results of a trial need to be interpreted and applied by therapists. Perhaps what we have failed to ask are the questions, 'What is the exact nature of therapeutic judgement, what realms of information are used to make that judgement, and who is to assess the legitimate outcome of that judgement?'

When controlled trials are carried out in a therapeutic setting then the benefit for the individual is set against the benefit for the group. The Declaration of Helsinki (1975) states: 'In any medical study, every patient – including those of the control group, if any – should be assured of the best proven diagnostic and therapeutic method.'

The clinical judgement of the therapist is on the side of the individual patient even if it means the corruption of a research project. When therapists, who are bound by contracts for treatment, take part in clinical trials then the dilemma is revealed, as we will see in a later chapter. Either they fulfil their individual contract for treatment with the patient, or they abdicate that contract and fulfil their obligations to the research contract which are concerned with group benefit. This raises further the conceptual issue for health care of whether 'health' is an individual or a societal concept. Are we as therapists committed to improving the health of individuals we see, or are we directed to improving the health of the communities we serve?

Meaning and Reality

A social science explanation of human behaviour has emphasized that human beings are not solely organisms responding to stimuli from the environment, or simply the sum of their interacting organ systems. The very difficulty of studying such behaviour is that people make sense of what they do, impose different meanings on to reality and alter their behaviour accordingly. When we try to understand social action we have to take into account that there are different available interpretations of that action. Furthermore, these actions take place as processes in natural settings and belong to social contexts. Not all patients have the same means of articulating their problems and concerns as do their therapists.

When a person consults a therapist and presents a problem, then that problem can be seen in varying ways according to the perspectives of the patient and the therapist. The presentation of that problem will have occurred

after previous discussions with other family members, and previously attempted health care activities. Similarly the choice of healer and the available
treatment is also part of a cultural context which embraces the therapist and
the patient.

Scientific medicine emphasizes one particular way of knowing. This
seems to maintain the myth that to know anything we must be scientists. If
we consider people who live in vast desert areas they find their way across
those trackless terrains without any understanding of scientific geography.
They also know the pattern of the weather without recourse to what we
know as the science of meteorology. In a similar way people know about
their own bodies and have understandings about their own lives. They may
not confer the same meanings as we do, yet it is those meanings and particular
belief about health to which we might best be guiding our research
endeavours. While as therapists we may help to bring about a change in
behaviour by technical means, it is the person whom we have to rely upon
to describe the meanings and implications of that change. This also leaves
out the burgeoning problem for us as scientists of explaining how a change
in meaning can bring about a change in behaviour.

The practical difficulty of researching subjective variables is they are not
accessible to quantitative methods, nor are they generalizable; they are indeed
subjective. To combat this difficulty and potential disruption of our knowledge we tend to ignore such data and reduce our variables to those which
are easily manipulated. To do so reduces the person to being simply a vessel
for the containment of a disease. When we include subjective variables such
as emotion, we treat them as if they could be weighed (Porter 1986).

When we intervene or treat persons in our research studies then we are
engaging in an activity which is not stable. Our intention is to bring about
change. This too poses a problem for generalizability beyond that seen in
the earlier section. Not only do we have to extrapolate from one group to
another, we have to induce meanings from a situation which is in a state of
flux.

In natural science studies objectivity is sought by separating the subject
from interference with the experiment. Some authors state that by doing this
the person is alienated from the study (Reason and Rowan 1981). Yet we
know that the attitudes and belief of the experimenter and the subject are
important, and that the experimenter and the subject interact with each other.
When we study health then we have to take into account biological,
psychological and social factors. They are not independent factors but factors
that interact with each other. It is we as researchers who separate the world

into categories, yet social life occurs in natural settings quite different from the artificial ones created for research.

Art and science

Research from this standpoint is not science in that it has no generalizable reference. The importance of such work is in its particular subjective and unconventional reference. While the aesthetic may appear to occupy a pole opposite to the scientific, we may propose that both poles are necessary to express the life of human beings.

Both art and science bring an appreciation of form and the expression of meaning. Maps, traces and graphs are articulate forms of an inner reality. So are the objects of art. They exist as articulate forms; they have an internal structure which is given to perception. However, while the graph is a regularized form whereby the individual, as content, is charted upon given axes, the object of art is both the expression and the axes of that expression, that is, form and content.

In expressive art sensory qualities are liberated from their usual meaning. While science requires the graph for regularity, art requires that forms are given a new embodiment; they can be set free to be recognized. In this way qualitative form can be set free and made wholly apparent in direct contrast to the questionnaire method where inner subjective realities are submitted to an external objective form. This is not to deny the use of the questionnaire, rather to emphasize the possibility of considering expressive forms when we wish to discover what the quality of life is. Sensual qualities then become of vital import to the whole, not to be rated on a scale, but intrinsic to the total gestalt.

In this way of researching we are concerned with showing rather than saying. For example, as we have read in Chapter Three, there are important factors in heart disease related to the Type A behaviour which can be discovered by interview. However, the picture of the individual gained from such interviews is rather negative and may be an artefact of the assessment method. A more neutral stance may be to allow subjects to improvise music.

Expression

The artistic symbol negotiates insight not reference. It expresses the feelings of the one from whom it stems and is a total analogue of human life. The symbol and that which is symbolized have some common logical form, i.e. they are isomorphic.

Science negotiates reference not insight. That which is within the individual is placed within a context.

Music and art are concerned not with the stimulation of feeling, but the expression of feeling. It may be more accurate to say here that feelings are not necessarily 'emotional state', more an expression of what the person knows as inner life, which may exceed the boundaries of conventional categorization. By encouraging non-verbal forms of expression we can learn and utter ideas about human sensibility. A reliance on verbal methods alone assumes that we can know and speak about all that we are. A reliance on machine expressions of our inner realities assumes that all that we are is measurable and material.

The art form presents the whole intelligible form as an intuitive recognition of inner knowledge projected as outer form: subjective is made objective but in the terms of the subject. In artistic expression we have the possibility of making perceptible an inner experience.

Research methods suitable for music therapy

As mentioned in the previous chapter, much valuable data, particularly in the field of music therapy research in psychiatry, for example, is wasted for want of a methodology. Such a lack of acceptable methodology highlights the difficulties in researching the arts therapies in general where artists are often coerced into using the language and methods of science. The axis of judgement 'health–illness' belongs to the world of medicine; music therapy must not necessarily restrict itself to such a world view. The parameters for music therapy assessment must include those of music itself. That music therapy is intended to have an effect in the context of clinical practice is evident, but the parameters of that effect and the way therapeutic change is described are made from an epistemology different from that of modern scientific medicine. What we are also challenged to ask of our therapeutic endeavours is, '*What meaningful change occurs for the patient, and their family; and for the clinicians and therapists involved?*' and '*How can this change be expressed and recognized?*' Thus the ascription of meaning also becomes a central issue in any research methodology applied to understanding health and illness.

Making sense: the pursuit of 'meaning' in researching therapeutic realities

And if you ask me for a recipe for speeding up this process, I would say first that we ought to accept this dual nature of scientific thought and be willing to value the way in which the two processes work together to give us advances in understanding of the world. (Bateson 1941, p.67)

Gregory Bateson was a leading thinker in the development of systems theory. He proposed the term 'ecology of mind' as a way of thinking about the ecology of ideas which bring about meaning (Bateson 1972, 1978). What we need in clinical research is to facilitate the emergence of a discipline which seeks to discover what media are available for expressing this ecology of ideas which we see as a person, and with which we engage as a therapist or researcher to discern the meaning of change. These media may be as much artistic as they are scientific.

The function of art is to acquaint the person with something he has not known before (Langer 1953). It is this acquaintance with the unknown which lies at the heart of the experience of illness. For the doctor or therapist there is the anxiety of facing death and 'failure'. For the patient in their journey into the unknown there is the anxiety of identity loss. However, this acquaintance is with a deeper aspect of self, and one to be welcomed. From this point of view symptoms become indicators of a struggle for an inner reality to find expression and part of an ecology which includes the patient, the family and the therapist. Symptoms then lose some of their pathological power, and can be seen as opportunities for development once given the opportunity to articulate their unspoken reality.

This acquaintance with the unknown operates both for the subject and researcher, therapist and patient. Consciousness becomes not a matter of 'I think that', but a matter of 'I can', not necessarily a spoken word, but a creative act. By working in this way we can be relieved of the tyranny of words and their imposed structure, and free to work dynamically. This 'I can' is the important element of intentionality which cannot be measured but can be heard, seen and demonstrated. To work in this way is to consider aesthetics; the essentials of pattern and form as expressed. For a research methodology in music therapy we cannot always revert to the questionnaire and a standard test. What we are challenged to develop is a way of presenting the work of art itself *as it appears in the context of therapy.*

Meaning

When studying human behaviour we must look at the context of which that behaviour is part, and the closely related phenomenon of the meaning of that behaviour. When we explain meaning we are mapping data on to what are already fundamental elements of our knowledge. However, the ultimate aim of what we are doing is to increase this fundamental knowledge. When we observe we are concerned with the basic act of induction. Yet these observations must be fitted within a framework. This is the framework of fundamentals.

The *dogmatic* approach in therapeutics requires a knowledge of the cause of disease, i.e. an underlying theory. Any therapeutic approach can then be derived by reasoning from this theoretical base and need not be validated by any other means. From this point of view I catch a cold because I go out with my hair wet, or fail to wear a vest in early spring. It was the dogmatic view which prevailed when the Catholic Church condemned the heliocentric system of Galileo.

The *empiric* approach requires the careful observation of clinical symptoms without any theoretical considerations. These symptoms can then be compared with what is already known from the clinical literature and various forms of available expertise. It is from this science of empirical observations that modern medicine has gained its strength. However, the notion of observation as a totally value-free atheoretical act is questionable. We see what we see from a theoretical standpoint. The choice of a measuring instrument for example, indeed the choice to measure, is made from the basis of an underlying set of fundamental theoretical premises. The starting point of observation is itself structured by a subject–predicate relation in the structure of language; i.e. deduction. This is not to advocate solipsism, rather to emphasize the need to chart a course between both errors, of empiricism and solipsism.

The mistake made by empiricists is to introduce sense data as objects as if they were isolated in time and space separate from an ecological niche. It is a pre-objective realm we have to explore in ourselves if we are to understand our experience and that of others. The question we have to ask is, *What are the fundamental elements of knowledge, that is, the ecology of ideas, which are being used at this time?* Further, there also exist the symptoms which are displayed by the patient. These represent another ecology of ideas and are often interpreted from the view of the therapist rather than the patient. However, yet another way exists. That is to allow the patient, or the subject of the research, to create a work of art with the therapist. The purpose of creation in this act is to make something known. What is made known can be interpreted on the basis of given fundamentals; but also exists as a new experience in and for itself.

Form

> The conservative laws of energy and matter are concerned with substance rather than form. Mental process, ideas, communication, organization, differentiation, pattern and so on, are matters of form rather than substance. (Bateson 1972, p.31)

Bateson tried to shift the thinking of behavioural scientists from the substantive metaphor of energy which he saw as misleading, to that of information. This 'energy' debate still continues in complementary medical approaches, and while it may be true of some therapies which use subtle energies, it is also vital to rethink our explanations of our therapeutic models. In Bateson's view the letter which does not arrive, and therefore imparts no energy, can have a dramatic effect on the waiting receiver, thus imparting information.

A principal feature of this thinking will be a consideration of consciousness. In our relationships we continually exchange information about unconscious processes. We tell each other what order of consciousness/ unconsciousness attaches to our messages. Art is a form of behaviour which perfects the communication about how to handle unconscious material. In addition it has the ability to express the fact that we are dealing with the interface between unconscious and conscious material. Consciousness talks about things or persons and attaches predicates to the specific things or persons which have been mentioned. In unconscious process the emphasis is on relationship between elements; that is, it is metaphoric. It is concerned with the self–other–self environment, about patterns of relationship – sometimes called feelings – and is the outward sign of a precise, often hidden, relationship.

The problem of iconic communication, as in the case of a headache, the closed fist or the flood of tears, is that it has no tense, no simple negative and no modal markers. Bateson uses the bared teeth of cubs as an example of such a communication: it looks like fighting but is play. What is often thought of as self-mutilatory suicidal behaviour is also an example of this iconic communication that has no simple negative. It is a communication about a life and death issue, about 'not dying' rather than living (Aldridge 1984; Aldridge and Rossiter 1984, 1985). These are the elements in communication which are more archaic than language and hence difficult to express verbally. No wonder that patients, whose communicative non-verbal language is that of symptoms, appear to be illogical when they are forced to express themselves in words. A verbal logic has no significant relation to their problems. We have to consider that sometimes we force our patients into inarticulacy by demanding verbosity. Music therapy has other expectations, that we perform isomorphically with the way that we are composed. The logic of improvisation may, then, mirror the logic of symptoms. If this is so, music therapy has a diagnostic relevance. Not only are patients made articulate, they are also understood in the very ground of their own being.

Bateson's explanation of how these problems become unconscious is one of habituation and learning. In the process of habit formation knowledge sinks down to less conscious and more archaic levels. This often contains painful matters which we do not want to inspect but also those things with which we are familiar. The economics of the system push organisms to sink generalities of the relationship, which remain permanently true, into the unconscious, keeping conscious the pragmatics of particular instances.

In his view habit formation is a major economy of conscious thought. It is not possible to be conscious or aware of everything in detail: note the relativity of time and space; focus on one and the other becomes less clear. Although economic, habit formation has its price in terms of accessibility. Many of our activities which we take for granted and are our unbidden responses to life's challenges are difficult to change or examine consciously; and thereby conservative. This conservatism is not necessarily a bad thing. In the face of continual perturbation and change it is important to have some central core of stability which does not require conscious decision making.

While these central processes are difficult to examine verbally or consciously, it is possible to express them artistically and musically. The skill of the artist, or rather the demonstration of his or her skill, becomes a message about those parts of his unconscious, but *not* a message from the unconscious. Our challenge then is to provide a vehicle for the expression and articulation of that which lies hidden.

The Corrective Nature of Art

Consciousness is necessarily selective and partial about the self. The total mind is an integrated network of propositions, images, processes, neural pathways; and consciousness is only a sampling of this network. Concentrating on what can be consciously reported is a denial of the integration of this whole. We see only arcs of what are really circuits. What art does is to allow us to appreciate the systemic nature of mind (Bateson 1978).

From a paper originally presented in 1967 Bateson (1978) writes:

> The point, however, which I am trying to make in this paper is not an attack on medical science but a demonstration of an inevitable fact:

that mere purposive rationality unaided by such phenomena as art, religion, dream and the like, is necessarily pathogenic and destructive of life; and that its virulence springs specifically from the circumstance that life depends upon interlocking circuits of contingency, while consciousness can only see such short arcs of such circuits as human purpose may direct. (1978, p.118)

Art then poses a question, 'What sorts of correction in the direction of wisdom would be achieved by creating or viewing this work of art?' Ironically a scientist of Bateson's stature found it necessary even then, some 33 years ago, to clarify that he is not attacking medical science. It is tempting to wonder what it is about medical science which is so weak that we must protect it so. Perhaps it only reflects our own hidden desires for certainty?

Pattern and relationship

Art, from a Batesonian perspective, requires skill and pattern. It is probably an error, he says, to think of 'dream, myth and art as being any one matter other than relationship'. 'Dream is metaphoric, and is not necessarily about the relata mentioned in the dream. In conventional interpretation, another set of relata, often sexual, is substituted for the set in the dream. There is no a priori reason for supposing that sexual relata are any more primary or basic than any other set' (Bateson 1978, p.123).

Rigid focusing upon a single set of relata (objects which are related) destroys for the artist the more profound significance of the work. It is about the relationship and not about the identifiable relata. The art work provides an experience which exposes errors in experience where one pole is chosen rather than another, because poles are mutually dependent.

It is important then to consider relationships first, and the relata as defined solely by their relationship. Bateson cites Goethe as setting an example of thinking about relata. A leaf in this way of thinking is not a flat green thing but related in a particular way to the stem (which itself is not a 'cylindrical thing') from which it grows and the secondary stem (or bud) which is formed in the angle between the leaf and the primary stem (Bateson 1972). We must look for an analogy between living things in the grammar of their structure, the relationship between their parts, as a classification of relationship. This is precisely what we find in the indexed musical analyses which music therapists make of their therapy sessions.

Analogic and symbolic language

Works of art do not point out the meaning directly, they demonstrate it by recreating pattern in metaphorical shape or form. In this way symptoms are an analogical symbolic communication. When symptoms are accepted as a form of expression, and part of a living ecology, then there is *no pathology*. Pathology is the observer's prejudice. What we see is indicative. This then changes the sign applied to behaviour from that of 'deviant' to 'accepted'.

From a modern scientific stance the body is to be manipulated according to the processes of classification and normalization. People are observed, classified and analyzed as 'cases' in relation to their deviance from a given norm. Disease becomes a category like any other rather than the unique experience which it is. Merleau-Ponty (1968) calls this the 'second positivity', that is, a normal human body against which any particular body can be measured. The dangers of this comparison are that the particular human being is then alienated from his or her body and his or her individuality. Furthermore, the epistemology of this normative process is that of natural science which emphasizes reason, constancy and predictability. In the face of death and disruption the imperative of health is to maintain continuity and control. Yet predictability and control are based on an ideal of conservatism. It is a philosophical assumption that what is here today will give ground for further instances tomorrow. There is no logical necessity which will safeguard our passage from past and present to future experiences.

Telling Stories and the Understanding of Narrative Form

When we each come to tell the stories of our lives they do not have the substance of conventional research reports, nor the quantified language of science. Our lives are best described in the dynamic expressions of a lived language. The essence of language is that of musical form, which is the vehicle for the content of ideas (Aldridge 1989,1989a, 1991d).

When we classify, codify and conceptualize from experience we are taking the classical approach to observation and experimentation. We see this in botany, meteorology and astronomy. The world is grasped through our senses or instruments designed specifically for the purpose of observation. This is the mode of explanation. However, whenever we seek the meaning of experience and wish to make that meaning manifest we can turn to modes of expression. This can be seen in the process of story telling.

The content of stories, like art, does not always make a point directly, they demonstrate by the form in which they come (hence the notion of epic poetry). Stories have a metaphorical shape and form which recreate a pattern of being, a pattern of being which symptoms also represent as a metaphorical, albeit restricted, reality. Stories then lend an understanding of pattern to our lives. They are a way of perceiving, feeling, relating and existing. Whereas scientific concepts are tied to nominalism, stories are connected to archetypal forms.

Our task as researchers is not to impose meaning on to stories, but to allow meaning to become manifest in reality. As Bateson says, it is not the relata which are important but the relationships between those relata and the interface between the unconscious and the conscious. This challenges the researcher as much as the subject, the therapist as much as the patient. We must develop means by which people can freely tell their own stories. Our task in therapy is to facilitate the telling; and then, in research, to understand that telling.

Stories are instruments of communication by their very form (Shah 1964). They cannot be unravelled by ordinary methods alone. It is no use trying to count words or correlate metaphors in a story with elevations in blood pressure and hope to extract any meaning, but it is possible to understand them as they are structured as a set of narratives. These narratives can be understood as being structured according to rules of construction, as are musical compositions.

A Descriptive Method

We can encourage people to creatively express the passage of their lives not only as patients in hospital, but in their daily living at home and at work. It is possible to have a descriptive science of human behaviour which can be based upon the aesthetic. In this way we can ask of our research that it expresses what it is to be human, what it is to be well and what it is to fall sick.

The advantage of the creative arts is that they allow us not only to express our pathologies, which many orthodox and unorthodox medical systems concentrate upon with their underlying moral condemnation, but they also allow the expression of potential. This tension between what we have become, and what we are becoming, can be reconciled within the context of the aesthetic as a created form. This is the meaning behind the aesthetic where the negative sign is transformed by the act of creation into the positive.

At the beginning of the next century there will still be the problems of chronic disease, death and suffering. Such is the human condition. What we may have to provide our selves, our students and our patients with is not the means to combat disease, an activity which has had only partial success, but the ability to help others creatively realize themselves. How we document this progress of those who come into our care, or those with whom we choose to journey, may be better expressed in works of art which are realized in the process of living and which bear the imprint of our sensuality and intuition rather than our rationality and technology.

We have properties which are concerned with a created knowledge. As clinicians and researchers our task is to ask of ourselves, and then of our patients, 'How can we create ourselves as a work of art?' (Rabinow 1986). The implications of this thinking for research practice is that we can encourage people to develop an articulacy of self based on their own expressive realizations expressed in the form of music, or pictures or stories. A major criterion, then, for assessing therapeutic change in the arts therapies will be that of the aesthetic.

Methods in music therapy will concentrate on comparing and analyzing expressed form. Thus we can compare accounts from the medical literature; parameters of musical playing; expressed form as photographs, paintings and drawings; and statements from patients, as diaries or journals or videotaped episodes of conversation, to discover correspondences between medical description, aesthetic expression, and patients' perceptions. This will entail a search for the grammar of underlying structures as the commonality in understanding human beings; that is, that we can classify change according to the relationship between parts, and that these relationships may be based upon particular rules of constitution and regulation.

However, music therapy research cannot solely be based on aesthetic changes. Music therapy is located in the context of the clinical practice of medicine and psychotherapy. Bridges must be built such that clinical change can be recognized by clinical practitioners in both medicine and the arts. Single case studies incorporating elements of both medical assessment and musical assessment can be an effective compromise, allowing for both individual treatment initiatives and consideration of scientific medicine. Small group trials can then be designed from understandings gleaned in the single case investigations which will elicit those parameters which are subject to measurement and assessment. Longitudinal studies, involving compared groups or matched controls, may be feasible at a later stage for comparing chronic problems which are either resistant to change or subject to long-term change.

It is essential that some form of standardized assessment for adult improvised music playing is developed, and that that standard is acceptable to a broad platform of music therapists from differing backgrounds. This will allow music therapists to validate their clinical findings by submitting samples of their research work to a panel of colleagues who can assess particular episodes according to common criteria.

Any research methods must allow for a follow-up period and compare previous clinical changes with those found at follow-up. Furthermore, most of the previous research published in the medical literature indicates, albeit indirectly, changes in the quality of life in patients and subsequent changes in depression. Music therapy studies could easily incorporate in assessment methods indicators of life quality changes and changes in depression using well validated clinical measures based on patient report, which would serve as a common preliminary base for clinical comparisons.

Methodological difficulties in music therapy research

As yet there is no established research methodology for music therapy. Many practising music therapists are wary of methodological suggestions from non-music therapists as those suggestions are often seen as unsuited to their work. Suggestions from psychologists and medical researchers are often considered as attempts to move the therapists away from the musical therapeutic experience, which interests them, and impose a restrictive alien structure on the research using a language developed from an altogether different epistemology, manipulating patients as subjects, in a way which music therapists find intolerable.

It is possible to find a way of working which satisfies music therapists, but this takes time. The advantage of developing a methodology with the therapists themselves is that the results of that work are seen as valid within the working group, and that research itself is used to promote further studies. These studies themselves begin to identify weaknesses in previous research initiatives such that the therapists themselves include those elements of rigour which are pertinent. Developing research methods in music therapy is a process of education; the epistemology, agenda, and timing of which are negotiated with and decided by the therapists themselves. However, when we speak of rigour it is important to emphasize that the rigour of scientific medicine will appear different from the rigour of social science, as it will from the rigour of aesthetic theory. Some medical scientists when they speak of human clinical research fail to see beyond their own methodology, mistaking method for knowledge, and become crippled by their own insecurity at not being able to tolerate ambiguity in ascertaining meaning. We see this reflected in the dilemma of working with two epistemologies; scientific as generalizable reference and *a priori* conventional, and the aesthetic as individual and *a priori* unconventional. A tolerance of both the scientific and the aesthetic is called for, with neither demanding predominance over the other, rather that each has something valuable to contribute as a facet of a greater understanding (Aldridge 1991a).

Creative arts therapists have criticized classical scientific research methods for failing to take into account several important features of their work (Tüpker 1990). One such feature is that of reliability; i.e. that another researcher can use the same method of music therapy with a group of matched patients and obtain the same result. The reply from the creative arts therapists is that in their mental make-up no two people are the same, and the same measure when applied to two or more people can never bring the same result. Music therapy is a transpersonal happening and what happens cannot be separated from the person of the therapist. Two therapists can apply the same therapy with quite different results. Similarly, in therapeutic art forms in which patients improvise music, paint pictures, make movements, no two improvisations, pictures, or movements will be wholly the same.

Moreover, it must be borne in mind that in psychotherapeutic and creative arts approaches people have histories and life stories which are taken into account, and also considered as playing an important part in treatment considerations. It is not possible to reproduce the same situation that occurs in one person in another person. Every therapist must start with the person as they are according to their individual biography. Each work produced as art will develop out of this history and contribute to this history. Works of art taken out of the context of the patient, i.e. an individual being with a personal history located within relational and cultural contexts, lose their validity as phenomena.

It is almost impossible to seek out objective measures in creative arts therapies when subjective factors play such a predominant role. Much so-called music therapy research has been concerned with the application of a series of tones to a passive receptive patient rather than active music making. The idea that particular tones and tonal intervals have an effect which can be generally determined within therapy is a weak and discredited idea. Furthermore, in the situation of improvising music it is impossible to separate out the influences of patient and therapist one from another. The improvisation is mutual. Attempts to objectify the process of therapy disturb the therapy such that it no longer represents that which is to be measured, thus countermanding any attempts at objectivity.

Assessment methods

There is no 'gold standard', i.e. a universally agreed and validated measure, for assessment in music therapy. Because creative music therapy relies upon individual interpretations of each patient, assessment methods have tended to be idiosyncratic, relying upon both the theoretical persuasion of the therapist and their experience with a given theory, which becomes a personal interpretation of that theory. Bruscia (1988) has suggested a set of standards for music therapy research emphasizing that assessment attempts to understand a patient's needs. Treatment and evaluation differ in purpose (see Table 5.2). Treatment intends to produce change. Evaluation documents that change.

Table 5.2 Forms of assessment and their implications for treatment (after Bruscia 1988)

treatment implications	*form of assessment*	
	general validity	*internal validity*
absent	diagnosis: defines and explains the patient's pathology focusing primarily on causes, symptoms and severity	description: describes the patient only in relationship to themselves according to phenomenological criteria
present	interpretation: the patient's problem is explained according to a particular theoretical background, and often includes prognosis	prescription: describes the patient with recommendations for treatment incorporated in a treatment plan

Music therapists emphasize that the basis of assessment should be musical parameters taken from their therapeutic epistemology, not those borrowed, or imposed, by medical science or psychology. Their work is *not* visual and spatial, unlike most medical observations, i.e. the graph, the EEG trace, the metre reading. Their work is aural and temporal. This shift in emphasis between the two major elements of modern scientific thinking is a crucial point. Observe one and the other becomes less precise. Concentrate on physical spatial measures and time factors become elusive; focus on time factors and spatial precision is lacking. What has been argued throughout the preceding chapters is that while modern medicine provides a spatial understanding, music therapy offers a complementary balancing understanding of the person he or she exists in time. It is this notion of time which is of importance in understanding problems in Western medicine in that the individual is caught in the contradictions of self-demand and societal demand, which for some people may become pathogenic (Helman 1987).

While medicine relies upon 'the Gaze' in a Foucauldian sense, music therapy relies upon 'Being' (Dasein) in an existential Heideggerian phenomenological sense. The sensory modality of music therapy, as it once was in medicine, is that of sound organized as music, and analyzed as musical parameters; rhythm, melody, harmony, phrasing, timbre, articulation. As form, and a therapeutic form which is art not science, each production/performance makes sense in itself and for itself. Our task in assessing persons is not judgemental according to a societal norm, but a creative act which attempts to understand the person as they create themselves moment to moment as individual beings, in relationship with another human being, in time. We attempt to make sense of how a person maintains coherence in their daily lives not in terms of discovering pathology and limitation, but in terms of potential.

Armstrong criticizes modern medicine in concentrating on the 'lesion' or biological abnormality where the patient is considered as an impediment to treatment (Armstrong 1987). The concept of disease with assumptions of normality based upon statistical evidence is a reflection of social judgements, not of biological norms. There are numerous criteria by which we can be judged as abnormal, only some of which are said to represent disease. This ascription of disease according to functionality is based on a particular theoretical background and epistemology of modern medicine which has at its core 'the ideal' or 'the social'. While there may or may not be a biological reality for a particular disease, there is always a social reality. By developing techniques of visual observation, such that the body was opened or penetrated to discover 'the lesion', what was hidden became apparent and acted as a focus by which the clinical experience could be rationalized. Music therapy assessment relies upon the performance of the person in the therapeutic relationship such that they define themselves as they are musically expressed in the moment. The criteria by which they are assessed are not normative.

We need a research approach which accepts the individual as they are, in performance, and attempts to discover correlations between what it is that patients expect of the therapeutic endeavour, what therapists expect of the therapeutic endeavour and how those expectations can be made evident when satisfied. That the work of art, painted, drawn, played or acted, is sufficient in itself is only a partial truth once it is brought into the framework of therapeutic activity. Therapy implies an expected change, that a change has occurred; and what has been instrumental in this change is the task of therapeutic research. Such assessments that change has occurred rely upon how varying phenomena are aggregated such that they have meaning. If a variety of descriptions are collected, then some commonality of understanding can be teased out.

Some Suggested Data Sets for Comparative Research

- *Musical playing parameters* would be tempo, metre, rhythm, harmony, melody, voice timbre, fluency, articulation, dynamic, responsiveness and adaptability, phrasing, and form.
- *Physical parameters* would include posture, movement, eye contact and relational proximity, range of movements.
- *Psychological parameters* would be mood state, attention, confusion and attitude.
- *Relational playing parameters* would be initiative taking, potential for exchange within the therapeutic dialogue, avoidance of contact, continuity of the relationship.
- *Journal descriptions* by the patient on a daily basis, semi-structured for content analysis.
- *Art therapy parameters* including drawing, painting and modelling where each 'product' is photographed after every session to record changes in form. In addition it could be possible to include videotapes of the process of modelling/painting/drawing.
- *Body form* as a standardized drawing.
- *Medical clinical* descriptions of the patient collected on a regular basis.

The development of appropriate methodologies

It is necessary to develop a research methodology and research strategy for creative music therapy, and the creative arts in general. At the centre of this work is the creative act. The creative act is aesthetic; it is concerned with expression and the articulation of form, and is best understood when expressed as an existential reality concerned with the individual. Therefore, the scientific perspective of modern Western medicine alone is not sufficient to understand the art of music therapy. However, as music therapy itself enters the arena of medical discourse (i.e. it is a clinical practice) certain elements of medical research can be incorporated into a research methodology *when appropriate*. As music therapy is concerned with people, and thereby relationships, understandings gleaned from social science research can play an important role in the development of a methodology.

Science and art can work together to give us an understanding of the person in the world. This does not mean counting the number of notes a person produces in a minute, and correlating that production with a clinical parameter controlled in a subject blind to the intention of the researcher and plotted on a graph. Furthermore, we demand of medical science that it pays more than lip service to this acceptance of art and actively incorporates such activities as complementary in understanding the way in which people live in the world and have their Being.

Understandings in medicine are linked to what is seen, and comparisons are made by reducing the individual to what is the 'same', that is, the process of normalization; whereas at the heart of creative arts therapies is an inherent existentialism which emphasizes the individuality of persons. Any research methodology which attempts to do justice to the creative arts therapies must be prepared to incorporate this individual perspective and live with the dilemma of maintaining a dialogue with Western medicine. Complementary to this understanding, Western medicine must accept that the power of scientific thought, while organizing our perceptions in such a manner that we can survive in the world, as we saw in the last chapter, has neglected the human body as an instrument of knowledge and as a vehicle for sensations as direct as ordinary sensory experience but as subtle as consciousness.

A critical feature in any future research designs will be the development of a 'time-based' methodology for establishing clinical change. This methodology will evaluate different modes of coping according to the monitoring of variables as they change during time periods. It is possible, using single case approaches, to propose and evaluate specific intervention strategies with individuals. Furthermore, with the development of statistical methods suitable for the monitoring of subjective, rhythmic or episodic data; methods can be developed that not only detect change but also discriminate between those changes, even when they occur in the 'normal' range. Thus, clinicians have an opportunity to further validate their clinical findings. What we must keep in mind is that the pattern of reactivity in the individual is something like a weather pattern; it constantly changes, never going to a steady state. This analysis is pertinent to the individual in that they are always compared to their own individual physiology.

Musical experiences are essentially those of form and order, which are continually creatively realized by the person. As a means of treatment, creative music therapy attempts to mobilize the creative potentials of the patient towards a restoration of the state we call 'health'. When we come to interpret what takes place in therapy as a goal of clinical research we can also rely upon artistic terms. However, we may be able to find correspondence at the next higher level of description which is that of structure, i.e. the elements of form, order, pattern, dynamics and orientation. This level of structural correspondence may provide the ground for a common therapeutic discourse (Aldridge, Brandt and Wohler 1990).

A time has come when we can judge our research on 'whether it makes a powerful and important contribution to the cumulative evidence' (Pringle 1984) on a particular issue rather than whether or not it formally proves a point. This recognition of subjective data is occurring at a time when an emphasis is being placed on the 'whole' patient rather than fragmenting the person into organ systems.

It is not solely scientific skills which help us to understand the patient fully. It is possible to have a descriptive science of human behaviour which can be based upon the aesthetic. In this way we can ask of our research that it expresses what it is to be human, what it is to be well and what it is to fall sick.

As modern living provokes ever more anxiety then the present search for scientific solutions based upon predictability, and the attempted control of nature by technology continues. This retreat from the anxiety of dying and its emphasis on the material prevents us from understanding the true process of living. How can we then offer hope and comfort to the sick and the dying (Aldridge 1987, 1987a, 1987b, 1987c)?

A phenomenological perspective on research concerns itself with the person as they are 'coming into being' rather than the verification of hypotheses which are predicated on observations of the past. To say that the future will be as the past was is a cultural artefact of our dominant scientific epistemology. From such a deterministic view of the past how can we account for change and all that is new?

The politics of medicine, and the technology of modern medicine which serves it, place the existence of the individual in question. Personal means of health are concerned with a subjective reality which is symbolic. As human beings we are capable of self-regulation, and the foundations of this regulation are not confined to objective criteria. In many cases we are mysterious to ourselves. We have properties which are concerned with a created knowledge.

As therapists and researchers, then, how are we to face the problem of how to constitute an ethics of existence not solely founded on a scientific knowledge of the self which is comparable to group norms, but one in which the principal act is creative? Our task is to ask of ourselves, and then of our patients, 'How can we create ourselves as a work of art?' (Rabinow 1986).

The implication of this thinking for research practice is that we can encourage people to develop an articulacy of self based on their own expressive realizations. These may be expressed in the form of music, or pictures or stories. We can encourage people to document their journeys through life not as the accumulation of material quantities of flesh and blood but in sounds, words and pictures. The documentary of life's journey through a chronic illness may be realized in a series of case notes. However, it can also be possible to document that journey as a series of photographs, which are far more eloquent for the travellers. The preservation of the values of humanity within our culture is as much in the hands of the clinician/researcher as artist as it is in the clinician/researcher as scientist.

Human behaviour cannot be studied from one point of view only. Within the total repertoire of psychological medicine it is necessary to have different approaches to understanding the world: the scientific and the aesthetic. This position, of multiple understandings, offers an acceptance of orthodox clinical trials together with a promotion of new understandings (Touw-Otten and Spreeuwenberg 1985). By doing so differing studies inform each other. In later chapters of this book, the reader will find that I am suggesting such an eclectic view. All too often quantitative research is set against qualitative research methods as if only one approach were valid. In music therapy we cannot really afford the luxury of such an argument. We have too little published research work, and a young, under-developed research tradition.

It is vital that we pursue academic rigour in our experimentation. But not by burying our heads in the sand. Rigour without imagination leads to stagnation just as imagination alone leads to anarchy. Modern clinical research can combine the two. A combination of rigour and imagination is necessary to meet the challenges of health care. Our intellectual endeavours should be astute enough to see that science can accommodate multiple viewpoints (Freeling 1985; Howie 1984; Rose 1984) and search for a reconciliation of difference within the framework of the *scientific*, which is Truth, and the *aesthetic*, which is Beauty.

As one possible solution to beginning research, in a way that offers a structure for either qualitative research studies or quantitative research methods, the use of single case designs appears to be a pragmatic compromise.

CHAPTER SIX

Single Case Research Designs
for the Creative Music Therapist

> The basic problem confronting therapeutic science is that the important therapeutic phenomena exist only in actual therapeutic contexts, and yet it seems impossible to test and verify causal theories of psychotherapy and therapeutic change in these settings. (Martin 1993, p.371)

We need an approach to music therapy research that stays close to the practice of the individual clinician; that is, the musician as therapist. As we have read in the previous chapter, each therapeutic situation is unique. Yet somehow, we have to use methods of research so that we can compare our cases and share our knowledge; the classical case of generalizability that we find in psychology. What I will be arguing for in this chapter is a common flexible structure that can be applied to clinical practice. The practice is allowed to remain true to itself, although any research endeavour, by the nature of its reflexivity scrutiny, alters practice. In doing research we ask questions of ourselves as clinicians, and when we involve our patients in the process, then they too will reflect about what is going on.

Single case research designs (Barlow and Hersen 1984; Hilliard 1993; Kazdin 1982; Kazdin 1983; Yin 1989) are a part of a whole spectrum of case-study research methods applied to the investigation of individual change in clinical practice. Such designs have the advantage of being adaptable to the clinical needs of the patient and the particular approach of the therapist. The designs are appropriate for the development of research hypotheses, testing those hypotheses in daily clinical practice and refining clinical techniques. Single case designs, if systematically replicated, can provide an ideal developmental collaborative research tool for uniting creative arts therapists from differing backgrounds. Most appropriately they allow for the assessment of individual development and significant incidents in the patient–therapist relationship. Whereas single case experimental designs in medicine can ascertain significant change in a physiological variable leading to timely intervention, psychotherapy studies concentrate on both changes in the symptoms that the patient displays and interactive events in the ongoing process of therapy.

Single case designs are particularly important for the creative arts therapies as they allow for a close analysis of the therapist–patient interaction (Aldridge 1992, 1993b; Jones 1993). Furthermore, within this approach there are possibilities for comparing differing sets of data throughout a course of treatment such that intra-individual comparisons can be made. Personal change is considered within the patient, not by comparison with a group norm. A music therapist can, for example, treat a patient over the course of a year and compare his or her findings (changes in the music), both with colleagues in other creative arts disciplines (changes in painting or movement) and with colleagues from psychological disciplines (changes in mood rating scales or personality inventories). These findings can then be compared with the timing, and reasoning, behind varying therapeutic interventions. Such process research allows the therapists to see, or hear, how the emerging phenomena of therapeutic change are related to their therapeutic activities, hence the emphasis on single case designs for the promotion of theory building based on clinical practice and in generating data to support new models of intervention (Moras, Telfer and Barlow 1993).

The folklore of single case study methods suggests that these designs emerged from the practice of experimental psychology and psychoanalysis. Such a myth ignores the simple fact that human ideas have been conveyed in story form for centuries. 'Once upon a time…' until 'They lived happily ever after' reflects this basic narrative form. Bruscia (1991) endorses this position in his book of 42 collected case studies of music therapy when he dedicates the book 'To the individuals whose stories are told in these case studies'. When therapists of whatever therapeutic persuasion gather together their clinical discussions, they focus on cases; whether these be diverse, difficult or dangerous. Even research scientists at conferences adopt a style, usually when away from the podium, which reflects the human story as epitomized by the single case. Indeed, patient narratives are being championed as a valid form of health care research (Hydén 1995).

Single cases bring an important facet to clinical research – that of personal application. While clinical medicine demands the study of groups as its research convention, it accepts single cases as special examples drawing attention to anomalies in practice, alerting practitioners to matters of urgent attention (in the case of dangerous side-effects, for example), or as falsifiers of a particular theory (Velanovitch 1992). In the creative arts we are looking for methods which say what happens when we do our therapy, and the reasons for doing what we do. Ideally as research practitioners, we would want to be so clear about what we were doing that another practitioner could try it in a similar situation. Such clarity of practice description leads to replication and is one way of conferring validity on what we do as individuals but also builds up the common research stock of our professional groups.

Single case study designs are an attempt to formalize clinical stories. These designs take as their basis the clinical process where the illness is assessed and diagnosed, a treatment is prescribed, the patient or client is monitored during the application of that treatment, and the success of the treatment is then evaluated (Aldridge 1993b).

However, the validity of this therapeutic 'success' is open to question. There may be a subjective bias influenced by the expectations of the therapist and the patient. Similarly, the patient may appear to improve through willingness to please the physician. In some medical cases, the disease may have run its course and improvement would have occurred without a therapeutic intervention. Furthermore, the initial assessment of the patient may have represented temporary extreme values which are lessened at a subsequent assessment; i.e. in statistical terms, a 'regression towards the mean'. The experimental approach in single case research attempts to accommodate these difficulties by 'systematically varying the management of the patient's illness during a series of treatment periods', using randomization of treatment periods and blind assessment (Guyatt et al. 1986, 1988; Louis et al. 1984). Randomization here means that treatment and control periods do not always occur in the same, or chosen, order. Blind assessment refers to the fact that the person assessing change does not know whether the patient was receiving treatment or not.

Single case research designs are not a unified approach. There are three differing levels of formality and experimentation; randomized single case study designs, often called N=I studies (Guyatt et al. 1986; McLeod et al. 1986); single case experimental designs (Barlow, Hersen and Jackson 1973); and case study research (Hilliard 1993; Yin 1989), which may include diary or calendar methods (Murray 1985), and traditionally includes qualitative data. As Hilliard (1993) says 'single case research is best viewed as a sub-class of *intra-subject* research' (p.373). Rather than considering a cross-section of a group of similar subjects, this approach looks at the variation of selected variables within one subject over time.

General Approach

A common feature of all these designs is that they stay close to the practice of the therapist. A further advantage is that there are no difficulties over recruiting large groups of patients, or having to collect and analyse large data sets. These methods are, therefore, feasible for the practitioner interested in beginning research. The problems of recruitment (finding enough willing subjects who satisfy rigorous inclusion criteria) are minimized, the study is cheap and the results are generally evident. Much research flounders because of the difficulties of finding large groups of patients with similar symptoms, a lack of resources (time, personnel and money), or an absence of clear statistical analysis which is often compounded by initial confusions in the methodological approach.

A criticism of group designs is that they mask individual change and the results of large-scale trials are not always easy to translate into clinical terms for the therapist, as we saw in the previous chapter. Improvement or deterioration is not evident for particular patients in a group. Single case designs highlight individual change in daily clinical practice, and allow the practitioner to relate those changes to therapeutic interventions. Furthermore the dilemma of clinical priorities or research priorities is minimized. This type of research is applied as part of the clinical treatment and is relevant to both therapist and patient. In some studies, patient and therapist are the researchers.

In this approach each person serves as his or her own control. Effective treatments are linked with specific patient characteristics which are immediately relevant to the therapist and the patient. Any decisions about the design of the trial, and the choice of outcome measures, can be made with the patient (Cook et al. 1993; McLeod et al. 1986). It is this practical co-operation which makes these designs favourable for the music therapist. The primary focus of the research is upon the treatment benefit for the individual, whereas conventional studies are more concerned with changes between groups of patients. (The word 'group' is being used here as an aggregate of patients for statistical purposes, not as in group therapy.)

A weakness of single case designs is that, while individual change is specific, it is difficult to argue for a general validity of the treatment. Hilliard (1993) counter-argues that the generalization of findings is addressed through replication on a case-by-case basis. For such replication to occur there has to be a formal level of research design applied to the case study, and it is this formal rigour, with the inclusion of specific assessment instruments, that extends a normal case history into a case study.

Randomized single case designs

The first step in this approach is to identify the target behaviour. This can be a symptom or physical sign, a result of a test, or an indicator suggested by the patient. This is negotiated with the patient and is understood by both therapist and patient as being appropriate and relevant to the patient's well-being or clinical improvement. A *critical feature* of this target behaviour is that it will be susceptible to rapid improvement when therapy begins.

This target behaviour then becomes the *baseline* measure in an initial period of observation. The initial period of observation is sometimes called the 'A' phase. The intention of this phase is to enable a stable pattern or trend to emerge. This is based on the natural frequency of the symptoms. Any treatment effects can then be seen clearly in contrast to this baseline. Barlow, Hersen and Jackson (1973) recommend a minimum period of three observation points in a given period of time.

It is important that the method of measuring the observed behaviour is specified accurately. There can of course be more than one form of assessment. The therapist may want to rely upon markers of physiological, immunological and biochemical status, or indicators of symptomatic, affective and behavioural change. The patient may devise a self-report index. Apart from its clinical value, the choice of measure has a secondary research value. If the case study is to be part of a systematic research approach the measure will need to be reliable, i.e. it will produce consistent, repeatable results. Similarly, if the research is also intended to speak to other therapists it is important to develop a measure which they too can validate, i.e. does the measure measure what it says it does?

The development of a specific evaluative index (Kirshner and Guyatt 1985), or battery of tests, is an important task which challenges the therapist to relate theory to clinical practice. The main requirement of such an index is that it will be sensitive to change over time and will include all the clinically important effects. It is important to be able to link those clinical changes to the treatment.

The next step is to introduce the agreed treatment, and there can be multiple treatment courses during this period. In the randomized case design these treatment courses are randomly assigned. For example, a selected piece of taped music may be used in the treatment period, and 'white noise' or therapeutically meaningless music used as the non-treatment phase. Such a design is strengthened when an external assessor is used who is 'blind' to the treatment period. An external assessor can also act as a monitor of the trial and halt the trial if it is in the best interests of the patient.

Single case experimental designs

Where the treatment variables cannot be randomized, single case experimental designs are used. The intention is to stay as close to experimental method as possible with an assessor blind to the treatment phase.

The initial baseline 'A' period is followed by a treatment period, 'B'. This is an improvement on the case history in that it offers comparative data in two clear phases. This design can be extended by an additional assessment 'A' phase after treatment. There are problems here in that a decision about when to stop treatment has to be made, and the treatment may not be continued to conclusion. This is compounded by the difficulty of ending on a 'no treatment' phase.

If a further treatment period is introduced, then an 'A.B.A.B' design occurs. The intention in these designs is to keep the length of the treatment phases identical.

These designs can become quite complex. An example of an 'AA.B. C.BB' design is demonstrated by Rose (1978). The 'A' refers to the baseline phase of the behaviour of a girl on a particular diet which contained no artificial flavours or colours, and no natural salicylates. 'The 'B' phase was another type of baseline and involved the introduction of an oatmeal biscuit which contained no additives. The 'C' phase included the introduction of an oatmeal biscuit which contained an artificial yellow dye. This artificial biscuit appeared to be the same colour as the other biscuit. The girl's behaviour was then observed by her parents and others who were blind to the introduction of the biscuit containing artificial colouring. In the 'C' phases of the experiment the girl became hyperactive, leading the author to conclude that artificial colouring led to her hyperactivity.

A further elaboration of this method is to introduce composite treatments. Parts of the treatment can then be omitted or included systematically. For example, after the baseline data are gathered, 'A', then a composite treatment is administered 'BC'. This could be a treatment which included a creative arts therapy and medication. In the following 'B' phase the medication could be withdrawn. The next phase returns to the composite treatment. This then becomes an 'A.BC.B.BC' design.

These composite designs are particularly useful when the therapist–patient relationship is assumed to be a significant part of the treatment. Anyone familiar with composing a rondo form will understand the underlying principles of such research designs.

Multiple baseline designs have been used to test some psychological behaviour approaches (Hanser 1995; Murphy, Doughty and Nunes 1979). The treatment variable stays the same, but there are multiple baseline target behaviours of differing duration. Ideally these target behaviours are specific and independent.

The application of the treatment variable is staggered. First, after assessment, the treatment is applied to one particular target behaviour. If the target behaviours are independent then the chosen target behaviour will change and the others remain stable. The behaviours are constantly monitored. Then the treatment variable is also applied to a second target behaviour which should demonstrate a change at the onset of therapy. This treatment may be administered by another therapist. The other target variables continue to be monitored and treated in turn.

Clinical applications of experimental and randomized designs

As might be expected of research methods that were formally developed from the field of psychology, the majority of the clinical literature has its origin in psychological or psychotherapeutic applications.

Single case studies have been used to assess the impact of behaviour therapy for the treatment of mental handicap (Hoefkens and Allen 1990); epileptic seizures (Brown and Fenwick 1989); infantile autism (Bernard-Opitz, Roos and Blesch 1989; Gillberg, Winnergard and Wahlstrom 1984); obsessive ruminations and compulsive behaviour (Salkovskis 1983; Salkovskis and Westbrook 1989); delusional experiences (Brett-Jones, Garety and Hemsley 1987); neurotic patients and pain (Bryant 1989; Fagen 1982; Lavigne, Schulein and Hahn 1986; Moss, Wedding and Sanders 1983); depression (Jones *et al.* 1993; Richter and Benzenhofer 1985); agoraphobia and panic disorders (Cottraux 1984); anxiety-based disorders (Hayes *et al.* 1983); and multiple personality disorder (Coons 1986). They lend themselves well to individual problems where diagnostic categories are broad yet symptoms are idiosyncratic, and where it is necessary to combine both behavioural and existential considerations (Butcher 1984).

These techniques are also seen as useful for encouraging structured learning. Milne (1984) used single case designs to introduce behaviour therapy techniques and skills to nurses. With their emphasis on methodological awareness (Lavigne, Schulein and Hahn 1986) and formal experimental decisions while retaining the patient as the primary focus of research, these approaches are particularly useful for teaching and developing research methods (Aldridge 1991).

In more recent years the field of neurology has also developed these single case approaches. In assessing the cognitive competence of patients following brain injury, and the effects of therapeutic interventions intended to remedy the effects of injury, it has been important to develop specific, often idiosyncratic, indices and treatment plans (as in the creative arts therapies). These methods have been applied to the study of aphasia (Karanth and Rangamani 1988); apraxia and alexia (Wilson 1987); problems after stroke (Edmans and Lincoln 1989); attentional difficulties after brain injury (Gray and Robertson 1989); and memory problems (McLean *et al.* 1987).

The study of individual brain damaged persons has also led to inferences about normal cognitive functions (Caramazza 1986; McCloskey, Sokol and Goodman 1986) although the validity of these assumptions has been challenged (Marshall and Newcombe 1984). The reasoning behind this challenge reflects both the strength and the weakness of the single case approach; namely, while arguing for the specific validity as applied to individual patients, it is not acceptable to argue for a generalized validity as applied to the group.

However, 12 patients were studied using single case designs to see how they coped with the stress of being diagnosed as having breast cancer (Wittig 1989). This design used standardized diaries during the first 90 days after diagnosis and surgery to obtain a multivariate description of individual mood states and coping responses. By using such a time-based approach, which evaluated different modes of coping, it was possible to propose specific intervention strategies for individuals, albeit with a common problem. The secret to understanding such studies lies in understanding what is common to the methodological approach and what is specific to the treatment intervention, what is common to the overall problem, and what is specific to the individual patient in the way in which he or she responds to such a problem. Unfortunately many arguments resolve around either the group or the individual, without realizing that there are intermediary levels; i.e. not all individuals behave idiosyncratically, or all the same, and there may be clusters of common responses.

Statistical analysis

In single case designs there are possibilities for a statistical analysis of each single study (Barlow and Hersen 1984; McLeod *et al.* 1986). The main appeal of working in this way is that daily measures are plotted on a chart and can be seen by eye. Clinical improvement can also be assessed by reports from the patient and various persons connected with the patient (spouses, relatives, experts) who can also suggest that the change is of applied significance.

Statistical analysis can be used where subtle significant changes occur in the data which are not immediately visually apparent, or where many variables are collected from an individual and need to be correlated one with another.

The most familiar tests are the t and F test depending on the number of different conditions or phases during treatment. The main difficulty in applying these tests is an artefact of the research design itself. The collection of data over time may mean that the data are serially dependent, that is, that each measure affects the next one. Serial dependence occurs when successive observations in a time series are correlated, and this dependence seriously violates the premise of analysis of variance. It is necessary in these studies to test data to see if they are auto-correlated.

If the data are serially dependent then it is possible to perform a *time series analysis* of the data (Jones *et al.* 1993; LeBlanc 1986; Moran and Fonagy 1987; Onghena 1992; Salkovskis 1983). Such time series analysis requires large samples of data points to select the processes within the series itself.

A difficulty which can arise in single case studies occurs when they are used following a period of standard treatment which has not worked. Some general improvement may occur which is nothing to do with the treatment being used but is a 'regression towards the mean', i.e. the tendency of an extreme value when it is re-measured to be closer to the mean. This can be overcome in studies where medication has been previously used for treatment, by including a 'washout' period between the former treatment and the time when the case study begins. The term 'washout' period is a phrase borrowed from pharmaceutical research and refers to a period when no treatment occurs, offering the opportunity for previous treatment effects to leave the body by natural means. Such a period would serve to establish the patient's eligibility for the trial and to discuss and plan the research approach together. Following this there would be a period in which baseline data are collected. In music therapy, there would be a period when the subject would be expected to be without any intended musical influence. As this is almost impossible to achieve, and suggests that somehow the people whom we treat do not learn, or develop, it is a technical device that owes more to the methodolatry or worship of science than to the intelligent application of a research method. These experimental single case approaches assume that music can be given in doses, and, once removed, cease to have influence. Our intention as artists, and that of the people with whom we work as patients, is to create something new or learn something as a discovery. Therapeutic change in this sense is not ephemeral. As human beings we really do have the capacity to learn from our experiences.

The consistent recording of longitudinal multiple data in these studies requires great perseverance on the part of the collector and the patient. This is mitigated by the fact that only one person is being studied. There may be a temptation by some researchers to lump together single case designs and treat them as a group. To do so contains all the pitfalls of *post hoc* hypothe-sizing, i.e. making up the ideas to support the results you get; loses the primary advantage of individual consideration; and means handling vast amounts of often disparate data.

Jones *et al.* (1993) describe the long-term psychotherapeutic treatment of a woman who was 35 years old when the treatment began. Their concern was to articulate the reciprocal influence processes between the patient and therapist during the course of therapy over a two-and-a-half-year period. Time series analysis was used to demonstrate the causal relationships between therapeutic phenomena; in this case, shifts in the nature of the therapy process, therapist acceptance, therapist activity, and patient symptom change. Such a method can be used to test whether the therapist influences the patient, the patient influences the therapist, there is a concurrent mutual influence, or that no influence occurs. Indeed, the authors conclude that therapist and patient mutually influenced one another, that the therapist used clearly identified techniques of support and expression which were related to specific stages in the therapy process and the dysphoric mood of the patient. What is impressive about this study is the battery of measures used in assessment, ranging from clinical evaluation rating scales, well validated patient self-report measures to the 100-item psychotherapy process Q-Set. (The Q-Set is a 'language and rating procedure for the comprehensive description, in clinically relevant terms, of the patient–therapist interaction in a form suitable for quantitative comparison and analysis' (Jones *et al.* 1993, p.384).) Furthermore, videotapes of the sessions were independently rated by two judges blind to each other's ratings.

Case Study Methods

The case study is perhaps characteristic of the single case approach in psychotherapy and has its roots in the traditional studies of psychoanalysis. In the following chapters we will see examples that are based upon this approach. A story is related about what happens without any efforts at quantification of given variables. Indeed, the general approach is qualitative, relying upon the passive description of identified variables as they change throughout the process of therapy. The researcher often selects specific parameters for therapeutic change, and identifies how such change would be expressed. This way of working would be similar to a hypothesis-con-firming approach. Other researchers may be convinced that setting hypothe-ses and indicators restricts them, allowing no room for new ideas to develop. A patient in this approach would be treated, observed and described quite freely without any attempt to set formal parameters. This way of working would be an exploratory approach.

Whatever the method used there has to be a way of recording data for analysis. Material is collected on audiotape, videotape, film, pictures or as written documents. One special way of collecting written data is the patient diary (Murray 1985). Not only does the diary bring the minimal element of formal structure to observations, it is culturally acceptable as a way of setting down thoughts and recording what has happened.

Although a research approach in itself, the patient diary can also be part of the evaluative index mentioned in the previous approaches. The patient diary is rather a 'catch-all' term. Some researchers will ask the client to collect personal data according to specific rating scales on a daily basis, and this technique could be more appropriately termed a calendar method. An extension of this technique of daily rating to include a brief subjective commentary would be appropriately called a diary method. The detailed daily recording of patient commentaries involving introspective accounts, and even dreams or fantasies, may be likened to a journal and is the least formal, in experimental terms, of the three methods mentioned here.

In diary studies the principal collector of data is the patient. One of the tasks of research scientists working in the field of clinical practice is to discover what happens in the context of the patient's daily life and to make some attempt to discover how his or her problem impinges upon his or her daily routine. Similarly, it is important to discover who in the family of that person is involved at the time of onset of the symptoms and in the management of those symptoms. The use of subjects making their own assessments of symptomatology is not new (Murray 1985), and offers a non-intrusive means of gathering data. Perhaps as significantly, the diary also offers the patient a neutral stance whereby the symptoms are assessed methodically and in accordance with a particular framework designed to be ultimately beneficial.

Health care diaries have been used to discern the content of clinical practice with all its diversity of complaints and problems (Beresford *et al.* 1977; Freer 1980; Robinson 1971; Scambler, Scambler and Craig 1981). Most symptom episodes are transient and limited in extent (Dunnell and Cartwright 1972; Horder and Horder 1954). Retrospective interviews cannot provide sufficient or precise data about the events which precede the onset of symptoms, or the details of the management of such episodes. A further addition from qualitative research approaches would be for the therapist as researcher to keep a diary, journal or personal log also (Bruscia 1995).

Clinical applications of case study methods

Bruscia's *Case Studies in Music Therapy* (1991) highlights the breadth of methods available even within this one approach. Most of these studies are qualitative and often reply upon the specific language relevant to particular musical and psychotherapeutic direction. Such richness in diversity makes for an interesting mix in papers intended to inform practice. For researchers, however, there is the constant problem of finding a common base from which one can build further replicative studies.

Clair (1992) describes the influence of 15 months of weekly group therapy with a man suffering from dementia. She uses videotaped analysis by a trained independent observer of five behavioural categories (communicating, watching, sitting, interacting with an instrument, and remaining seated without restraint). Despite the man's cognitive and physical deterioration, he chooses to respond to music and musical stimuli. In quite an elegant little paper, Clair brings to the simple case study an extra dimension of validity resulting from independent observations pertinent to her criteria of what is valuable in therapeutic assessment.

In the same volume of studies, and from a psychoanalytical perspective, is a stunningly impressive case report of a boy showing signs of autism. Lecourt (1992) takes us through an overview of 88 sessions of music therapy. Her case descriptions focus on the structuring of the boy's experience of sounds and relationships. From such a focus she elicits examples of principles relevant to understanding the process of therapy itself. In this way the case study maintains its cardinal position amongst psychotherapeutic research methods. What is necessary for the single case study to work as a piece of informative research, as is exhibited in this example, is the ability to weave a number of behaviours together with therapeutic insights such that therapy makes sense to both the therapist and the reader at a number of different levels.

The ability to analyse material at a higher level, to see the connections between themes and to discern the emerging meanings in therapeutic process, is to engage in a meta-level analysis. Lett (1993) utilizes this form of analysis in the supervision of three female counsellors over ten weeks. He illustrates this work through the medium of a single case study basing the reports on Pam, one of the counsellors. Each session is videotaped and the participants write their own texts of their impressions regarding their feelings towards a particular client. From the resulting transcripts, both the supervisor and the counsellors select themes and significant incidents relating to feelings and occasions of learning. Apart from transcripts of the texts there are also opportunities for the counsellors to express themselves in a combination of arts modes, and Lett uses a variety of visual images to illustrate his paper.

Lett argues powerfully for a phenomenological approach which abdicates a prejudged analytical system and returns to the 'least contaminated' condition of therapeutic supervision (1993, p.383). Given the explanatory power of such work when it appears formally as a paper, it is difficult to argue against the method for the experienced practitioner/researcher. However, for the novice researcher, or the inexperienced practitioner, springing to the conclusion of 'no method other than the practice' can be a disguise for aimlessness and lack of focus in the research. Unfortunately the rigour which Lett and Lecourt bring to their work is assumed by some researchers who lack the background of experience and who read the politically correct material about research methods without having actually done the practice. In some ways this received knowledge of 'no system' has led to the paucity of research in the creative arts therapies, where practitioners have carefully rehearsed the arguments against adopting a scientific method, and thereby have done nothing.

Some music therapists, with psychotherapeutic colleagues, have attempted to forge new methodological ground. Langenberg (Langenberg, Frommer and Tress 1992) uses a method of audiotape evaluation which includes the assessments of the patient, independent describers and the therapist herself. These descriptions are qualitative in that they attempt to define both the qualities of what is heard as content (Quality 1) and the feelings or emotional experiences released by what is heard (Quality 2). In addition the taped material is assessed to discover what thematic motifs occur in the individual accounts, and as each motif is identified then the accounts are compared to see if there any motifs in common. In addition a musical analysis of the improvisation is carried out by two composers. While this research approach is only in its preliminary stages, the richness of the data based on musical phenomena and therapeutic descriptions is proving to be a valuable research tool which has resonance with other psychotherapeutic practitioners.

A benefit of the single case approach is that it generates empirical data suitable for proposing further work. Stanley and Miller's (1993) paper about short-term art therapy with an adolescent demonstrates how such a brief approach can bring about significant positive changes in self-esteem and an improvement in the adolescent–parent relationship as measured by a recognized self-esteem instrument. Similarly, in evaluating the quality of the child–parent relationship using structured observations from dance and drama therapy, Harvey and Kelly (1993) succeed in weaving both quantitative observations (time spent in interaction) with qualitative evaluations (avoidance, resistance, proximity seeking, use of transitional objects).

The phenomenological approach is of value for other arts therapies too in that it helps in understanding the client's experience during the therapy. Quail and Peavy (1994) wanted to overcome the tendency to focus on the art object apart the person. They used tape-recorded narratives of the client's retrospective descriptions of her own art works as created in previous art therapy sessions. The recordings were made of unstructured interviews which elicited descriptions about the art therapy process itself, the relationship between the art work and art therapy and everyday life and the experience of the art work in the current context of the research interview. Descriptions, rather than interpretations or explanations, were sought. The audiotapes were transcribed, read several times, and categorized in terms of the meanings inherent in the texts which led to the recognition of specific themes of 'temporality, spatiality, deep connection and contact, motivation, being visible and vulnerable, increasing awareness, and intense emotion and energy' in the client's account of the therapeutic process (p.55). For the music therapist, such recorded narratives can be made about the played music.

Personal Validity and the Construction of Meaning

As mentioned earlier in this chapter, we need to consider how the research we do with our patients singly can be generalized to working with others, and that we really are doing what we say we do. Validity is a general term used in scientific research to establish the truthfulness of a piece of work. Within our culture, the word 'valid' is used to comment on whether something is correct, either correct in its conclusions, or correct in the way in which those conclusions are reached. In some forms of research, notably the quantitative approach, this term has relatively strict meanings and is divided into sub-categories related to internal validity and external validity associated with both the way in which the work is carried out, and the meanings that are argued from the methods. Within qualitative work, the word validity has come to be represented by establishing trustworthiness and credibility (Koch 1994).

The way in which I choose to use the word validity, here, leans towards methods found in qualitative research (Denzin and Lincoln 1994; Lincoln and Guba 1985) and attempts to return to the archaic meaning of the word. The old root of the word stems from the Latin roots of *validus* = robust, and *valere* = to be strong. In this way, the validity of a piece of work rests upon a strong, robust argument, and the strength of that argument is to establish the premises upon which that argument is based. The basis of establishing validity as trustworthiness, in its sense in qualitative research, is to show that the work is well grounded, to make transparent the premises that are being used, to develop a set of sound interpretations and relevant observations, and to make these interpretations credible. Although it appears that we are questioning the nature of the data, and the interpretations that are being made of it, we are often also questioning the credibility of the researcher. While we may pretend to be asking purely methodological questions, much of what goes on in methodological debate is a questioning of the credibility of the researcher, not the data.

One step in establishing credibility is to state what the researcher's own perspectives and biases are. I shall present here some ways of looking at how two experienced therapists consider their own work, and the dialogue between a student and her teacher. This work can only be subjective. It is about how they consider their work in relation to the way in which they see, or rather hear, their clients.

There are two main questions for us concerning generalizability and validity. First, is there is anything from this work that we can learn for our own practice? In formal terms this would be expressed as 'Is there anything that is generalizable from this work?', and is a question of external validity. Second, we can ask the question, 'Are there any blind spots that the music therapist has herself towards her own playing?' This would be more concerned with internal validity. One of the ways of finding out is to discuss with a sympathetic listener, or more formally, in clinical practice, a supervisor. Bruscia (1995) refers to this as part of the process of self-inquiry referring. The supervisor's role is that of consultant thereby removing the hierarchical overtones often associated with supervision. A conversational paradigm is being used here to draw out the researcher's understandings about their own work, and the structure of those understandings that are not immediately apparent in everyday life. From this perspective such work is hermeneutic; that is, it is concerned with the significance of human understandings and their interpretation.

Many of the terms that are used in qualitative research – trustworthiness, credibility, legitimacy – are value judgements and it is therefore difficult to separate out the results from the investigator. We are really attempting to find out the bias of the person doing the research and how this influences what they do. Such work is therefore, inevitably, subjective. It is the premises for subjectivity that we need to discover. The task is not to establish the legitimacy of the person as researcher – we must accept that the researcher is acting in good faith – but to clarify the bias with which the data is gathered and interpreted. Meaning is not inherent in the data, it is influenced by the way in which the researcher interprets reality and that interpretation may differ from situation to situation (Dzurec 1989). Once that interpretation bias is made clear, then we as readers are able to discern how that work resonates with our own premises of interpretation and, indeed, our own bias.

A strength of qualitative research is that it concerns itself with interpretation. It is hermeneutic (Moustakas 1990), and therefore has a resonance with the very processes involved in music therapy. A first step, in this qualitative way of working, is to investigate how the therapist understands his or her patients. It is important to note here that I am working from the premise that therapists invest their practice with an element of deep personal meaning. As the music semiologist Nattiez (1990) himself remarks, 'the musicologist's persona is present behind his or her own discourse' (p.210).

Personal construct theory

The personal construct theory of George Kelly (1955), and the repertory grid method that is allied to it, were designed specifically to elicit such systems of meaning. This approach does not concern itself with identifying a normative pattern, rather it makes explicit idiosyncratic meanings. However, while each set of meanings is personal, and therefore unique, there is built into the theory awareness that we live in shared cultures and that we can share experiences and meanings with others. The personal construct theory method allows us to make our understandings, our construings, of the world clear to others such that we can identify shared meanings. As Kelly (1955) devised this conversational method for teaching situations, counselling and therapy, we can see the potential relevance for the creative arts therapies and for supervision. Indeed, Kelly discusses human beings as having a scientific approach. He proposes that we develop ideas about the world as hypotheses and then test them out in practice. According to the experiences we have, we then revise our hypotheses in the light of what has happened. Our experiences shape, and are shaped by, our construings. Each situation offers the potential for an alternative construction of reality. The personal construct approach allows us to elicit meanings about specific natural settings as we have experienced, or can imagine, them.

Qualitative methods, and particularly those proposed by Lincoln and Guba (Denzin and Lincoln 1994; Guba and Lincoln 1989; Lincoln and Guba 1985), present themselves as being constructivist. Therefore, there should be a historical link with Kelly's personal construct theory. However, nowhere in any of the major books related to qualitative research cited above do we find any reference to Kelly. It is only in Moustakas (1990) that we find a reference to Kelly in terms of 'immersion' where, during the collection of research data, the researcher as 'subject' is asked what he or she thinks is being done. Some commentators have found Kelly to be rather cognitive in his approach, but this may be due to the way in which he is taught. A reading of Kelly himself stresses the application of beliefs about the world in practice, and that the words that are used to identify constructs are *not* the constructs themselves. He argues that we each of us have a personal belief system by which we actively interpret the world. We create and change the world along with our theories. While we may be charged with bringing those beliefs into the realm of words and conscious expression, it does not mean to say that those beliefs are verbal, or necessarily conscious. This is an important point for the music therapist, who is often asked to translate his or her musical experiences and understandings into the realm of verbal expression. Knowing that some slippage occurs between these realms is an important stage in our understanding. Finding an acceptable way to accomplish such verbalization is a primary task of the research endeavour in this book.

The purpose of the work presented here is to find out how the music therapists organize their world of musical experience in one particular realm of activity, the understanding of a selected group of patients. Making clear constructions of the world is important for establishing credibility. We can see how her world is constructed. The therapist can reflect upon her own construction of the world of clinical practice. Such understandings are discovered when we talk to each other, sometimes called the 'conversational paradigm' (Thomas and Harri-Augstein 1985). Each person has their own set of personal meanings that can be communicated, but these meanings can be shared with another person. In this way of working, the personal construing of the world is primary in evaluating the world, and leans towards the narrative methods of qualitative research. Sharing those meanings with others must be negotiated and is, therefore, a social activity. To establish our credibility and trustworthiness as researchers, we need to make explicit our understandings of the world in some form or other. The repertory grid approach is one such way of formally presenting such understandings.

Eliciting constructs

Music therapy researchers were asked to select individual patients currently being worked with in clinical practice to elicit their personal meanings associated with those patients. In technical terms, meanings are described here as constructs and the patients as elements. Each therapist was asked to select patients who had some relevance for him as a practitioner. The selection could be a group of patients that the therapist was currently working with or had recently worked with. This request was not worded as a specific expectation regarding personal meaning in terms of emotions about patients, nor as an anticipation of intellectual associations. The statements were expected to be spontaneous expressions that came forth concerning significant patients in terms of practice. By choosing such patients, significant to the practitioner according to his criteria, there is the likelihood that patients who are challenging or rewarding are chosen, and these bring out contrasting poles of relevant constructs. An advantage of this way of working, as Kelly himself proposed, is that it elicits verbal labels for constructs that may be pre-verbal. In terms of a researcher's understanding, and bias, the explications from a musico-therapeutic realm of experience into a verbal realm may be of benefit for practice, supervision, and research. The verbalization of musical experiences is one step on the way to establishing credibility by getting the practitioner to say what she means in her own words.

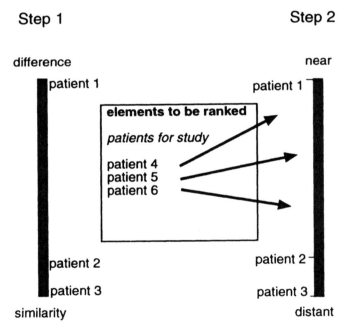

In Step 1 the construct poles are differentiated according to contrasted elements (Patient 1, who is different, and Patients 2 and 3, who are similar).

In Step 2 the construct poles are now labelled (near and distant) and the patients are rank-ordered on the construct 'near-distant'.

Figure 6.1 The labelling of construct poles and the ranking of elements

The numbers within the rectangle are the ratings for the constructs as made by the therapist and are converted digitally to a scale from 1-15. The degrees of the scale are given by the researcher.

The numbers at the top and the bottom of the rectangle are the element numbers referring to the order in which the elements were identified. Diane was the first element, number 1 and David was the last of the six elements, hence number 6.

The numbers to the left and the right, and outside, of the rectangle are the reference numbers of the constructs as they were elicited. 'Easier to talk to' was the first construct that was elicited, number 1 and 'Fluid musically-perseverates musically' was the last of the sixteen elicited constructs, hence number 16.

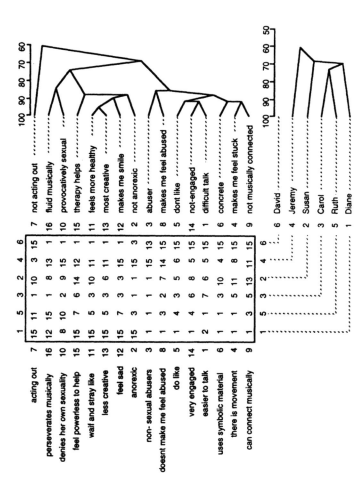

Figure 6.2 A focus grid analysis of a therapist's construing of child clients

Constructs are elicited by comparing three of the selected patients and asking how one patient is different from the other two. The practitioner is then asked how the other two patients, or clients, are similar (see Figure 6.1). Constructs are assumed to be bi-polar; for example 'good–bad' is a construct of worth with 'good' at one pole and 'bad' at the opposite pole.

In Figure 6.2 we see the names of the children being discussed in the lower right corner. Each name is an element in the grid and is rank ordered on the elicited bi-polar constructs; 'acting out–not acting out', for example. This process can be computerized and the RepGrid (RepGrid 2 V2.1b, Centre for Person-Computer Studies, Calgary, Canada) program is used here to prompt the constructs and to analyse the data. When the person being interviewed can find no further significant similarities and differences between patients, the data is analyzed.

There are two principal forms of data analysis and presentation. One is in the form of a principal components analysis that shows a spatial conceptual structure of the data (see Figures 6.3, 6.5, 6.7, and 6.9). The other is in the form of a Focus analysis that shows an hierarchical conceptual structure of the constructs (see Figures 6.2, 6.4, 6.6, and 6.8). Each can be displayed graphically. Both displays offer ways of presenting the data for further analysis with the practitioner or student. The discussion of the presented data is a part of the technique. It is not a finished analysis in terms of unequivocal results. Like all methods of research, the results demand interpretation. The clinician is then asked if this presentation makes any sense to her and any interpretations are noted. In Figure 6.10, we see how, in the far right column, interpretations made by the therapist are connected to construings. It is important to note here that the construings and their interpretations are always made in the words used by the therapist. An advantage of this method is that a phrase can also be used to represent the pole of a construct; for example, 'I liked them – I didn't like them'.

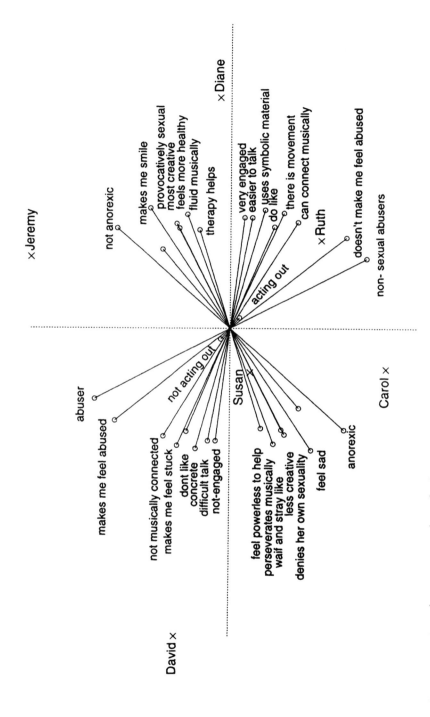

Figure 6.3 A principal components analysis of a therapist's construing of child clients

The numbers within the rectangle are the ratings for the constructs as made by the therapist and are converted digitally to a scale from 1-13. The degrees of the scale are given by the researcher.

The numbers at the top and the bottom of the rectangle are the element numbers referring to the order in which the elements were identified. Edith was the first element, number 1 and Aaron was the last of the eight elements, hence number 8.

The numbers to the left and the right, and outside, of the rectangle are the reference numbers of the constructs as they were elicited. 'Not resistant in the imaging' was the first construct that was elicited, number 1 and 'I liked them' was the last of the nineteen elicited constructs, hence number 19.

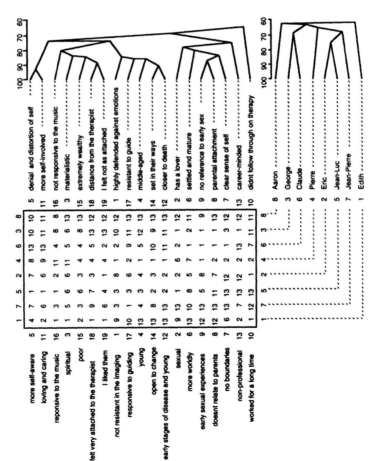

Figure 6.4. A focus grid analysis of a therapist's construing of adult clients

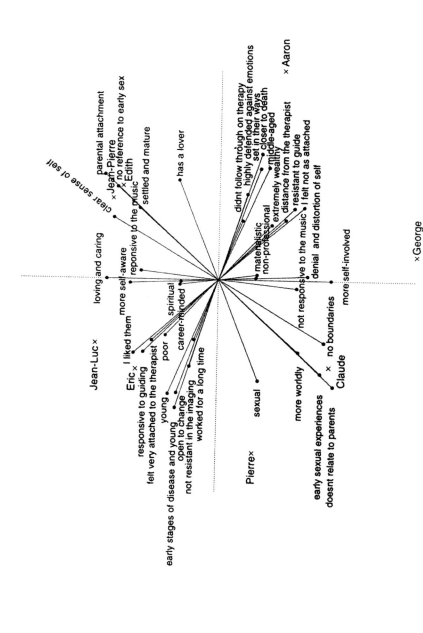

Figure 6.5 A principal components analysis of a therapist's construing of adult clients

U refers to the construct being unrated.

The numbers within the rectangle are the construct ratings. The numbers outside the rectangle, at the top and the bottom, are the element identification numbers. The numbers outside the rectangle, at the right and the left sides, are the construct identification numbers.

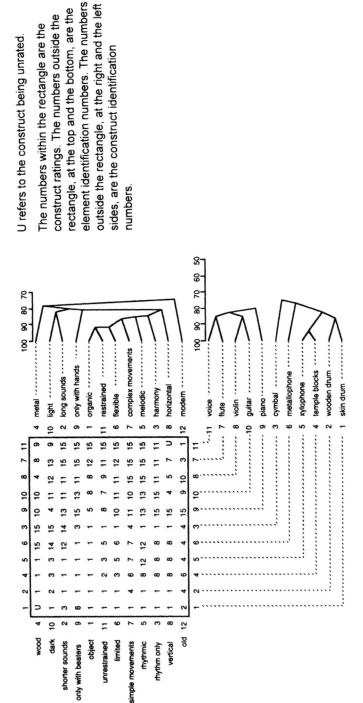

Figure 6.6 A focus grid of musical instruments as construed by a student

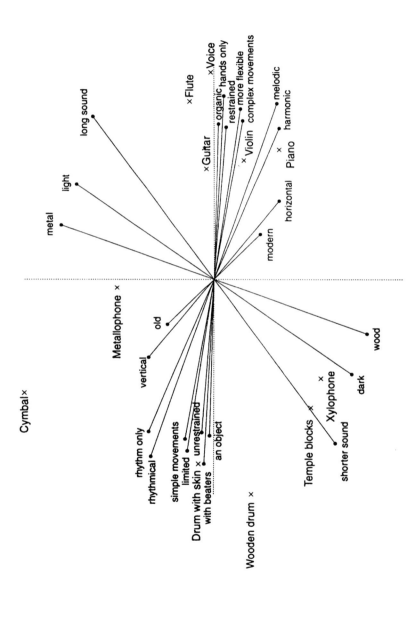

Figure 6.7 A principal components analysis of musical instruments as construed by a student

The numbers within the rectangle are the construct ratings. The numbers outside the rectangle, at the top and the bottom, are the element identification numbers. The numbers outside the rectangle, at the right and the left sides, are the construct identification numbers.

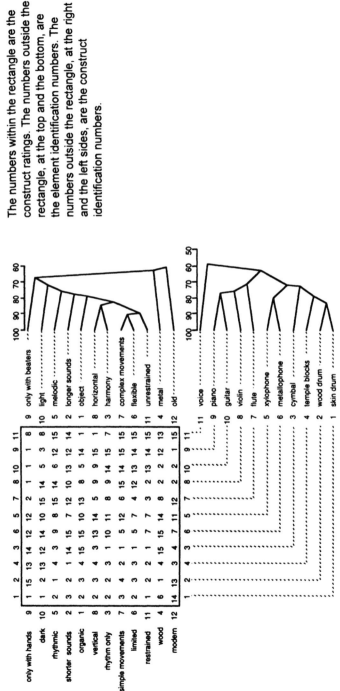

Figure 6.8 A focus grid of musical instruments as construed by a supervising tutor

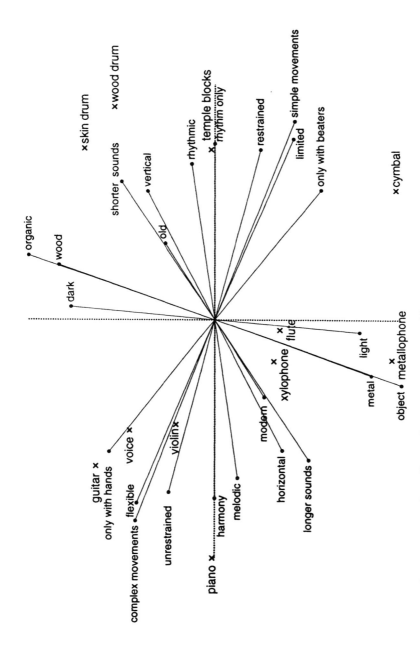

Figure 6.9 A principal components analysis of musical instruments as construed by a supervising tutor

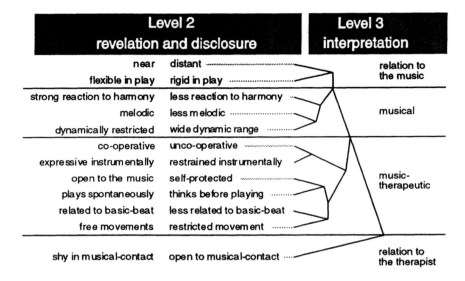

Level 2 revelation and disclosure		Level 3 interpretation
near	distant	relation to the music
flexible in play	rigid in play	
strong reaction to harmony	less reaction to harmony	musical
melodic	less melodic	
dynamically restricted	wide dynamic range	
co-operative	unco-operative	music-therapeutic
expressive instrumentally	restrained instrumentally	
open to the music	self-protected	
plays spontaneously	thinks before playing	
related to basic-beat	less related to basic-beat	
free movements	restricted movement	
shy in musical-contact	open to musical-contact	relation to the therapist

Level 1 would be the experience of the practice itself as a musical/therapeutic phenomenon.

Figure 6.10 Disclosed constructs related to therapy and their groupings as interpretations

The supervisor or consultant can then also suggest the patterns that she recognizes within the data that make sense for her too. This negotiating of a common sense is a part of the supervisory activity and the ground for establishing validity in a qualitative paradigm. In Figure 6.11 we can see how this negotiation is taken one step further and specific construings are discussed from the student's perspective. It is possible to see graphically where two people are agreeing and where they are of a different understanding.

The computational analysis is to take the values of the construct as they are assigned to the elements, as if they represented points in space. The dimensions of that space are determined by the number of elements involved. The purpose of the analysis is to determine the relationship between the constructs as defined by the elemental space. The computation is looking for patterns in the data, and organizes the constructs and elements until patterns are found. This is termed clusters analysis, in that cluster of similar data are organized together. What we see is how similar the constructs are when they are plotted in space. Two constructs that appear close together may be being used in the same way. Other constructs may not be equivalent and will influence the whole of the data as a constellation. Indeed, the principal components analysis of the data presents such a stellar appearance (see

The darker squares in the grid indicate a greater difference between construct ratings. The numbers to the right of the figure reflect the percentage of agreement between the constructs and elements. There is least agreement about the construct 'restrained-unrestrained' and 'object-organic'. Similarly, there is a difference in the way in which percussion instruments are perceived. There is an agreement of more than 80 per cent for the construing of the piano, metallophone and violin.

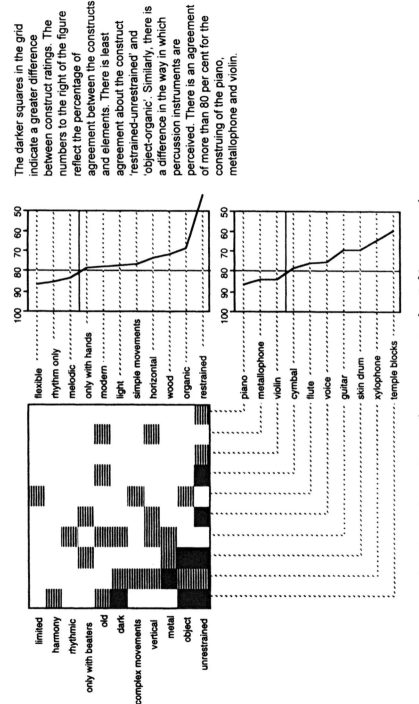

Figure 6.11 A comparison of two therapists' construing using the same constructs and musical instruments as elements

Figures 6.3, 6.5, 6.7, and 6.9). Here the two principal components of the data are used as axes onto which the constructs are projected. This allows the researcher to gauge the major dimensions on which the experiences of clients are being construed. These two axes appear as horizontal and vertical dotted lines in the figures.

The Focus analysis structures constructs and elements that are closest together in the dimensional space into a linear order. These are then sorted into matching rated scores and mapped according to their similarity (as percentages). Clusters of constructs are then computed by selecting the most similar ratings and presented as a hierarchical tree diagram that shows the linkages between groups of constructs (see Figures 6.4, 6.6, and 6.8). In the figures, similar constructs are arranged together so that we have a visual display, albeit two-dimensional, of how meanings are linked together. 'Feels more healthy–waif and stray like' is rated as a construct similarly to 'less creative–most creative' in Figure 6.2, and we may want to assume that in this therapist's thinking health and creativity are closely linked.

The results of both forms of analyses are then presented to the subject to see if indeed any such sense emerges from the analysis. An academic supervisor, using this method, could also suggest relationships that appear, to see if they have any relevance for the researcher. At this stage the researcher can be encouraged to find labels for construct groupings and these labels themselves represent constructs at a greater level of abstraction. These labels are a step in finding categories for use in analysing case material in qualitative research. There are analogies here with the process of category generation in grounded theory methods and are based on empirical data. For pheno-menological research, such categories, once they have been articulated in this way, could be bracketed out of the analysis. We see this in Figure 6.11 where overarching interpretations are presented based on specific construings.

Therapists and their construings

In Figures 6.2 and 6.3 we see the graphic analysis of a music therapist's constructs concerning her work with abused children. While most of the children share common characteristics, David is a child who stands apart in the therapist's construing (Figure 6.2). He is, according to the way in which the constructs are rated, a boy whom the therapist does not like. He makes her feel abused and stuck, without any musical connection, and that it is difficult to talk to him. She feels sad and powerless to help him. As a clinical supervisor it would be tempting to ask her if it might not be a good time to consider not working with him further.

From Figure 6.3 we see in the right-hand quadrants that Diane and Ruth are easier to talk with: they are engaged in the therapy, they demonstrate some therapeutic engagement related to their musical responsiveness, and they are also liked. Jeremy is a little different. He is a child who makes the therapist smile, who is 'musically fluid', for whom therapy works and, albeit provocatively sexual, is 'most creative'.

Susan and Carol are clients who make the therapist feel sad and powerless to help. They are less creative too. Such an analysis gives us a basis to discuss how a therapist sees her clients, either in terms of clinical supervision, or in terms of the relationship between personal perceived qualities and musical responsiveness as a research topic. For this researcher both her main topics concerning engagement (talkativeness, liking and the use of symbolic material) and health (creativity, amusement and sexual provocation) are connected with musical themes; that is, the clients can 'connect musically' or are 'fluid musically'. It would be a further step to discover what the qualities of musical connection are, and what it is in fluid musical playing that signifies health but not necessarily connectedness.

Another therapist, in construing his clients, presents a set of constructs that also reflect responsiveness of the client to the therapist and whether or not he likes them (see Figures 6.4 and 6.5). By looking to the right of the construct list in Figure 6.4, we consider how the constructs are linked together in a 'tree diagram'. These linkages signify how one construct is related to another, how they form small clusters that are themselves further linked at a higher level of abstraction. Thus we see linkages between constructs 5 and 11 where being 'more self-aware' and 'loving and caring' are very similar in rating (at a 94% level). 'Worked for a long time–didn't follow through on therapy' is a construct of a higher order of abstraction and related to several other sets of constructs, but quite separate in the way in which it is rated.

Moving to Figure 6.5, where the dotted lines represent the two main axes on which the constructs are plotted, 'loving and caring–more self-involved' is seen as a principal construct, as is 'working for a long time'. We see that the middle-aged Aaron appears to be resistant, and distant, to his therapist, highly defended against emotions and closer to death. However, the younger Eric and Jean-Luc are more responsive to the therapist, are open to change, feel attached to the therapist and work for a long time. Above the horizontal axis we have the loving-caring clients with a clear sense of self. Below the axis, we distinguish clients who are less responsive to the music, sexually worldly, likely to deny and distort their own self-images.

For the clinical supervision process such a grid would offer the opportunity to discuss transference and counter-transference issues in the therapeutic relationship. As a research tool, we have categories of construing regarding relationship and responsiveness, either musical or therapeutic, that can be compared with the previous examples from the therapist working with children. We might collect further examples of therapeutic construings to discover how other therapists construe their clients. For example, in Figure 6.10 we also notice that relationship to the music and relationship to the therapist are significant higher-order constructs for assessing clinical practice. While each construct grid is idiographic, it is possible to compare construings from several therapists and look for commonalities. While this is indeed normothetic, it does provide us with some knowledge that we have a commonality of interests as therapists, even when working from different music therapy training backgrounds. George Kelly referred to this shared commonality in his social corollary. We have our individual meanings, but we are also linked to shared meanings in a common culture. The power of the personal construct is that it allows for individual meanings to emerge, but commonalities are also preserved.

Objects as subjective elements

The previous examples have focused on how therapists perceive other people. However, it is possible to comprehend how objects are perceived. In Figures 6.6 to 6.9, we can discern how a teacher and a student, from differing cultural backgrounds, construe the same set of musical instruments.

In Figure 6.6 we observe how 11 chosen instruments are separated distinctively into two main groups that are further reflected in Figure 6.7. Voice, flute, guitar violin and piano are grouped as an organic constellation requiring more complex and restrained movements. This organicity is contrasted with the 'object' quality of the drums where movements are simple, limited and unrestrained. The cymbal and metallophone are light, metal and have long sounds. Xylophone and temple blocks, in contrast, are wood, dark and have shorter sounds.

The purpose of this grid elicitation was to help a student with her diploma thesis. What she was looking for was a way of structuring her work that related to her own experience of the instruments rather than the European basis that was offered to her. She used the personal construct approach that used the musical instruments as elements. This approach generated a series of categories by which she could write about her own experiences of the instruments. For the academic supervisor, it helped him recognize how, as a staff group, there were sometimes differing interpretations regarding the students' case study descriptions and their own understandings. To highlight this contrasting experience, the tutor used the student's constructs, which she had elicited according to the instruments, and rated them from his own experience using the same instrumental elements. This is literally using her words to describe his own experiences of common instruments; trying to see it her way, in fact.

If we look at Figure 6.8, voice is construed separately from the constellation 'piano–guitar–violin–flute'. Xylophone and metallophone, as tuned percussion instruments, are construed as similar, and the other percussion instruments form a separate, yet linked, group. Exactly what we would expect from a conventional European academic! Turning to Figure 6.9, the main axis of the analysis is that of 'harmony–rhythm' as typified by the contrast between piano and temple blocks. Another principal axis is that of 'dark', which relates to organicity and wood, and 'light', which relates to metal objects. We can see here that it is in the literal translation of 'object', as in the metallophone as a metal object, that the student and the tutor differ. Her notion of an object is at the contrasting pole of organicity in a vocal, breathy, sounding-board sense found in the flute and guitar. For the tutor the flute is a metal object. For the student the flute is an organic instrument with a voice.

It is possible to compare the two grids formally using the computer program mentioned earlier. Essentially, the differences between the rated constructs are plotted for their percentage of agreement. Figure 6.11 shows how our construing of the piano, metallophone and violin is similar. However, when we consider the skin drum, xylophone and temple blocks, there is an increasing lack of agreement. As percussion instruments form a significant part of the music therapy approach the student uses, then this discrepancy in mutual construings produced difficulties of understanding in clinical supervision. Part of this discrepancy lay in the tutor perceiving the xylophone as metal and the student construing the xylophone as wood. However, it is in the playing qualities of the musical instruments, unrestrained or restrained, that the biggest difference resided. While the voice, guitar, violin and piano are unrestrained for the tutor; for the student, they are restrained. It is in the precise elicitation of these differences that such a technique brings its benefits for supervision, and in the generation of suitable categories of understanding that benefits research.

The territory of understanding

The value of working in this personal construct way is that both researcher, as subject, and supervisor become aware of the way in which the world of practice-meaning is constructed by the researcher. This construing is mutual and elicited through shared conversation. The grid data, when presented as a Focus analysis or principal components analysis, are maps of the same territory; the meaning that the elements, patients or instruments, have for the researcher/clinician. However, these constructs are not the territory itself. What we have are verbal constructs plotted in space and presented as artefacts open to discussion. In being made presentable and conscious, then they are open to negotiation and, thereby, validation. It is this perspective of consciousness that Giorgio (1994) claims is the starting point for phenomenological research. We see what the researcher's perspectives and biases are. The supervisor comes to know what the researcher means through the process of construing. This is a means of establishing internal validity.

In the next chapter I will be referring to three differing levels of interpretation. Musical expression occurs at the experiential level 1; construing occurs at level 2, at a phenomenologically reduced level as revelation and disclosure; the higher levels of interpretation where coding and categorization occur would be level 3 ·(see Figure 6.10). The verbalization of constructs is descriptive, yet stays close to the musical phenomena, in this case how therapists construe their patients or clients, or describe musical instruments. By using such a method we have a means of handling ideas and meanings as if they were objects themselves. The reason for emphasizing these levels of description is that in phenomenological and qualitative research it is the lived experience that we are trying to describe, and knowing at what level of description we are working helps us to understand how such terms and categories relate to the meanings discovered.

The construct method is flexible, accommodating the needs of both partners, therapist and consultant, while offering a structure in which to work. It is possible to refine the process further and develop the appropriate questions according to the stage of research. We could just as well work with patients' construings of the music using excerpts from sessions, or elicit their construings of the therapist in comparison with other significant persons in their lives.

The benefit for qualitative research is that from the research data itself it is possible to generate categories according to the researcher's perceptions, that themselves can be compared to existing categories. Furthermore, as qualitative research takes time, and researchers become more conversant with their topic, the repetition of the grid elicitation allows researcher and supervisor to see how the researcher has changed. If reality is constantly being revised according to our knowledge of the world, then it is pertinent to plot any changes as they occur during the passage of time (Seed 1995). Indeed George Kelly used this personal construct approach not only to understand the world of the client, but to see how that world of construing changed during the process of therapy.

One of the difficulties with using repertory grid theory is that although the process can be computerized, the elicitation may become mechanical. Like any system it is open to abuse and therefore in the hands of those without experience it simply becomes a blunt tool and the results are both coarse and meaningless. In any procedure that seeks to understand meaning, the process of eliciting that meaning has to make sense to those involved, and can only be as refined as the participants who use it. A perhaps more important critique is that the computer analysis is being made as a mathematical computation and thus based on a scientific principle that seeks to reduce human behaviour to mathematics. Again, the resolution lies in the hands of the user. What these analyses are proposing is a way of organizing the ideas as they are marked on particular constructs as they appear in two-dimensional space. For the researcher, supervisor or clinician, this organization is a proposal based on what has been given. It can be challenged, and in the challenging new insights can be gleaned. The initial step is that something concrete is generated that can later be negotiated and discussed. At the end of the next chapter we will read how such construings and interpretations at different levels can be woven together to formalize a clinical narrative.

The construct method can be used as a form of qualitative self-inquiry where the researcher continually checks out her understandings throughout the study period. As a form of research consultancy it allows two researchers to work together as equals, rather like the model of co-counselling (Reason and Rowan 1981). Subjective research means that the researcher herself is questioned as to her credibility. While we may try to hide behind a stance of 'questioning the validity of the data', the experience for the researcher is that his or her credibility is being questioned. What I am proposing here is one method for establishing credibility. By establishing some of the concepts that the researcher is using in her work, she offers others a view on how conclusions about practice are reached. In a classical construct technique, the same methodology is used to understand how the patient sees his world. As such, the technique is an important method for offering structure within a single case design. While a questionnaire has structure too, it also has an implicit content related to the world-view of the researcher. The construct grid, while being structured, has a content related to the subject. Thus, a conservation of structure can be made while allowing for an idiosyncratic content.

The Value of Single Case Designs

In our work we are trying to understand what is going on during therapy, or as a result of therapy. To achieve this we must ask the people involved at differing stages during the process. What we have to be continually aware of is that the process of asking may itself promote awareness. A research method seeks to provide a strategy for asking and a structure for answering. In some cases this will be a strategy for playing and a structure for responding as the essence of an expressive approach. Indeed, the forming of the musical answer will be the response indicative of the healing process.

The use of single case research designs, by concentrating on symptomatic relief and the possibility of immediate observable improvement, may promote clinical insights too. Single case experimental methods are generally reliant upon a stable baseline period in the 'A' phase. This means that they are not particularly relevant to acute or labile problems. With their emphasis on change over time within one person, these methods are appropriate for the study of chronic problems, or patterns of recurring behaviour, that have become stable over time, and this is often the case for the patients and clients who are referred to music therapy.

The advantages of single case research designs are their flexibility of approach and the opportunity to include differing levels of rigour. Such designs are appropriate for therapists wising to introduce research into their own practice, and particularly for developing hypotheses which may be submitted for other methods of clinical validation at a later date. Moreover, single case research captures the natural context in which therapist and patient interact, making explicit the mutual influences of both (Jones *et al.* 1993).

Case study methods broaden the spectrum further, with exploratory studies using standardized measures and descriptive data, to the full-blown phenomenological investigations which allow the modes of creation themselves to dictate form and content. When standardized measures are discarded then most researchers either refer to an overarching theoretical structure at a meta-level, or they utilize the technique of triangulation, by involving independent colleague observers, or a supervisor who analyses the material. Such steps are necessary to lend some element of validity to what we do when we call our work research.

For the creative arts therapist as well as the music therapist there is the possibility to use the artefacts of his or her own discipline as they emerge in time, as we shall see in the next chapter. Paintings are not always finished in one session and it is possible to describe both the way in which a painting develops, and the way in which it may fit into a series of paintings. Combined with a diary account written by the patient, a series of structured therapeutic process observations on the part of the therapist, and an analysis of these paintings, there would be a wealth of data sufficient for an exploratory case study. Similarly, in music therapy we may hear a restriction in the patient's ability to play rhythmically and an ability to paint rhythmically. Using musical examples and graphical illustrations throughout the therapeutic process, and including patient and therapist accounts, it is possible to demonstrate a common link between therapeutic modalities and therapeutic change (Aldridge, Brandt and Wohler 1990). As the reader will realize, such a collection of data is not too far removed from the usual practice of therapy. What is required is either a formal framework by which the data can be interpreted, a standardized evaluative instrument suitable for assessment and for replication, or a panel of clinical assessors to validate findings.

For those therapists working in psychiatric, psychotherapeutic or medical settings where there are opportunities for the implementation of formal measurement instrument and rating scales, there is the possibility of comparing the significance of varying phenomena as they occur over time, perhaps using time series analysis. Where mixed therapeutic endeavours occur, it is possible to see what individual contributions make to therapeutic regimes. The single case approach, given a framework of consistent assessment procedures, allows for flexibility in treatment while challenging our intellectual rigour and fostering the relationship between theory and clinical practice.

CHAPTER SEVEN

Shared Meanings

> The question for art [and] for theory…is, 'how is all this – which devolves upon a "subjective" point of view – to be demonstrated in a way which is intersubjectively valid and productive; how is it to be (re)constructed in (re)presentation?' (Burgin 1989, p.198)

As music therapists we believe that it is important for our work that we learn a language which unites us so that we can work together (Moreno 1988; Schmais 1988). Within our research programme we have been discovering that language as it is based in clinical practice, that is, in the studio and the therapy room. It is hoped that the patient, who is the focus of our work, benefits from our common endeavour. Our intention is to be able to share a common currency of ideas both among ourselves as creative artists and with our medical colleagues as therapists. In the last chapter we read how the same musical instruments can be differentially construed; some similarly and others quite differently, even when the same words are being used. It is important for mutual understanding to explicate these differences. This process of explication takes us beyond the words themselves into the phenomena that those words describe. When we come to describe human feelings, such an understanding is necessary for clinical practice and of the utmost relevance for research.

In this chapter the work of two creative arts therapists will be used to illustrate how expressive forms can be used to negotiate a common language. One is a trained music therapist using an evolved form of music therapy with adult patients developed from the creative music therapy approach originated for children by Nordoff and Robbins (1977). The other is an art therapist working from an anthroposophical approach based on the teachings of Rudolf Steiner. This work came together in the treatment discussions of a patient with whom they were both working.

As we saw in Chapter Two, there is a congruence between musical form and the self. Musical experiences are essentially those of form and order which are continually being creatively realized by the person. As a means of treatment, creative music therapy in this context attempts to mobilize the creative potentials of the patient towards a restoration of the state we call 'health'.

Anthroposophical medicine recognizes that many illnesses and problems arise when a person is estranged form his or her own creative capacities (Barfield 1978; Fulder 1988). Illness occurs when we become literally out of time, out of touch and out of tune with ourselves and others. A lack of harmony, or loss of rhythmical co-ordination, can be expressed in artistic activities; in movement and dance, in drawing, painting and sculpting, in speech, drama and story telling and in the processes of creating and playing music.

The art therapies use different expressive faculties but the source of these expressions is an underlying commonality of form and pattern. A feature common to these treatment approaches is a that they are based upon the creative process. In drawing and painting therapy it is the processes of drawing or painting that are important. Similarly, in music therapy it is the creative playing of improvised music that is important for recovery. In medical treatment it is also the use that the patient makes of medication that is of vital importance to the therapeutic success. In the approach taken here, it rests with the creative arts therapists and the doctor responsible for the patient to decide together what therapies are to be used in treatment; however, the patient shares the responsibility for treatment in his willingness to participate creatively in the healing activity. Such a stance does not blame the patient for his lack of recovery, but does emphasize the participatory nature of the healing contract. While therapeutic responsibility for treatment decisions remains with the clinicians, this is relativized, and democratized, by the inclusion of the patient's view.

Creative arts in the context of scientific medicine
Research within a hospital setting must take into account the perspective of modern scientific medicine. Our work is complementary to a scientific research approach and is concerned with the subjective experience of the individual patient, and of the therapist. From this standpoint creative arts research is not science in that it has no generalizable reference. The importance of such work is in its particular subjective and unconventional reference.

While the aesthetic may appear to occupy a pole opposite to the scientific, I have proposed in earlier chapters that both poles are necessary to express the life of human beings. This is not to deny that scientific approaches can be applied to the creative arts therapies, rather to emphasize that there are complementary methods of research. My perspective is that it is important to redress the balance in research activities concerned with the healing arts from the scientific towards the aesthetic. Both art and science bring an appreciation of form and the expression of meaning. If we imagine the construct 'forms of research', then 'aesthetic' would occupy one pole and 'scientific' the other, in my view of the world. This means that both can be accommodated within a research perspective, and while there are extremities, there are also positions between the poles. We could understand music solely according to aesthetic theory, at one pole, or analyse music in terms of physical frequencies, at the natural science pole. Between these two poles we will have opportunities for clinical research. Qualitative studies regarding meanings inherent in the music, and related to the patient's health, will veer towards the aesthetic pole. Quantitative outcome studies relating music therapy to quality of life measures and standardized clinical assessments will tend towards the other.

As the musical events described below occur in a mutually creative therapy, in that patients and therapist perform a joint activity – creating music together – then we must face the duality of personal meaning and cultural meaning. Such a debate is taking place in the study of language and the emotions, to which we will return later.

Musical Intervals and Psychology

Later in this chapter we will read of a young woman suffering from depression. This raises the thorny issue of music and the emotions. While music must be regarded itself as a phenomenon that can stand for itself, as soon as we engage in a therapeutic debate – that is, music used for the purpose of healing an 'emotional' problem in a therapeutic context – we must consider the ramifications of music as related to human emotions and expressivity. In the example here, it is a young woman who has identified and labelled her own problem, who has admitted herself for treatment in a hospital ward, which is publicly recognized as specializing in 'psychosomatic' problems, and who wants music therapy as part of the treatment initiatives. While it is necessary to consider her as a co-musician in the aesthetic project of performance, it would be a massive denial of both a personal reality, for her, and the social realities of the situation, to pretend that music therapy should have no corresponding medical or therapeutic outcome other than making music.

Music intervals have been linked to particular emotions and, like tones and their relationship with colours, have differed according to particular systems of interpretation. What confounds such hypotheses, particularly when arguing from a historical background, is that often tone/colour relationships are taken out of context. Most healing initiatives using applied sound, sometimes as music, locate that practice within a broader healing epistemology and cosmology. To separate out one particular strand of relationships is to disrupt the philosophical fabric of the whole garment. Furthermore, to argue from the influence of pure sound on emotions as expressed verbally is to assume that all emotions can be brought into the realm of speech and accurately identified lexically. This is precisely the argument which music therapists make against premature verbalization of their work; that is, it seeks to identify and concretize with relatively coarse lexical labels that which is subtle, elusive and perhaps outside the realm of verbalization. But not outside the realm of expressive performance. This accords with other forms of psychotherapy that emphasize the necessity not to verbalize change too soon.

Ironically, aesthetic theory in music has long challenged the idea of definitive relationships between intervals and emotions, realizing that each individual is influenced in a different way. Unfortunately, neither psychological science, nor some systems of music therapy, seem to be aware of these discussions and findings.

Maher (1980) set out to investigate the proposition that musical effects have different psychological effects (see Table 7.1). As he says, 'the experimental literature…can provide little in the way of support for the proposition that musical effects have different psychological effects since most researchers in the area have taken this for granted' (p.310).

Maher (1980) played a series of sounds, as musical intervals, to 16 (non-music) students individually. They were then asked to rate the intervals on given scales which incorporated: evaluative components (happy–sad, pleasing–displeasing); uncertainty components (familiar–unfamiliar, stable–unstable, simple–complex); arousal potency scales (active–not active, restful–restless); and psychophysical scales (quiet–loud, one tone–too many tones). Although musical intervals were never clearly discriminated one from another, certain correspondences appeared which were generally consistent with popular notions concerning the effects of musical intervals. These were that the major third is rated as more *happy* than the minor ninth; the seconds were judged to be more interesting, unstable, complex and restless than the octave; seconds and sevenths were rated as more displeasing than the fifth. The seconds and minor ninth were widely discriminated from other intervals and are generally considered as dissonances, which Maher suggests is the result of component tone frequencies. Intervals ranging from the minor third

Table 7.1 Musical intervals and their correspondence with expressive function

Interval name	Symbol	Sample notes	Theoretical status	Expressive function
unison	1	C–C	perfect consonance	emotionally neutral
minor second	2-	C–C#	dissonance	spiritless anguish
major second	2	C–D	dissonance	pleasurable longing
minor third	3-	C–Eb	imperfect consonance	stoic acceptance, tragedy
major third	3	C–E	imperfect consonance	joy
perfect fourth	4	C–F	perfect consonance	pathos
augmented fourth	4+	C–F#	dissonance	devilish and inimical forces
perfect fifth	5	C–G	perfect consonance	emotionally neutral
minor sixth	6-	C–G#	imperfect consonance	active anguish
major sixth	6	C–A	imperfect consonance	pleasurable longing
minor seventh	7-	C–Bb	dissonance	mournfulness
major seventh	7	C–B	dissonance	violent longing, aspiration
octave	8	C–c	perfect consonance	
minor ninth	9-	C–c#	dissonance	

Table 7.2 Musical intervals and their influences in Nordoff–Robbins music therapy

Interval name	Influence
single tone	an inward experience of absolute rest and inactivity
minor second	an inward experience, a tendency to movement, inner activity
major second	the inward experience becomes more active and searching within the self
minor third	the beginnings of inner balance which may recede to the major second
major third	a positive statement of inner balance and stability
perfect fourth	a movement outward towards others and the environment
augmented fourth	ambiguity and unrest; the possibility of withdrawing to the self or moving towards into the world of the perfect fifth
perfect fifth	extroverted, standing in balance with the external world
minor sixth	the movement of self towards the other
major sixth	a definite step out into the world beyond oneself and towards others
minor seventh	the beginnings of a tension between self and environment
major seventh	an experience of stretching and quivering outside of the self in unresolved tension
octave	the ultimate experience of ego in relation to the external world

to the major sixth were never discriminated one from another, although high-pitched stimuli were consistently rated as 'happy', as opposed to low-pitch stimuli.

Nordoff–Robbins music therapy has also incorporated the concept of musical intervals, adapted from Rudolf Steiner's recommendations for eurhythmy, and its effects in therapy (see Table 7.2). For an improvisational model of therapy such a seemingly deterministic system of musical interval relationships is paradoxical, and is not always adhered to by therapists from that system; some use it as a guide to therapy; some use it when they find that they are playing the same chords over and over again with a patient; others reject it outright saying that each person has an individual reaction to these intervals. This rejection is made on both intellectual grounds, i.e. that aesthetic theory indicates that what is dissonant in one epoch is consonant in another and what is stirring to one person is calming to another; and pragmatic grounds, i.e. people respond variously to musical intervals. As such it reflects the 'universalist'/'culturalist' debate concerning language and the emotions.

Bonny (1975, 1978, 1983, 1986, 1989; Bonny and McCarron 1984), working as a music therapist, has also suggested correspondences between moods and music for the relief of stress and for personal creative enrichment. She suggests particular compositions which are compatible with mood groupings and arranges them as a 'mood wheel'. Opposing emotions are located in opposing positions on the wheel. She suggests that for a solemn mood Brahms' Fourth Symphony, third movement and Gounod's 'Ave Maria' are appropriate. In opposition stand humorous pieces represented by Bach's Brandenburg Concerto and Elgar's *Enigma Variations*.

The matching of mood and music, or musical intervals, while superficially attractive to a general music therapeutic method, is rather crude psychologically. Individuals differ in their responses to music; mood responses are not generalizable. The same piece of music can soothe one listener, yet irritate another in its crassness and superficiality. While one listener may delight in dissonance, another may find it disturbing. While music evidently has an influence on personal emotion, the labelling of that emotion will vary from individual to individual, from circumstance to circumstance. Furthermore, a music may have a particular response at a certain time in a person's life, but later be heard quite differently. Again, we have the discrepancy between the idiographic and the normothetic approach. Yet, as we saw in the last chapter, the challenge is to discern what the differences really are and what commonalities remain. We share some cultural attributes, and doing so binds us together; it does not remove our individuality. However, categorizing individual expression can render us as objects open to manipulation and work against personal understanding. Differentiating personal and cultural is an important activity in clinical and research process.

Expression as the Function of Art and Science

We have seen earlier that the function of art according to Suzanne Langer (1953) is to confront the person with something which they have not known before. Both science and art are activities which attempt to bring certain contents of the world into cognition and, thereby, confrontation. The contention of this chapter is that when we study human behaviour both forms of acquaintance, as confrontation, are necessary for research in therapeutic practice. Thus science and art bring us face to face together with the contents of expression and the activity of that expressive experience.

The artistic symbol, as we saw in the previous chapter, negotiates insight not reference. It expresses the feelings of the one from whom it stems and is a total analogue of human life. The symbol and that which is symbolized have some common logical form, i.e. they are isomorphic. Science negotiates reference not insight. That which is within the individual is placed within an already defined and prescribed context of the conventional. Thus we have lexical labels applied to feelings that are ethnocentric. Looking back to the student and the tutor in Chapter Six, we saw how a word like 'object' is differentially interpreted and this has ramifications for a wider understanding.

Music, drama and visual art are concerned not with the stimulation of feeling, but the expression of feeling. It may be more accurate to say here that feelings are not necessarily 'emotional state', more an expression of what the person knows as inner life, which may exceed the boundaries of conventional categorization. By encouraging non-verbal forms of expression we can learn and utter ideas about human sensibility. A reliance on verbal methods alone assumes that we can know and speak about all that we are.

The art form presents the whole intelligible form as an intuitive recognition of inner knowledge projected as outer form: subjective is made objective but in the terms of the subject and thereby unconventional. In artistic expression we have the possibility of making perceptible an inner experience. I am not saying that there are no commonalities. We do have the ability to understand people from cultures other than our own, even when no language is available. Indeed, a general premise underlying this writing is that a fundamental element of human communication is non-verbal. As seen in the last chapter, the descriptions that the therapists made of their patients and clients, while subjectively different and from differing music therapy therapeutic cultures, had some understandings in common regarding musical and personal relationships.

European tradition: Der Blaue Reiter

> Art does not reproduce the visible, rather it makes visible. Formerly we used to represent things visible on earth, things we either liked to look at or would have liked to see. Today we reveal that reality that is behind all living things, thus expressing the belief that the visible world is merely an isolated case in relation to the universal, and there are many more latent realities. – Paul Klee (quoted in Grohmann 1987).

In the tradition of Western modern art, music and the graphic arts have shared an impulse for similar vocabularies. 'Der Blaue Reiter', a group of artists, poets, writers, dramatists, dancers and musicians who gathered together around 1911 in Munich, were interested in a synthesis of the arts based upon a spiritual idealism (Budde 1989; Gollek 1989; Hall 1977; Vergo 1977). They shared a community of interests where inner striving was a critical factor. This inner experience represented a mysterious reality which lay beyond the appearance of things. Their belief was that such complex and universal visions of the mysterious might require several artistic media as vehicles for their revelation, and these media were often presented together in the form of theatrical pieces.

Table 7.3 The underlying correlations between musical tones and colour in the work of Skryabin

C	Red	G	Orange-rose
D	Yellow	A	Green
E	bluish white	B	similar to E
F	dark red	F#	Blue, harsh
D♭	Violet	A♭	Purple violent
E♭	Steely with metallic lustre	B♭	similar to E♭

Source: a translation of the 'colour feelings' attributed to Skryabin as published in *Der Blaue Reiter* by Leonid Sabanejew, the Russian composer and music writer (Lankheit 1989, p.112).

Their first annual year book (Lankheit 1989) compiled essays about primitive art, dramatic productions, poetry, new songs and an essay on the relationship between the arts and writing by the composer Schoenberg (himself an amateur painter). Kandinsky, a founder of the group with Franz Marc, recognized that there was a parallel between his own painting and the musical ideas of Schoenberg. Through the influence of Skryabin, Kandinsky was stirred to produce an amalgam of music, movement and light in 'Der Gelbe Klang' (literally 'The Yellow Sound'). Schoenberg also conceived and designed a stage piece, *Der Glückliche Hand*, which included original words, scenic design, costumes, music, and detailed instructions for lighting closely correlated with the music.

An important idea in this group was that of the correspondence between particular colours and musical tones. Skryabin's work included a *clavier à lumières* which projected light not sound according to a system of notation as part of his composition 'Prometheus' (see Table 7.3). The idea was that the playing of particular keys would bring light not sound into the concert hall.

Table 7.4 Inner associations and colours of different writers and artists

	Steiner	*Kandinsky*	*Schoenberg*
Blue	The lustre of the spiritual	Solemn, above earthly inspiration, heavenly	Hope, fortune and inspiration
Yellow	The lustre of the soul and emotional life	As sharp trumpets	Sunlight, activity and the colours of the day
Red	The lustre of the living, the 'vital', life body	Energy, vivacity, reminiscent of flames and blood	Temptation and strong desire
Green	The physical body without its 'vitality'	The colour of serenity, wordless, soundless and immovable	Annihilation and destruction
Black	Death	Silence and death	Night and death

Synaesthesia, the hearing of colours and the seeing of sounds, was not a new phenomenon. Various healing traditions have also attempted such correlations between qualities, colour, and music (McClellan 1988). The problem of such correlation is that each tradition has its own idea of what colour corresponds with which musical tone (see Table 7.4). This highlights the problem for us as creative arts therapists seeking a commonality of language. At which level will we find correspondence? At too concrete a level we find that there is no generalizable significance, i.e. at the level of corresponding tones, whether they be colour or sound. However, we may be able to find correspondence at the next higher level of description which is that of structure, i.e. the elements of form, order, pattern, dynamics, and orientation. I suggest below that it is this level of structural correspondence that may provide the ground for a common therapeutic discourse, as it was demonstrated in the last chapter where individual differences in therapist construings were reconciled at another level of interpretative categorization. Thus are individual and cultural meanings integrated.

KLEE

Paul Klee, a painter and member of Der Blaue Reiter, claimed that in his painting such formal structural elements and their mutual relationships were analogous to musical thought. He saw the mystery of creation as the secret key to the source of all Becoming. Each work of art becomes a symbol of creation as the terrestrial life represented the cosmic (Grohmann 1987).

He puts forward a fourfold way of studying nature which includes the artist, the object, the earth and the universe. The artist explores the object's inner being; its cross-sections (anatomy), its vital functions (physiology), and the laws governing its life (biology); its ties with the earth as a static, concrete object; and its ties with the universe as a whole as abstract dynamic form.

The creative forces in the universe are seen reflected in the artist; the artist becomes both creator and creative where the world becomes both object and state of mind. He takes from Goethe, whose writing greatly influenced anthroposophy (Barfield 1978), the principle that the totality of cosmic laws is reproduced exactly in the tiniest leaf as the laws governing the universe are reproduced in the artist.

Klee sought, like the other artists in the group, a liberation from representation in the arts. This represented a European spirit of idealism where the inner life of depth gave rise to images on the surface. The formal elements of painting, and the relationships between those elements, were analogous to musical thought.

This thinking was developed by other Bauhaus artists at this time who were not interested in teaching painting as such, but the understanding of form. The rhythm of structure and pattern as repetition of form were seen as common elements in the grammar of this form in the creative arts. Variety within repetition was a natural form common to botany, as it was to modern music and the paintings of Klee. The notion of interval within a field was an abstract component which could be realized in various expressive forms, i.e. musical intervals as sound and chromatical intervals as colour.

In the following case example we will see how such comparisons of form and relationship are central to descriptions of the therapeutic process. The creative arts therapies presented here then lie within a continuing tradition within the arts.

Case Study

I want to introduce a case study here to illustrate how creative art products are interpreted such that the two therapists involved find a common way of talking about therapy together. More importantly, we notice that the therapists talk as much about the producing as about the product.

Maria was 36 years old when she first came for therapy. From her early childhood she had to bring her alcoholic father home from the pub because he was often drunk. Her parents had little money and she was forced to find a job as a clerical assistant while she was still young. Between the ages of 19 and 23 she suffered epileptic fits and this condition led to frequent job changes because she was ashamed to face her colleagues.

At the age of 28 years Maria married, and then had two children. In her marital relationship she felt herself to be unimaginative, nagging and without initiative. She was excessively perfectionist about housework. There appeared to be no balance within her life and work. She felt unable to develop any sustained interests. This created a deep-rooted problem of self-esteem which in turn fed the current moods of depression she experienced. At the time of her stay in hospital she was diagnosed as suffering from nervous depression. Her hospital therapy, from which the following examples are taken, occurred over a period of five weeks.

Art therapy

The patient had one-hour sessions of art therapy daily.

In the sessions of free painting the patient applied the watercolour paints so thickly that no play of light and dark was generated. As a result, the colours appeared to be lifeless and dull with no tension between dark and light areas. There was a great disorientation in the way in which she handled the paint. This was seen in the rapid undirected actions of the abrupt movements with the brush away from her body. These brush movements increased when she was nervous and the completed picture appeared turbulent and restless. She often kept to the corners of the sheet of paper, which offered some points of orientation, becoming lost towards the centre of the picture. Furthermore, the structure of the painting into top and bottom was difficult. No colour focus or visual centre appeared within the picture itself.

Maria was reliant on external stimuli from the therapist and could only be induced to pause and observe by continual encouragement. It was difficult for her to prepare the next stage of painting by looking at her picture and absorbing the qualities of the colours; thus the rhythm of observing and painting was seldom established. If left alone she appeared to be applying paint rather than painting as a creative activity.

When offered a structure by the therapist, in the form of a repetitive carefully oriented task, she became calmer and more ordered in her movements. Her stereotypical movements became relaxed. It was through the use of intensive structured therapist intervention that she found a centre of focus and the awareness of the need for an inner base from which she could work to achieve personal security.

Music therapy

The patient was seen for half-hour sessions weekly.

In the first few sessions the following characteristics emerged from her musical activity. Maria played in a heavy, fast and disordered way on the small drum. This playing was interspersed with occasional recognizable rhythmic patterns that bore little musical relationship to the music the therapist was playing on the piano, although the therapist was trying to mirror Maria's playing. Her tempo was basically fast and she was unable to vary it under her own initiative. As in the activity of painting, or more appropriately, applying paint, she had a tendency to become set in her musical playing. This was also visible externally in the movements she made while playing. When playing the drum, the ends of the sticks remained on the drum skin so that individual sounds could not develop freely. This is also partially indicative of not listening to what one is doing oneself. It is almost as if some people start an activity, painting or making sounds, and continue in that activity without any further awareness of what they are doing or that that process can be influenced. My argument is that the same process occurs too in emotional expression. A process is set in motion – anxiety or depression – and the sufferer then becomes locked into the process itself. Rather than being an emotional expression that is meaningful for the person themselves, in that anxiety is sometimes useful, it becomes habitual without any relevance within the expressive context of the person's life. The delicate ecology of expression is disturbed.

When asked to play on two instruments together, for example, a large and small drum, or with two beaters together she played in an unconnected way with no relationship to the music offered by the therapist.

During the first session her lack of receptivity to current external experiences was evident in her too rapid, unbalanced reactions. This was noticeably clear in her melodic playing. Any sustained melodic lines were interspersed quick sequences of notes which disturbed the overall context. In her own melodic arrangements on the xylophone or glockenspiel she lost any direction in her melodic playing. This loss of direction was also evident if there were gradual increases in volume or tempo. In the context of her life, she too recognized such a 'loss of direction' as the source of her problems. Here loss of direction may be interpreted as not being able to find a way from one point to another. However, loss of direction can also be interpreted as loss of direction in the way that a play for the theatre needs direction. While feelings were available, it was a performed direction that would bring some expressive form to her life and so enable some meaning to appear.

It was possible to stabilize her playing by musical means. Uniform consecutive chords played quietly brought a musical coherence to her playing, which by the end of the therapeutic period was free of incoherent sections. She was able to reproduce rhythmic patterns in a clear and conscious way and sustain these over a longer phrase.

In dialogic playing a fluent interplay was created between the therapist and the patient. Within this musical form she attempted to generate new sound possibilities and effects such as playing with her fingertips and playing at the edge of the drum.

A sense of security seemed to appear within the joint musical activity which was expressed by her being able to sustain a recurring rhythmic figure in various musical contexts with only minimal musical accompaniment from the therapist at the piano.

A feature of the therapeutic success was in drawing her into a quiet slower tempo and maintaining this over time. This gave her the opportunity for a greater perception of the musical processes and an inner receptivity to experience. She experienced and produced intervals and caesuras, she could sing alone with melodic lines and complete them alone when the therapist left her to do so. Thus the patient was able to construct her own melodic phrases forming a logical melodic line. The random and uncontrolled aspects of her playing were increasingly replaced by a consciously structured and directed way of playing, resulting in logically structured improvisations with greater stability of form.

Comparisons

The therapeutic changes in Maria over the five weeks of her stay were also confirmed in the medical report of her general condition. It was noticeable that the patient manifested similar behaviour in both types of therapy. These were seen in her limitations in handling form as expressed in colour and sound. Her inability to relate to what she did, which was expressed on the ward at times as extreme disorientation, could also be seen in her painting and heard in her playing.

Both therapists were struck by the patient's basic receptivity, her willingness to participate in artistic activity and her strength of will which led her to attempt to overcome her limitations in both art forms. Her outer willingness was in stark contrast to her inner inflexibility and emptiness. In both forms of therapy her actions were reinforced and moved quickly into a stereotypical sequence as soon as she had to continue on her own without considerable support from the therapist.

As far as expression was concerned both the paintings and playing showed no internalization and hardly any expression of feeling came to the surface. However, despite the seeming rigidity, changes took place. The decisive factor in the development of the therapy was an experience of her own disorientation. Maria perceived that what she did was repetitive and had no direction to it. With this realization she struggled to find a personal order to her existence. She was encouraged to do this within the ordered forms of painting and musical improvisation. Although she could express herself, these expressions were muddled, formless, without a centre or focus and, for her, unsatisfying. So too was her daily life. Once she realized this pattern, then she could be open to forming her experiences anew; that is, her life achieved an aesthetic that was satisfying. We can use the word realize in the sense that the pattern was made real either in the action of painting or the activity of music.

Her confidence grew as she handled sound and colour largely through repetition and imitation. The next stages in the therapeutic progress would have been to encourage her such that she would be moved from within herself to perform creatively, although the first signs of such an impulse were emerging. We might propose then that the process of artistic creation offered her opportunities for a new orientation and new directions in life. As Suzanne Langer writes:

> What it [art] does to us is to formulate our conceptions of feelings and our conceptions of visual, tactile and audible reality together. It gives

us forms of imagination and forms of feeling, inseperately: that is to say, it clarifies and organizes intuition itself. (Langer 1953, p.397)

It is quite clear from these descriptions that there common elements in both of the languages (see Table 7.5). These elements are mainly concerned with formal structure: form, pattern, orientation within time and space, dynamic qualities, repetition, the way in which the patient performs, and expressive qualities. There are other elements concerned with commonalities related to the therapeutic experience, the relationship to the medium, relationship to the therapist, and relationship with self.

Table 7.5 Some common elements of description in therapeutic usage

Art Therapy Elements	Music Therapy Elements
quick, abrupt	fast and slow: tempo
repetition	repetition
pattern	pattern
fixed in her way of painting	set in her playing
brush stroke movements	drum stick movements
relationship to the medium	relationship to the medium and reactions to the experience
develop an idea	play a melodic line
disorientation in handling the paint	disorientation in the music
sustained development of an idea	music sustained over a phrase
new creative possibilities	new creative possibilities
relationship between elements	musical intervals
structure and form	structure and form
dynamic; light and dark	dynamic; loud and soft
lifeless and dull colours	qualities of musical expression
internal/external	internal/external
prepare for the next stage	construct melodic phrases from what has gone before
orientation; centre of focus	orientation within the music

A Common Language

> It is probably an error to think of dream, myth and art as being about
> any one matter other than relationship...rigid focusing upon any
> single set of relata destroys for the artist the more profound
> significance of the work... In a word, it is only about relationship and
> not about any identifiable relata. (Bateson 1978, p.123)

In our Western culture time and space are major axes of construing in both
science and art. However, in modern scientific medicine the usage of time
and space is regularized into objective qualities subjected to measurement.
While this physical objectivity may be challenged within the realms of
quanta, relativity is not a feature of everyday scientific discourse. However,
in the arts, space and time have no fixed reference: they are relative to the
moment, the place and the person. Hence the differing notions of *chronos*
and *kairos*, mechanical time and timeliness discussed in Chapter Two.

There are also fundamental differences in the language which we use to
understand science and that which we use in the arts. Science is based upon
empirical data and a written language which exists 'out there', as does this
page for the reader. This language is built upon a grammar which orders
subject, object and predicate and thereby influences understanding. The
content of understanding is always subjected to a given linguistic form for
objectification. Written language is based upon nouns which become fixed
(Bateson 1978); creating artistically is a dynamic activity, fluid, and often
not amenable to verbal expression.

The arts are based on verbs and doing is all-important. Arts as performed
are predicated upon quite different grammars; those of dynamics, of process,
of becoming and being in action. There is a difference between the grammar
of psychology, for example, and the grammar of dance. What the arts offer
is a common grammatical structure based upon performance where space
and time are lived and experienced directly often out of the verbal realm.
Showing rather than saying. When words are used in the arts they are
sometimes used in a different dimension according to another grammatical
structure, i.e. as in the case of poetry, improvised drama or singing. Importantly for the therapeutic descriptions it was the 'performing' that was
significant, not solely the 'product'. In this way we realize what we are; that
is we make ourselves real, and this is demonstrated through creative activity.
Through playing music with a therapist who mirrors what the patient is
doing, perhaps Maria heard herself as she was.

In our attempts to find a common language then it is also important to
emphasize that talking about therapy is always at several steps removed from

the actual activity in which we partake. Dancing, painting, singing, acting, doing therapy are different activities from talking about dancing, talking about singing, talking about painting and talking about doing therapy.

We need to emphasize that there are different levels of reporting, as remarked in the last chapter.

Level 1: Experience – Here we have the phenomenon as it is experienced. This is what transpires in the therapy session. It lives and exists in the moment, and is only partially understood. It cannot be wholly reported. We can see, feel, smell, taste and hear what is happening. These are the individual expressive acts themselves.

Level 2: Revelation and description – We can talk about what happens in the therapeutic situation in the particular terms of our artistic disciplines. These descriptions are accessible to verification and they emerge into consciousness with lexical labels. For example, we can talk about the particular notes and rhythms in music therapy and the particular colours and patterns in art. We can play our recorded tapes or show our pictures. This is the shared element of language that is available for systematic study and is part of our common everyday discourse and is what Nattiez (1990) would regard as the trace or the neutral level of understanding. Whereas Level 1 would be 'sounds', Level 2 is already perceived as music, therefore demanding a description, which is itself based on a theory implicit to the listener.

Level 3: Interpretation and discourse – When we come to explain what happens in terms of another system, i.e. to transpose the musical changes into terms of academic psychology, psychotherapy or a system of medicine, or to say what the relationship between the activity is and the process of healing, we are involved in interpretation. For the musicologist Nattiez (1990), this would be the level at which poiesis and esthesis take place; that is, conclusions are drawn about the music.

It is only our hubris which attempts to say that we know what the process of healing in therapy is. In medicine it is possible to know how to bring broken bones together in the correct position to heal, but impossible to describe the actual process of healing.

At the level of performance, what passes in the therapeutic session exists for itself. Everything else is an interpretation and depends upon language and is therefore an imposition of a subject–predicate grammar upon a dynamic activity. However, as therapists working together with patients we do need to talk to each other about what happens and what we do. Knowing

Table 7.6 The relationship between Nattiez's analytic situations, music therapy interpretations and constitutive and regulative rules

Analytical situations after Nattiez	Music therapy interpretations	Constitutive and regulative rules
	The music therapy session	**Constitutive rules** **Level 1** the sounds themselves, the experience as itself, the performance as phenomenon
I Immanent analysis, neutral ground of the music the physical corpus being studied, the trace	the score as a description of musical events	**Level 2**
II Inductive poietics	the music therapy index of events	revelation and description descriptions of what happens in the therapeutic situation
III External poietics	clinical reports from other practitioners, drawing from art therapists	
IV Inductive esthesics	music therapy meanings, interpretations of therapeutic significance	**Level 3** interpretation and discourse, the relationship between the musical or clinical activity and the system of interpretations
V External esthesics	sampling methods from psychology or expert assessment of chosen episodes as part of a research methodology	
VI A complex immanent analysis relating the neutral ground of the music to both the poietic and the esthesic	therapeutic interpretation from a fixed point but intuitively used in the therapeutic explanation	**Regulative rules**

at which level we are talking will aid our discussion and prevent confusion. My contention is that we can use construct methodology to find a common language at Level 2, which is based upon descriptions of the artistic process yet not too far removed from the activity of therapy itself. This is the level where personal construings emerge as revelations, where we put a name to what is going on. It is a level of description. By doing so, we can then discern when the therapeutic process is being described at Level 3, i.e. that of interpretation and inference, where there may be a unity in the grammar of verbal discourse. At this level we begin to find commonalities between individual discourses, as in the last chapter where we read how therapists began to talk about musical relationship and therapeutic relationship. This is a step forward on the road to establish the meaning of events in clinical practice. There may indeed be further levels of interpretation. Take, for example, the various schools of psychoanalytic therapy, or the different humanistic approaches; each will have a varying interpretation system that may find some commonality at a meta-level of interpretation.

Nattiez (1990, pp.140–142) gives examples of varying relationships between the description of the music and the interpretations of meaning that those descriptions hold for the researcher. These relationships can be translated into the music therapy situation, and the music therapy research approach. In Table 7.6 we see in situations III and V the inclusion of external interpretations of the therapeutic events that will include more than the music itself. Note that Nattiez as a musicologist is willing to include in an analysis more than the musical events themselves. We have a similar situation in music therapy in clinical settings where not only is the music available as a tape-recording (situation I) enhanced by a commentary form the therapist (situation II), but there are also clinical reports available from other practitioners (III). What significance those descriptions and interpretations have for practice will then be assumed under situations IV and V, inductive and external esthesics.

Rules for the Making of Sense

Understanding levels may not be enough in itself. A critic of the construct approach is that it is rather static and does not bring that dynamic horizontal level of linking in time that music has; that is, performance. In trying to make sense of what people do, we can look at how they construct those understandings in a vertical sense, which is seen in Levels 1, 2, and 3, based on a constructivist perspective. But we can also see how sense is actively made by linking those construings in a horizontal form. An everyday example of this is when we question someone about why they have done something (reasons) and then ask them what they did next (action). We seek an understanding, and then we want to know what the consequent action was. A formalized approach can be made in terms of constitutive and regulative rules based upon personal construings (Aldridge 1993a).

A number of authors suggest that 'making sense' is rule based (Harré and Secord 1971; Pearce, Cronen and Conklin 1979). These rules can be separated into two forms (Pearce and Cronen 1980). One, there are rules of constitution. A constitutive rule would be invoked when we say: this behaviour (a sore throat) counts as evidence of another state (a cold). Figure 7.1 shows a formula for constructing such a rule. Two, there are rules of regulation (see Figure 7.2. A regulative rule would be invoked when we say: if this behaviour (a sore throat) counts as evidence of a particular state (having a cold), then do a particular activity (go home to bed).

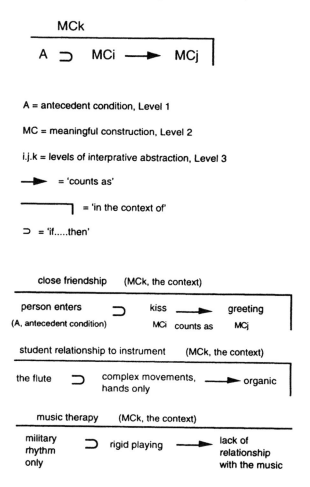

Figure 7.1 A formula for constructing a constitutive rule and three examples

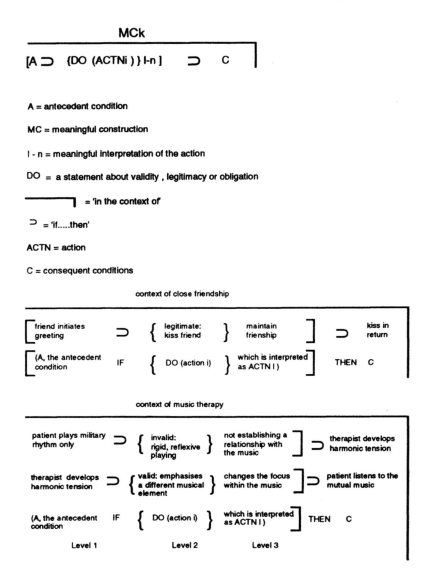

$$\overset{\textstyle \text{MCk}}{[\text{A} \supset \{\text{DO (ACTNi)}\}\,\text{I-n}]\quad \supset \quad \text{C}}$$

A = antecedent condition

MC = meaningful construction

I - n = meaningful interpretation of the action

DO = a statement about validity , legitimacy or obligation

⌐ = 'in the context of'

⊃ = 'if.....then'

ACTN = action

C = consequent conditions

context of close friendship

| friend initiates greeting | ⊃ | { legitimate: kiss friend } | maintain frienship | ⊃ | kiss in return |
| (A, the antecedent condition | IF | { DO (action i) } | which is interpreted as ACTN I) | THEN | C |

context of music therapy

patient plays military rhythm only	⊃	{ invalid: rigid, reflexive playing }	not establishing a relationship with the music	⊃	therapist develops harmonic tension
therapist develops harmonic tension	⊃	{ valid: emphasises a different musical element }	changes the focus within the music	⊃	patient listens to the mutual music
(A, the antecedent condition	IF	{ DO (action i) }	which is interpreted as ACTN I)	THEN	C
Level 1		Level 2	Level 3		

Level 1 refers to the musical experience as phenomenon
Level 2 refers to the level of construing as revelation.
Level 3 refers to interpretation.

Figure 7.2 A formula for constructing a regulative rule and examples

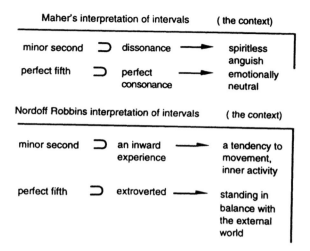

Figure 7.3 An example of constitutive rules relating to two differing interpretations of common intervals from Tables 7.1 and 7.2

We can use constitutive rules to compare various forms of reasoning as they occur in context. In Figure 7.3 we can see how information taken from Tables 7.1 and 7.2 can be reconstructed to demonstrate how meanings are constructed. Here the same intervals, the minor second and the perfect fifth, are differentially understood according to context.

If constitutive rules then are generally concerned with meaning, regulative rules are concerned with process and the linking of meaning and action. In Figure 7.4 we see how rules of regulation can be linked to piece together behaviour in a music therapy session. In the upper half of the diagram we see a sample of text taken from a case description. Key words are highlighted and noted as relevant constructs. We can read that personal connection is important, and that there are certain behavioural indicators such as posture and the positioning of the limbs that can be interpreted as indicators for the music therapy.

In the lower half of Figure 7.4 these constructs have been assembled into regulative rules, albeit using more detailed information than can be incorporated in the figure. Nevertheless, we see how textual data from clinicians' reports can be assembled according to a hierarchy of understandings to demonstrate at what level the musical behaviour is being described, and how those descriptions are further interpreted. Thus we have an indicator of the complexity of the music therapy discourse that is taking place. This allows music therapists to explicate both what is taking place and their under-

TEXT	CONSTRUCTS
A prominent feature of the way in which these patients play music is that they appear to have no **personal connection** with what they are playing.	personal connection
They appear to play with a '**distance**' from what they are playing. This distance is evident in their **posture**.	distance posture
When they are strong enough to stand their **posture** is often such that both feet are **not firmly on the ground**, i.e. **their legs are crossed**.	not firmly on the ground legs are crossed
The drumsticks are held loosely in the hands with the **inner wrist uppermost**, and they play from the wrists without involving the whole body.	inner wrist uppermost
This seemingly **uncommitted** posture make it difficult to play a clear beat on the drum.	uncommitted
Any **drum beats are loose**.	drum beats are loose
Beaters are allowed to fall and rebound rather than being used in a **directed intended beating movement**.	directed intended beating movement
Such texts can then be used to generate constitutive rules below	

Figure 7.4 Constitutive rules generated from a clinical description by one therapist regarding the improvisation of patients with chronic bowel disease

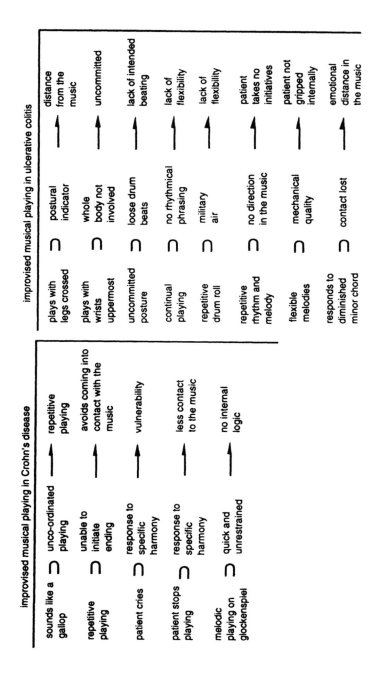

improvised musical playing in Crohn's disease

sounds like a gallop	∩	unco-ordinated playing → repetitive playing
repetitive playing	∩	unable to initiate ending → avoids coming into contact with the music
patient cries	∩	response to specific harmony → vulnerability
patient stops playing	∩	response to specific harmony → less contact to the music
melodic playing on glockenspiel	∩	quick and unrestrained → no internal logic

improvised musical playing in ulcerative colitis

plays with legs crossed	∩	postural indicator → distance from the music
plays with wrists uppermost	∩	whole body not involved → uncommitted
uncommitted posture	∩	loose drum beats → lack of intended beating
continual playing	∩	no rhythmical phrasing → lack of flexibility
repetitive drum roll	∩	military air → lack of flexibility
repetitive rhythm and melody	∩	no direction in the music → patient takes no initiatives
flexible melodies	∩	mechanical quality → patient not gripped internally
responds to diminished minor chord	∩	contact lost → emotional distance in the music

Figure 7.4 Constitutive rules generated from a clinical description by one therapist regarding the improvisation of patients with chronic bowel disease (continued)

standings related to what is taking place. There could of course be other interpretations of the same behaviour, and these could be useful to engage in a comparative discourse, as we have seen in the comparison between grids relating to the same set of instruments.

Such an approach gives a way of formally charting what meanings are associated with therapeutic activity and change. Meanings cannot be counted or measured, but they can be expressed and analyzed (Aldridge 1993a, 1993c). In our development of a methodology suitable for music therapy, also applicable to the creative arts, we can incorporate an element which attempts to understand the person as they present themselves as their own expressions; these may be played, painted or told. What these expressions may have in common is a formal structure and rules of relationship.

Our languages in the arts have commonalities. They are those of pattern and interval, which are based upon the logics of time and space. Rhythmic repetition and the notion of pattern go hand in hand, one in time the other in space. There is the embracing notion of form which in the abstract is that of an underlying essence, but when expressed is that of the concrete reality of the piece as performed, whether this be a painting, a play, a poem or a partita.

We can also talk in structural terms of melodic lines or themes, of dynamics and tempo, of articulation and expression, of timbre and tonal changes. In therapeutic terms we have the ideas of form expressed in terms of seemingly random behaviour, as loss of coherence in the forming of the piece; initiation and innovation, activity and passivity; the ability to orientate the form within the prescribed space or time; the relationship between the patient and the therapist in the dialogue between patient and therapist in terms of listening and acting, openness to new ideas.

CHAPTER EIGHT

Music Therapy
and Inflammatory Bowel Disease

Introduction

A basic strategy of the research approach has been to generate under-standings between clinical practitioners. In this way I have not been so concerned with abstract theorizing but with a specific purpose of promoting co-operation in clinical practice, as we saw in the last chapter; and with a way in which music therapists and doctors can interpret what they have in common. This chapter presents, for a clinical dialogue, two comparative views of inflammatory bowel disease that have arisen. One is from the general medical literature, the other is that of a music therapist who has played extensively with patients who have the disease. The music therapist was unaware of the medical descriptions of the disease when she made her descriptions of the musical improvised playing of such patients. This was deliberate in that we wanted to see what spontaneous matchings occurred without any adjustments being made by either practitioner, for under-standings to become compatible.

Inflammatory bowel disease is a term which refers to a collection of diseases affecting the bowel. These diseases are characterized by the presence of chronic inflammation of the gastro-intestinal tract which cannot be ascribed to any specific cause. The most common of these diseases are ulcerative colitis and Crohn's disease. Both diseases have a common, insidi-ous onset resulting in chronic symptoms which may include severe episodic diarrhoea, colicky abdominal pain, weight loss, nausea and vomiting, and pus, blood or mucus in the stool.

While there are common symptoms in inflammatory bowel disease, Crohn's disease is distinguished from others as it generally affects the terminal ileum and the right colon, sometimes the whole bowel (Calkins and Mendeloff 1986), but rarely the entire digestive tract, although it can affect any part of the alimentary canal (Strober and James 1986). Ulcerative colitis always affects the rectum, and sometimes the entire colon.

Although these are not generally highly fatal diseases, they are important for public health concerns in that their incidence is early in life, therapy often involves surgery, there is a risk of developing intestinal cancer in later life and there are enormous social costs involved in chronic illness (Sanderson 1986). These diseases cause great personal embarrassment and discomfort for the patient, often resulting in a restricted lifestyle and a miserable existence (Robertson et al. 1989). Any therapeutic endeavours then must attend to enhancing the quality of life of the patient.

Epidemiological factors

The aetiology and pathogenesis of both Crohn's disease and ulcerative colitis have not yet been clarified. Diagnosis of the specific disease is difficult. A significant time may elapse between the first onset of symptoms and a definite diagnosis. As the diseases share similar symptoms then diagnosis is problematic (Bruce 1986; Shivananda et al. 1987). The incidence of ulcerative colitis appears to be more frequent in modern Western society and is increasing (Calkins and Mendeloff 1986).

The primary age ranges for the incidence of the disease in both sexes are between the ages of 15 and 25 years, and between the ages of 55 and 60 (Calkins and Mendeloff 1986; Shivananda et al. 1987). Children under 6 years of age appear to be resistant to the development of Crohn's disease. Between the ages of six to ten years ulcerative colitis occurs with increasing frequency, but not Crohn's disease.

There is an increased frequency of inflammatory bowel disease in families of patients with the disease, with a mixture of both Crohn's disease and ulcerative colitis. This has suggested a genetic basis for the disease (Sanderson 1986; Strober and James 1986) that remains as yet undiscovered. Although there is no genetic basis for these diseases, they do appear to run in families.

Diet

Because of the nature of the disease, dietary intake has been considered as one of the most important environmental exposure factors of the digestive system. Among patients with Crohn's disease, one possible causative factor is increased sugar consumption. Dietary fibre, increased milk products, carbohydrate, protein and total calorie consumption have also been implicated (Persson and Hellers 1987).

These studies have proved to be problematic, because either dietary exposure may have occurred many years prior to the diagnosis, or the prolonged onset of the disease itself may lead to the alteration of dietary practice. For example, patients may increase their consumption of refined sugar in an attempt to compensate for loss of energy or weight as a consequence of the disease.

Liquid 'elemental' diets developed for the space programmes in the United States have been used for the treatment of Crohn's disease. Although the efficacy of such a diet is not known (Sanderson 1986) the effects are shown to be as effective as high dose steroids for the remission of small bowel Crohn's disease in children. Children treated in this way experience an acceleration of growth.

While the use of nutritional supplements may have a small role to play in helping extremely sick children to obtain some calories, this approach is seen as beneficial only in the short term (Clark 1986). Patient enthusiasm for the diet wanes in the long term because the diet is unpalatable. Bruce (1986) also comments that an elemental diet worsens the difficulties of young people with the disease by placing them in a regressed position which allows the mother to exercise absolute control, as she did when they were infants.

What is lacking in dietary studies is any perspective that it is not necessarily the content of the food which is important. The way in which it is eaten, the situation in which it is eaten, and the conditions in which it is digested are important. The preparation of food, the way it is eaten and the way that waste products are disposed of are also closely patterned by culture. The offer of food, and acceptance of that food, are also of great symbolic value (Helman 1985; Kleinman 1978).

Immunological factors

As it has been difficult to establish an infectious cause for inflammatory bowel disease some researchers have sought an immunological basis (Kett, Rognum and Brandzaeg 1987; Strober and James 1986; Trabucchi *et al.* 1986; Van Spreuuwel, Lindeman and Meijer 1986). Crohn's disease begins as the product of an underlying inflammatory process. The presence of increased numbers of macrophages and mast cells appears to be an important feature of the disease. While the specific physiological function of mast cells remains unknown, they are known to contain inflammatory mediators such as histamine and may play a role in allergic reactions. Although a pathogen has not been found, somehow the patient becomes sensitive to the constituents of his or her own gut flora, which has widespread negative effects on the entire immune system. The patient reacts negatively to their own body, a rejection of a part of their very own 'self'.

Modern researchers have taken the old idea that emotions influence the health status of the person and developed the sciences of psychoneuroimmunology (the study of the effects of psychological factors on the immune system) (Baker 1987; Blalock and Smith 1985), and of neuroimmodulation (the study of the mechanisms whereby the nervous system modulates the activity of the immune system) (Baker 1987; Stein, Keller and Schleifer 1985; Trabucchi *et al.* 1986). Emotions influence health status as disturbances to the immune system by specific interactions between the nervous system, immune and endocrine systems. This subtle combination of physiological mechanisms is designed to recognize and deal with 'non-self' or altered material. What is 'self' and 'non-self' are crucial decisions isomorphic with the physiology and psychology of the person and the family with whom they dwell.

Chronic stress has also been shown to alter the immune system (Baker 1987; Patterson 1988; Stein, Keller and Schleifer 1985) and thereby recovery. Immunological descriptions of inflammatory bowel disease also suggest a similar process, a transient infection provoking an immune response which is exacerbated by psychological factors. Strikingly, patients with bowel disease often attribute the onset of their disease to a stressful event (Robertson *et al.* 1989). This is literally a 'gut' reaction to a significant life event.

Psychological factors

There has been a long history of associating somatic symptoms and emotional disturbance. If inflammatory bowel disease is, as some authors believe, a motility disorder of the gut, then that motility is sensitive to the emotional state of the person. Highly anxious patients may produce symptoms at times of emotional distress (Lask 1986).

Although psychiatric illness and psychopathology are no more prevalent in patients with inflammatory bowel disease (Clouse 1986), there does appear to be some evidence of depression in patients with Crohn's disease (Tarter *et al.* 1987) but this appears to occur only in patients with persistent disease activity (Robertson *et al.* 1989). High levels of neuroticism (a score of more than 12 on the Eyesenck Personality Inventory) are associated with these patients, and patients become more introverted as the disease progresses (Robertson *et al.* 1989).

The search for causative psychological factors has been in vain, principally because of the insidious onset of the disease. While most authors accept that psychological difficulties are sequelae of the disease and that stress and emotional difficulties exacerbate the disease, no factors appear to be causative.

Traditionally ulcerative colitis has been regarded as a psychosomatic illness. Psychoanalysis has taken the view that such illness has its origins in the mental mechanisms used to cope with the emotions. From this perspective the disease represents a reaction to a real or threatened loss of the mother, or someone else that the patient is dependent upon. Patients with ulcerative colitis are seen as rigid, controlling and dependent. Recent psychoanalytic approaches have observed that patients with inflammatory bowel disease have a tendency to somatize their problems, and that such patients have difficulty in expressing emotions and feelings with words (Bruce 1986; Stanwyck and Arnson 1986). This state is termed 'alexithymia'. To spare themselves emotional pain these patients project those problems into bodily functioning; hence the situation in which some patients with bowel disease appear to be coping well with difficult life situations.

In children there appears to be a clearer link between abdominal pain and emotional upset (Bruce 1986). Abdominal pains are common in children and the gut appears to 'mirror' the emotions better than any other body system. Furthermore, those clinicians working with children with bowel disease remark that abdominal pain appears to be a common occurrence in the repertoire of distress management in the families of those children (Bruce 1986; Lask 1986). There appears to be a vicious circle where the physical symptoms of the disease lead to stress and behavioural problems. These problems then provoke physical symptoms and aggravate pre-existing organic pathology. The child and the family are affected. If the family cannot cope, and there is a family repertoire of distress management by an escalation of physical symptoms then the symptoms of the child are further exacerbated.

Lifestyle Factors and the Patient's View

In the literature patients with inflammatory bowel disease have been described in a negative and limited way. They are seen as dependent, restricted in their relationships, sexually and emotionally inadequate, depressed, isolated, demanding, angry and lacking in self-confidence (Joachim 1987). A lack of self-confidence is hardly surprising given that there is such a negative perception of the patient by practitioners, combined with the difficulties of the disease itself. A number of authors have attempted to present the patient's view of the problem. As both a nurse and a sufferer, Neufeldt (1987) says that the most difficult part of the disease is its unpredictability, and that the symptoms themselves frequently cause depression. The bouts of nausea, vomiting and diarrhoea lead to loss of sleep, listlessness and nutritional deficiencies. The combination of embarrassing symptoms, and the randomness of onset of those symptoms, are socially disruptive for the working life and home life of the patient.

Joachim and Milne (Joachim 1987) investigated the impact of inflammatory bowel disease on the lifestyle of patients. Patients said that overall their disease greatly influenced their satisfaction with life in a negative way. Yet, paradoxically, those patients reported a minimal influence on a day-to-day basis. This appears to represent the observation frequently made by clinicians that these patients appear unwilling to complain about specific problems, or they deny that problems exist in the face of evident personal and relational turmoil.

In an attempt to understand the relationships between biological, psychological and social phenomena, Helman (1985) examined the self-perceptions and explanatory models of patients with ulcerative colitis. He found that most patients had a multi-causal holistic model of their disorder. Tension, anger, frustration, stress and uncertainty were seen as attacking the body and were separate from the 'self'. Similarly, where their own personalities were seen as contributory to the chronicity of their condition, that 'personality' was seen as separate from the self. These causal attributes, he argues, are learned from various medical encounters and are part of the culture. This notion of 'non-self' was also applied to organs of the body. Weakness in an organ could be hereditary, constitutional or acquired. Somehow the weak organ was separate from the self, but responsive to interactions with other people. The disease or organ then becomes a public interface between the 'self' and the environment, and is responsive to 'outside' forces separate from the 'inside' self.

In Helman's view the image a person has of the disease is a natural symbol whereby the physiological process of the disease is understood:

> the symbol organizes both social and emotional experiences, and helps define certain emotions, thoughts, personality traits, and parts of the body as either 'self' or 'non-self'. Defining some of these as 'non-self' can bring the patient's self image closer to the normative order of contemporary life – to social values of independence, fitness, youthfulness, contentment and social success and control the bodily functions and emotions. (1985, p.15)

Not only does this image that the person has affect their physiological state, it may also affect the way that they perceive and are perceived by members of their family (Aldridge 1990, 1992).

Family perspective

A family systems perspective of bowel disease emphasizes that the functions of the gut, the patient, the family and the treatment system evolve together (Bloch 1987; Stierlin 1989). In this view the process of chronic illness begins by a 'random disequilibrating event'. This could be a transient infection or a stressful life event. Pain ensues. This event occurs in the context of a relationship. The patient has a family, and the event is given meaning by the patient and the family. We know that in the case of some viruses they do not kill the host cell but transform it such that it has an altered function, particularly in terms of immunocompetence (Bloch 1987).

A similar situation occurs in the family context where a disease event is handled in a particular way (Aldridge 1990). Experiences surrounding gut pain are organized around a set of beliefs about what the cause of the pain is, what it means, and how it is to be handled, that is, a repertoire of distress management. Not only do the patient and the family of the patient share the similar meanings about an illness, and what counts as disease, they also share a similar immune context. In this way a random event such as an infection may find that its host is not only the patient *but the immunocompetence and beliefs of the family milieu.*

Approaches to treatment

It would appear that inflammatory bowel disease is best approached from a holistic perspective which integrates different understandings. While surgical interventions will still be necessary it is important to remember that the sequelae of surgery are not only physical. Surgery can be traumatic, leaving the patient with a sense of anger and resentment, feeling both anxious and depressed, and having to adapt to a new lifestyle. These psychological and social consequences may best be handled by a team approach which includes people who comprehend the day-to-day living situation of the patient within their relational setting.

Lask (1986) and Bruce (1986), in their work with children, approach their treatment from such a family systems perspective and recommend the use of a physician, surgeon, psychologist, social worker, nurse and stoma therapist. Stress management techniques can be used to reduce anxiety and communication skills, while psychotherapeutic activities can be used to control excessive worry (Freyberger *et al.* 1985; Milne, Joachim and Niehardt 1986; Svedlund *et al.* 1983).

A feature common to many reports about the treatment of inflammatory bowel disease is that the disease is intractable to therapeutic endeavours. Furthermore, the patients themselves are described quite negatively, which may be in part because of their inability to communicate in verbal terms about their emotional distress. What is often ignored is that the communication medium for these patients is essentially non-verbal. Symptoms are the form of communication which symbolizes the distress of these patients. For practitioners dependent primarily on forms of communication which are predominantly verbal, there is a disparity between modes of communication. Music therapy, which requires no verbalization but demands expressivity, would appear to be a viable medium.

Implications for Music Therapy

There are no psychological factors which are necessary or sufficient to cause intestinal disease in susceptible individuals. However, it is also clear that there are certain psychological or social factors which can either influence the course of the disease, or provide a context for the disease to develop. The presence of beliefs about 'self' and 'non-self' appear to be fundamental in these patients linking immunocompetence, individual psychology and familial status.

While psychological factors may not be causal, they are important for recovery. Our therapeutic endeavours may be better directed to actively stimulating the immunocompetence of the patient. If the mind does influence the immune system then we have a battery of therapeutic interventions. As the main mode of communication about distress for these patients is non-verbal, then non-verbal therapies would appear to be an essential part of a co-ordinated therapeutic approach.

Music therapy which stimulates positive emotions, enhances coping responses and is isomorphic with the form of physiological systems would appear to be an ideal therapeutic medium. The motility of the gut is rhythmic and it would seem reasonable that music therapy could restore, or promote, rhythmic flexibility. Similarly the processes of the immune system too are rhythmic in their ultradian cycle. Music may provide the substrate for entraining various physiological sub-systems. As I have suggested earlier, essentially music can 'tune' the communicational context which unites the central and peripheral nervous systems and the immune system.

It has been shown that positive experiences such as laughter, when incorporated into a coping style, have a beneficial influence on the immune system (Dillon 1985). If this is true of laughter then we might expect that the greater range of positive experiences available in creatively playing music, if incorporated as a coping style, will have a healing effect via the immune system. Note that the word 'incorporated' literally means taken into the body. It may also be necessary for clinicians from other disciplines to communicate with their patients non-verbally if symptomatology is the currency of communication (Aldridge 1989a, 1991a, 191d).

Finally we must attend to the symbolic aspects of the disease for these patients such that they are no longer separated from the self which feeds them. In this sense the playing of improvised music gives the disease itself an objective appearance as a played reality. The patient is then offered a chance to change in the concrete sensual realm of their own existence.

Musical Playing by Patients with Bowel Disease

As we saw in the previous chapter, my task has been to build bridges between the work of medical practitioners and creative arts therapists (Aldridge 1989a, 1991d). One way to promote a dialogue between practitioners is to compare differing realms of description. First, I will put forward some observations made about musical playing by patients with bowel disease. In the following sections I will compare the features of improvised musical playing with the features that we find in the medical literature.

Ulcerative colitis

A prominent feature of the way in which these patients play music is that they appear to have no personal connection with what they are playing. They appear to play with a 'distance' from what they are playing. This distance is evident in their posture. When they are strong enough to stand their posture is often such that both feet are not firmly on the ground; for example, their legs are crossed. The drum sticks are held loosely in the hands with the inner wrist uppermost, and they play from the wrists without involving the whole body. This seemingly uncommitted posture makes it difficult to play a clear beat on the drum. Any drum beats are loose. Beaters are allowed to fall and rebound rather than being used in a directed intended beating movement. The drum is also played with alternate hands (right, left, right, left) and there seem to be difficulties for these patients in co-ordinated playing using both hands together.

This unco-ordination is reflected in their rhythmical playing, which has a limited range and often occurs as typical rhythmical patterns. Often the playing is on the upbeat before the bar starts and begins with a small drum roll, giving the music a military air. The playing itself goes on and on without any rhythmical phrasing. This lack of flexibility in the rhythmical playing is reflected in the tempo of the musical playing, where there are constant attempts to return to a fast tempo.

Generally there is an intolerance for strong harmonies in the playing, and contact becomes lost particularly when diminished minor, fifth or augmented chords are played. The therapist believes that this is indicative of an emotional distance in the music; and with an increase in musical tension, for example, patients stop playing before a musical climax is achieved.

However, in the construction of melodies these patients are flexible and full of imagination. Even these melodies have a mechanical quality, as if the playing was an intellectual exercise and never really gripped the patient internally. While able to construct and copy melodies there is an inability to sustain a melody. There is, as in the rhythmical playing, the impression that the same music could go on and on repetitively without any direction to it and without the patient taking any initiatives.

Crohn's disease

These patients appear to be very stiff in their upper body movements. They too have difficulties in co-ordinating their hands and mostly alternate between left and right handed playing on the drum. Because of these co-ordination difficulties their playing often sounds like a gallop. Similarly the rhythmical structure is disordered and gives the impression of going on and on without end. Like the previous patients there seems to be no means of initiating an end to this repetitive music, and consequently they appear to avoid coming into contact with the music. This is also reflected in their inability to respond to tempo changes, giving the musical playing a quality of immovability.

When using specific harmonies, notably the sixth and diminished chords, their response is one of vulnerability. Sometimes they cry; sometimes they stop playing altogether, walking away from the instruments; or they continue to play indifferently and mechanically with even less contact to the music.

Melodic playing on the xylophone or glockenspiel is quick rhythmically, unsustained, and appears to have no internal logic. The intervals between tones are chaotic, that is, wide then narrow. This melodic playing, like that of the colitis patients, is generally quiet. There is an overall feeling of emotional distance in their playing while they give the impression that they are totally at the mercy of the situation.

Overall both groups of patients have a similar lack of dynamic to their playing which is limited and rigid; a feature which is reflected in the activity of their gut. These patients are also described as 'not being gripped internally' by the expressive form. Such a description reflects an apparent emotional distance without, seemingly, any bodily commitment. Either these patients lack the ability to integrate their feelings with their bodies, or a body that has become so painful is eventually dissociated from any feelings.

Generally these patients require many sessions before any improvement is apparent. The co-ordination problems disappear and there is more stability and control of the hands. The rhythmical playing becomes more definitive and there is an apparent form to the phrasing and tempo. Overall there is less rigidity in the playing and the patient appears to sense the bigger musical form in which they are playing. However, what remains is the impression that the patient never really comes to grips with the music and that they still play with an empty passivity, as if they were not tuned to their own bodies. Finally the musical give-and-take in the therapeutic relationship is difficult for these patients and they appear isolated from their musical partner, the therapist.

Linking understandings between clinicians

There are correlations between findings in the literature which describe patients with inflammatory bowel disease and their musical playing (see Table 8.1).

While the patients themselves say that they have fun playing there remains an underlying intractable emotional distance within the playing and within the therapeutic relationship. Any therapeutic endeavours with these patients must then take into account the personal and relational difficulties of these patients, which would suggest that an early therapeutic contact be made in the process of treatment. If the basis for the patient presenting himself is that of somatic problems, then music therapy would appear to be an approach isomorphic to this presentation and make therapeutic sense. As patients are renowned for having difficulty in expressing themselves verbally, music is an important means of expression, as it is not lexically dependent, and would seem to offer a valuable tool. Music therapy is firmly based upon rhythmic playing, and we know from a variety of sources (see Chapters Three and Four) that music therapy also promotes relaxation, so there are further arguments to sustain such an adjuvant treatment approach. However, it may be that music therapy only clarifies diagnoses reached from other clinical perspectives. As a treatment form it remains questionable unless combined with some form of therapy that will combine relations between emotional expressivity and bodily awareness. Perhaps music therapy is a preparatory stage for psychotherapy.

Table 8.1 A comparison of two sets
of descriptions of bowel disease

Descriptive elements from the medical literature	Elements of the musical playing
separation of self and 'non self'	not tuned to themselves, unco-ordinated
lack of gut motility	lack of rhythmic flexibility, unresponsive to tempo changes and lack of rhythmical phrasing
increasingly introverted	quiet playing with no personal contact within the playing
restricted in their relationships	difficult to contact in the musical relationship
difficultly expressing feelings	intolerant of particular harmonies
appear to be coping well with life in the face of internal turmoil	appear to be going along with the music but an underlying chaotic structure
dependent	no initiatives within the music and dependent upon the therapist
intractable to change	difficult to treat, requiring many sessions

In research terms we have found a way to reconcile two clinical languages (see Table 8.1). The language of clinical medicine is linked to the language of music therapy practice such that practitioners can talk about their mutual construings. The idea that this mutuality is not an isolated case will be pursued in the next chapter. As a form of analysis we can use the rules of constitution mentioned in the last chapter as a means of analysing clinical texts. We see in Figure 7.4 that various postural activities like playing with crossed legs, playing with the wrists uppermost and musical events like repetitive playing are interpreted as to their meaning for clinical practice. Using such a method we have an idea of how a music therapist builds her clinical reasoning based upon specific events in the course of the therapy.

Note that I am not proposing that such rules exist like rules written in a rule book. Just as such lexical construings are one step removed from the actual activity of the musical playing, then these proposed 'rules' as structured meanings are also only crude representations of what really happens. However, they are a form of structuring clinical knowledge and can be used with the clinician to discover if such a formulation approximates to her understanding. Furthermore, these rules are specific to the therapist and to the patients she has worked with. They are not meant to be generalized rules. For our research purposes we could develop a sense of clinical under-standings that we could further discuss and share in clinical practice with various practitioners: such as the relationship of fixed rhythmical playing and its implications for therapeutic practice in the musical playing; its relationship to gut function and peristaltic rhythm, from a medical perspective; and flexibility in structuring the day and contact with other practitio-ners, from a social psychological perspective.

CHAPTER NINE

Music Therapy with the Elderly

We have seen in the previous two chapters that it is possible to build a bridge between music therapy understandings and art therapy understandings, between music therapy and medicine. Furthermore, I have proposed a way in which we can analyse how music therapists construct their clinical understandings regarding the way that patients play. This chapter continues in the same vein, addressing the pressing problem facing modern Western society of dementia in the elderly. First, the scene is set in terms of the problem of dementia within the broader health care community. Then, a music therapy understanding is presented that compares the problem as it is seen in individual therapy. We will read that music therapy has something significant to offer in terms of treatment in what is often regarded as a hopeless problem. Indeed, as we will see in the next chapter, which deals with music therapy with HIV and AIDS patients, the diagnosis of the disease and the reactions of both patients and practitioners to such a diagnosis often compound the negative aspects of the disease itself. A form of therapy that introduces some element of hope, when grounded in a reality that all parties can agree upon, is an important step forward in treating such chronic problems.

Dementia is an important source of chronic disability, leading to both spiralling health care expenditure among the elderly and a progressive disturbance of quality of life for the patient and his family. In the United States of America the cost of institutional care for patients with dementia is estimated at over $25 billion a year (Steg 1990). If 4 per cent to 5 per cent of the North American elderly population suffer from dementia, then 1.25 per cent of the total population are suffering with the problems of severe dementia. Other estimates of the same population suggest that 15 per cent of those over the age of 65 will have moderate to severe dementia with projections to 45 per cent by the age of 90 years (Odenheimer 1989). Current estimates are that over 60 per cent of those cases of dementia result from Alzheimer's disease (Kalayam and Shamoian 1990). With anticipated increases in the population of the elderly in Europe,[1] it is timely to find treatment initiatives in the Western world which will ameliorate the impact of this problem.

Dementing illnesses, or acquired cognitive disorders, have been recognized for centuries, but little progress was made in specific diagnoses until the evolution of the nosological approach to disease and early clinical descriptions of neurosyphilis and Huntington's chorea in the 1800s. Such descriptions were further supported by concurrent understandings that suggested the influence of the brain on behaviour. The first histopathological characterizations of cognitive disorders were enabled by developments in the optical microscope. Thus, Alzheimer (1907) was able to see the neuronal degeneration and senile plaques in the brain of a 55-year-old woman with progressive memory impairment, and identify the disease which today bears his name.

While cognitive impairment is evident from behaviour, and neurohistopathy can recognize neuronal degeneration, the diagnosis of Alzheimer's disease is prone to error[2] and authors differ as to the difficulty of making a precise diagnosis (Odenheimer 1989; Steg 1990). In the early stages of the disease the symptoms are difficult to distinguish from those of normal aging, a process which itself is poorly understood. To date there exist no normative established values of what cognitive impairment or memory loss are, or what neurochemical and neurophysiological changes accompany normal aging. It is therefore extremely difficult to establish criteria for determining abnormal changes from a normal population, and the researcher/clinician must in part rely upon within-the-subject designs to indicate progressive deterioration.

A second source of error in diagnosing Alzheimer's disease is that it is masked by other conditions (see Table 9.1). Principal among these conditions is that of depression, which itself can cause cognitive and behavioural disorders. It is estimated that 20 per cent to 30 per cent of patients with Alzheimer's disease will have an accompanying depression (Kalayam and Shamoian 1990), thereby compounding diagnostic problems further.

---

1   Between 23 per cent and 25 per cent of the national populations aged over 65 by the year 2040 (Aldridge 1990).
2   Estimated in a range from 10 per cent to 30 per cent error in the general medical population (Steg 1990).

Table 9.1 Differential diagnosis of Alzheimer's disease

Differential diagnosis of Alzheimer's disease

Multi infarct dementia and other forms of cerebrovascular disease

Parkinson's disease

Progressive supranuclear palsy

Huntington's disease

Central nervous system infection

Sudbural haematoma

Normal pressure hydrocephalus

Multiple sclerosis

Seizure disorder

Brain tumour

Cerebral trauma

Metabolic disturbance

Nutritional deficiency

Psychiatric disorder

Substance abuse or overmedication

Clinical Descriptions of Dementia

The clinical syndrome of dementia is characterized by an acquired decline of cognitive function which is represented by memory and language impairment. While the term dementia itself is used widely to describe cognitive impairment it is specifically applied in medical literature to two conditions: dementia of the Alzheimer's type (DAT) and multi-infarct dementia.

The course of Alzheimer's disease is one of progressive deterioration associated with degenerative changes in the brain. Such deterioration is presented in a clinical picture of episodic changes and a pattern of particular cognitive failings which are variable (Drachman *et al.* 1990). Mental status testing is one of the primary forms of assessing these cognitive failings, which include short- and long-term memory changes, impairment of abstract thinking and judgement; disorders of language (aphasia), and difficulty in finding the names of words (anomia); the loss of ability to interpret what is heard, said and felt (agnosia); and an inability to carry out motor activities, such as manipulating a pen or toothbrush, despite intact motor function (apraxia). When such clinical findings are present then a probable diagnosis can be made; a more definite diagnosis depends upon tissue diagnosis (see Table 9.2).

Table 9.2 Diagnostic evaluation of dementia

Diagnostic categories

Complete medical history

Mental status examination

Complete physical and neurological investigation (including investigation for infection of central nervous system if suspected)

Complete blood count and blood chemistry tests (including vitamin B12 levels)

Thyroid function tests

Serology for syphilis

Computerized tomography (CT) or magnetic resonance imaging (MRI), electroencephalography (EEG), or positive emission tomography (PET) scanning

While dementia of the Alzheimer's type begins after the age of 40, and is considered to be a disease of the elderly, the influence of age on prognosis is not as significant as the initial degree of severity of the problem when recognized (Drachman *et al.* 1990). Disease severity, as assessed by intellectual function, appears to be the most consistent predictor of the subsequent course of the disease, particularly when accompanied by a combination of wandering and falling, and behavioural problems (Walsh, Welch and Larson 1990). However, the rates of decline between sub groups of patients are variable and a patient's rate of progression in one year may bear little relationship to the future rate of decline (Salmon *et al.* 1990). Some authors (Cooper, Mungas and Weiler 1990) suggest that an as yet unproven factor, other than declining cognitive ability, may also play a part in the associated abnormal behaviours of anger, agitation, personality change, wandering, insomnia and depression which occur in later stages of the disease.

Clearly Alzheimer's disease causes distress for the patient. The loss of memory and the accompanying loss of language, before the onset of motor impairment, mean that the daily lives of patients are disturbed. Communication, the fabric of social contact, is interrupted and disordered. The threat of progressive deterioration and behavioural disturbance has ramifications not only for the patient themselves, but also their families, who must take some of the social responsibility for care of the patient, and the emotional burden of seeing a loved one becoming confused and isolated.

Assessment of dementia

A brief cognitive test, the Mini-Mental State Examination (Folstein, Folstein and McHugh 1975), has been developed to screen and monitor the progression of Alzheimer's disease. The test itself is intended for the clinician to assess functions of different areas of the brain, and is based upon questions and activities (see Table 9.3). As a clinical instrument it is widely used and well validated in practice (Babikian *et al.* 1990; Beatty and Goodkin 1990; Eustache *et al.* 1990; Faustman, Moses and Csernansky 1990; Gagnon *et al.* 1990; Jairath and Campbell 1990; Summers *et al.* 1990; Zillmer *et al.* 1990). As a bedside test the MMSE is widely used for testing cognition and is useful as a predictive tool for cognitive impairment and semantic memory (Eustache *et al.* 1990) without being contaminated by motor and sensory deficits (Beatty and Goodkin 1990; Jairath and Campbell 1990).

Table 9.3 Mini-Mental State Examination

Item	*Component*	*Score*
Orientation for time	year, season, month, date and day	5
Orientation for place	state, county, city, building and floor	5
Registration	Subject repeats 'rose', 'ball' and 'key'	3
Attention for calculation	Serial subtraction of 7 from 100 or spell 'world' backward	5
Recall	'Rose', 'ball' and 'key'	3
Naming	Pencil and watch	2
Repetition	No ifs, ands, or buts	1
Three-stage verbal command	Take a piece of paper in your right hand, fold it in half, and put in on the floor	3
Written command	Close your eyes	1
Writing	A spontaneous sentence	1
Construction	Two interlocking pentagons	1
Total		30

Source: after Folstein, Folstein and McHugh (1975).

Elderly patients scoring below 24 points out of a possible total score of 30 are considered as demented. However, this scoring has been questioned on the grounds of its cut-off point of 24 as the lower limit, particularly for early dementia (Galasko *et al.* 1990); and that it is influenced by education (Gagnon *et al.* 1990). Poorly educated subjects with less than eight years of education may score below 24 without being demented.

Further criticisms of the Mini-Mental State Examination (MMSE) have been that it is not sensitive enough to mild deficits, but it could be augmented by the addition of a word fluency task and an improvement in the attention–concentration item (Galasko *et al.* 1990). In addition, the MMSE seriously underestimates cognitive impairment in psychiatric patients (Faustman, Moses and Csernansky 1990). An important feature neglected by the MMSE is that of 'intention' or executive control (Odenheimer 1989), which refers to the ability of the patient to persevere with a set task, to reach a set goal or to change tasks.

The items which the MMSE fails to discriminate (minor language deficits), or neglects to assess (fluency and intentionality), however, may be elicited in the playing of improvised music. A dynamic musical assessment of patient behaviour, linked with the motor co-ordination and intent required for the playing of musical instruments used in music therapy, and the necessary element of interpersonal communication, may provide a sensitive complementary tool for assessment.

We see in Table 9.4 how medical elements of assessment can find their correlates in musical parameters. As we have seen in the chapter related to bowel disease, both languages share similar terms, and it is possible to build a conceptual bridge between two forms of practice. By doing this neither practice is reduced to the other, but we do have a valuable conceptual tool for proposing commonalities in the practice. We can take all the elements demanded in a medical assessment and translate those into terms that are applicable for music therapy. Conversely, we can translate what happens in music therapy and demonstrate its applicability to medical practice. What is important to take from the music therapy assessment is that the idea of intention (which is behavioural as much as it is cognitive) can be demon-strated in an activity that offers a situation in which intentionality can be achieved. The problem with assessment tests is that they are so often reduced that they become unnatural and totally divorced from the context of the person's life. How we behave in laboratories and consulting rooms is often somewhat different from our behaviour in our own homes and with friends. Music therapy, too, is no natural context; but embedding an assessment of intentionality within the context of musical playing is less clumsy, and more flexible, than a specific test.

Table 9.4 Features of medical and musical assessment

Medical elements of assessment	Musical elements of assessment
continuing observation of mental and functional status	continuing observation of mental and functional status
testing of verbal skills, including element of speech fluency	testing of musical skills; rhythm, melody, harmony, dynamic, phrasing, articulation
cortical disorder testing; visuo-spatial skills and ability to perform complex motor tasks (including grip and right–left co-ordination)	cortical disorder testing; visuo spatial skills and ability to perform complex motor tasks (including grip and right–left co-ordination)
testing for progressive memory disintegration	testing for progressive memory disintegration
motivation to complete tests, to achieve set goals and persevere in set tasks	motivation to sustain playing improvised music, to achieve musical goals and persevere in maintaining form
'intention' difficult to assess; but considered important	'intention' a feature of improvised musical playing
concentration and attention span	concentration on the improvised playing and attention to the instruments
flexibility in task switching	flexibility in musical (including instrumental) changes
mini-mental state score influenced by educational status	ability to play improvised music influenced by previous musical training
insensitive to small changes	sensitive to small changes
ability to interpret surroundings	ability to interpret musical context and assessment of communication in the therapeutic relationship

Music and Dementia

Late in adult life, at the age of 56, and after completing two major concertos for the piano, Maurice Ravel, the composer, began to complain of increased fatigue and lassitude. Following a traffic accident his condition deteriorated progressively (Henson 1988). He lost the ability to remember names, to speak spontaneously and to write (Dalessio 1984). Although he could understand speech he was no longer capable of the co-ordination required to lead a major orchestra. While his mind, he reports, was full of musical ideas, he could not set them down (Dalessio 1984). Eventually his intellectual functions and speech deteriorated until he could no longer recognize his own music.

However, the responsiveness of patients with Alzheimer's disease to music is a remarkable phenomenon (Swartz *et al.* 1989). While language deterioration is a feature of cognitive deficit, musical abilities appear to be preserved. This may be because the fundamentals of language, as we have seen in previous chapters, are musical, and prior to semantic and lexical functions in language development.

Although language processing may be dominant in one hemisphere of the brain, music production involves an understanding of the interaction of both cerebral hemispheres (Altenmüller 1986; Brust 1980; Gates and Bradshaw 1977). In attempting to understand the perception of music there have been a number of investigations into the hemispheric strategies involved. Much of the literature considering musical perception concentrates on the significance of hemispheric dominance. Gates and Bradshaw (1977) conclude that cerebral hemispheres are concerned with music perception and that no laterality differences are apparent. Other authors (Wagner and Hannon 1981) suggest that two processing functions develop with training where left and right hemispheres are simultaneously involved, and that musical stimuli are capable of eliciting both right and left ear superiority (Kellar and Bever 1980). Similarly, when people listen to and perform music they utilize differing hemispheric processing strategies.

Evidence of the global strategy of music processing in the brain is found in the clinical literature. Morgan and Tilluckdharry (1982) tell how singing was considered to be a welcome release from the helplessness of being a patient, allowing thoughts to be communicated externally. Although the 'newer aspect' of speech was lost, the older function of music was retained. Berman (1981) suggests that recovery from aphasia is not a matter of new learning by the non-dominant hemisphere but a taking over of responsibility for language by that hemisphere. The non-dominant hemisphere may be a reserve of functions in case of regional failure. If singing gives a glimpse of this brain plasticity, then music therapy has a potential for working with dementia patients.

Little is known about the loss of musical and language abilities in cases of global cortical damage, although the quality of response to music in the final stages of dementia is worth noting (Norberg, Melin and Asplund 1986). Any discussion is necessarily limited to hypothesizing, as there are no established baselines for musical performance in the adult population (Swartz *et al.* 1989). Aphasia, which is a feature of cognitive deterioration, is a complicated phenomenon. While syntactical functions may remain longer, it is the lexical and semantic functions of naming and reference which begin to fail in the early stages. Phrasing and grammatical structures remain, giving an impression of normal speech, yet content becomes increasingly incoherent. These progressive failings appear to be located within the context of semantic and episodic memory loss illustrated by the inability to remember a simple story when tested (Bayles *et al.* 1989).

Musicality and singing

Musicality and singing are rarely tested as features of cognitive deterioration, yet preservation of these abilities in aphasics has been linked to eventual recovery (Jacome 1984; Morgan and Tilluckdharry 1982), and could be significant indicators of hierarchical changes in cognitive functioning. Jacome (1984) found that a musically naive patient with transcortical mixed aphasia exhibited repetitive, spontaneous whistling, and whistling in response to questions. The patient often spontaneously sang without error in pitch, melody, rhythm and lyrics, and spent long periods of time listening to music. Beatty (Beatty *et al.* 1988) describes a woman who had severe impairments in terms of aphasia, memory dysfunction and apraxia, yet was able to sight read an unfamiliar song and perform on the xylophone which to her was an unconventional instrument. Like Ravel (Dalessio 1984), and an elderly musician who could play from memory (Crystal, Grober and Masur 1989) but no longer recalled the name of the composer, she no longer recalled the name of the music she was playing.

Swartz and his colleagues (Swartz *et al.* 1989, p.154) propose a series of perceptual levels at which musical disorders take place:

(1) the acoustico-psychological level, which includes changes in intensity, pitch and timbre

(2) the discriminatory level, which includes the discrimination of intervals and chords

(3) the categorical level which includes the categorical identification of rhythmic patterns and intervals

(4) the configural level, which includes melody perception, the recognition of motifs and themes, tonal changes, identification of instruments, and rhythmic discrimination; and

(5) the level where musical form is recognized, including complex perceptual and executive functions of harmonic, melodic and rhythmical transformations.

In Alzheimer's patients it would be expected that while levels (1), (2) and (3) remain unaffected, the complexities of levels (4) and (5), when requiring no naming, may be preserved but are susceptible to deterioration.

It is perhaps important to point out that these disorders are not themselves musical; they are disorders of audition. Only when disorders of musical production take place can we begin to suggest that a musical disorder is present. Improvised musical playing is in a unique position to demonstrate this hypothetical link between perception and production.

Rhythm is the key to the integrative process, underlying both musical perception and physiological coherence. Barfield's (1978) approach suggests that when musical form as tonal shape meets the rhythm of breathing there is the musical experience. External auditory activity is mediated by internal perceptual shaping in the context of a personal rhythm. When considering communication, rhythm is also fundamental to the organization and co-ordination of internal processes, and externally between persons (Aldridge 1989, 1989a, 1991d).

Music Therapy and the Elderly
Much of the published work concerning music therapy with the elderly is concerned with group activity (Bryant 1991; Christie 1992; Olderog Millard and Smith 1989) and is generally used to expand socialization and communication skills, with the intention of reducing problems of social isolation and withdrawal, to encourage participants to interact purposefully with others, assist in expressing and communicating feelings and ideas, and to stimulate cognitive processes, thereby sharpening problem-solving skills. Additional goals also focus on sensory and muscular stimulation and gross and fine motor skill preservation (Segal 1990).

Clair (1990, 1991; Clair and Bernstein 1990, 1990a) has worked extensively with the elderly and found music therapy a valuable tool for working in groups to promote communicating, watching others, singing, interacting with an instrument, and sitting. Her main conclusions are that although the group members deteriorated markedly in cognitive, physical, and social capacities over an observation period of 15 months, they continued to participate in music activities. During the 30-minute sessions the group members consistently sat in chairs without physical restraints for the duration of each session, and interacted with others regardless of their deterioration. This was the only time in the week when they interacted with others (Clair and Bernstein 1990a). Indeed, for one 66-year-old man was it is the sensory stimulation of music therapy that brought him out of his isolation such that he could participate with others, even if for a short while (Clair 1991).

Wandering, confusion and agitation are linked problems common to elderly patients living in hostels or special accommodation for Alzheimer's patients. A music therapist (Fitzgerald Cloutier 1993) has tested singing with an 81-year-old woman to see if it helped her to remain seated. After 20 singing sessions, the therapist read to the woman to compare the degree of attentiveness. While music therapy and reading sessions redirected the woman from wandering, the total time she sat for the music therapy sessions was double that of the reading sessions (214.3 mins vs 99.1 mins), and the time spent seated in the music therapy was more consistent than the episodes when she was being read to. When agitation occurs in such elderly women, then individualized music therapy appears to have a significantly calming effect (Gerdner and Swanson 1993). In terms of reducing repetitive behaviour, musical activity also reduces disruptive vocalizations (Casby and Holm 1994).

The above conclusions are supported by Groene (1993). Thirty residents (aged 60–91 years) of a special Alzheimer's unit, who exhibited wandering behaviour, were randomly assigned either to mostly music attention or to mostly reading attention groups, where they received one-to one attention. Those receiving music therapy remained seated longer than those in the reading sessions.

One of the central problems of the elderly is the loss of independence and self-esteem, and Palmer (1983, 1989) describes a programme of music therapy at a geriatric home designed to rebuild self-concept. For the 380 residents, ranging from those who were totally functional to those who needed total care, a programme was adapted to the capacities and needs of individual patients. Marching and dancing increased the ability of some patients to walk well; and for the non-ambulatory, kicking and stamping to music improved circulation and increased tolerance and strength. Sing-along sessions were used to encourage memory recall and promoted social interaction and appropriate social behaviour. (Palmer 1983, 1989). It was such social behaviour that Pollack (Pollack and Namazi 1992) reports as being accessible to improvement through group music therapy activities. It is the participative element that appears to be valuable for communication, and the intention to participate that is at the core of the music therapy activity, which we will see in the following section.

Music therapy has also been used to focus on memory recall for songs and the spoken word (Prickett and Moore 1991). In ten elderly patients, whose diagnosis was probably Alzheimer's disease, words to songs were recalled dramatically better than spoken words or spoken information. Although long-familiar songs were recalled with greater accuracy than a newly presented song, most patients attempted to sing, hum, or keep time while the therapist sang. However, Smith (1991) suggests that it is factors such as tempo, length of seconds per word, and total number of words that might be more closely associated with lyric recall than the relative familiarity of the song selection.

In a further study of the effects of three treatment approaches, musically cued reminiscence, verbally cued reminiscence, and music alone, on the cognitive functioning of 12 female nursing home residents with Alzheimer's disease, changes in cognitive functioning were assessed by the differences between pre- and post-session treatment scores on the Mini-Mental State Examination. Comparisons were made for total scores and sub-scores for orientation, attention, and language. Musically cued and verbally cued reminiscence significantly increased language sub-section scores and musical activity alone significantly increased total scores (Smith 1986).

Music therapy with an Alzheimer's patient

Nordoff–Robbins music therapy is based upon the improvisation of music between therapist and patient (Nordoff and Robbins 1977). The music therapist plays the piano, improvising with the patient, who uses a range of instruments. This work often begins with an exploratory session using rhythmic instruments, in particular the drum and cymbal; progressing to the use of rhythmic/melodic instruments such as the chime bars, glockenspiel or xylophone; developing into work with melodic instruments (including the piano); and the voice. In this way of working the emphasis is on a series of musical improvisations during each session, and music is the vehicle for the therapy. Each session is audiotape-recorded, with the consent of the patient, and later analyzed and indexed as to musical content.

In the case example below music therapy is used as one modality of a comprehensive treatment package. The patient is seen on an outpatient basis for ten weekly sessions. Each session lasts for 40 minutes. She is unable to find her way on public transport and is brought to the hospital by her son.

Edith was a 55-year-old woman who came to the hospital for treatment. Her sister had died of Alzheimer's disease, and the family were concerned that she too was repeating her sister's demise as her memory became increasingly disturbed. She began playing the piano for family, friends and acquaintances at the age of 40, although without any formal studies, and, given this interest, music therapy appeared to have potential as an intervention adjuvant to medical treatment.

The patient was referred initially to the hospital when she, and her son, became aware of her own deteriorating condition, although the disease was in its early stages. At home she was experiencing difficulties in finding clothing and other things necessary for everday life. She could not cook for herself anymore and was unable to write her own signature. While wanting to speak, she experienced difficulty in finding words. It may be assumed that given the family background and her own understanding of her failings, the cognitive problem was exacerbated by depression.

Characteristics of the musical playing
RHYTHMIC PLAYING

In all ten sessions Edith demonstrated her ability to play, without the influence of her music therapist, a singular ordered rhythmic pattern in 4/4 time using two sticks on a single drum. This rhythmical pattern appeared in various forms and can be portrayed as seen in Figure 9.1. Example 1.

A feature of her rhythmical playing was that in nearly all the sessions, during the progress of an improvisation, the patient would let control of the rhythmic pattern slip such that it became progressively imprecise, losing both its form and liveliness. The initial impulse of her rhythmical playing, which was clear and precise, gradually deteriorated as she lost concentration and ability to persevere with the task in hand. However, when the therapist offered an overall musical structure during the course of the improvisation, the patient could regain her precision of rhythm. It could well be that to sustain perception an overall rhythmical structure is necessary, and it is this musical gestalt, that is, the possibility of providing an overall organizing structure of time, which fails in Alzheimer's disease.

The patient reacted quickly to changes in time and different rhythmic forms, and incorporated these within her playing. Significantly, she reacted fluently in her playing to changes from 4/4 time to 3/4 time, often remarking, 'Now it's a waltz...' With typical well-known rhythmical forms, e.g. the Habaner rhythm, in combination with characteristic melodic phrases, she laughed, breathed deeply and played with stronger, more thoughtful intent.

These rhythmical improvisations, using different drums and cymbals, were played in later sessions on two instruments together. The patient had no difficulty in controlling and maintaining her grip of the beaters. Similarly she showed no difficulty in co-ordinating parallel or alternate handed

Example 1

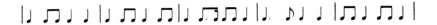

Example 2

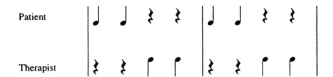

Example 3

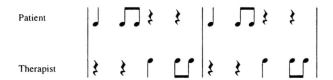

Example 4

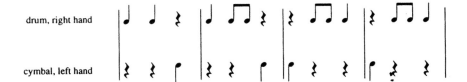

Figure 9.1 Examples of musical playing

playing on a single instrument, although she played mostly with a quick tempo (120 beats per minute). However, the introduction of two instruments brought a major difficulty for the patient, who stood disorientated before the instruments, unable to integrate them both in the playing. It was only with instructions and direction from the therapist that the patient was able to co-ordinate right–left playing on two instruments; changes in the pattern of the playing were also difficult to realize (see Figure 9.1, Examples 2 and 3).

Throughout the improvisations the inherent musical ability of the patient, in terms of tempo (ritardando, accelerando, rubato) and dynamic (loud and soft), was expressed whenever she had the opportunity to.

MELODIC PLAYING

Melody is an expression of motion which arises and decays from moment to moment. In this motion the size of the intervals provides a melodic tension which itself has a dynamic power. The experience of melody is itself an experience of form. As a melody begins there is the possibility of grasping a sense of the immediacy of the whole form, and preparing for the aesthetic pleasure of deviations from what is expected. This element of tension between the expected and the unpredictable has been at the heart of musical composition for the last two hundred years. In addition, it is melody that leads the music from the rhythmical world of feeling into the cognitive world of imagination.

When Edith played her melodies were always lively. She knew many folk songs from earlier times and was able to sing them alone. After only a few notes played by the therapist on the piano she could associate those notes with a well known tune. However, when she tried to play a complete melody on the piano or other melody instrument, it proved impossible. Although beginning spontaneously and fluently she had difficulty in completing a known melody.

Melody instruments like the metallophone and the xylophone, which were previously unknown to the patient, remained forever strange. At the introduction of a new melody she would often seek a previously known melody rather than face the insecurity of an unknown improvised melody. When the therapist sat opposite her and showed her which notes to play she was able to follow the therapist's finger movements. When presented with a limited range of tones she also had difficulty in playing them, which may have been compounded by visuo-spatial difficulties, in that it is easier to strike the surface of a drum than the limited precise surfaces of adjacent chime bars.

At the beginning of the very first session after entering the therapy room, Edith set her eyes on the piano and began spontaneously to play 'Happy is the Gypsy Life'. She easily accompanied this song harmonically with triads and thirds. The second song which she attempted to play proved more difficult as she failed to find the subdominant, whereupon she broke off from the playing and remarked '…that always catches me out'. This pattern of spontaneously striking up a melody and then breaking off when the harmony failed was to be repeated whenever she tried other songs like 'Happy Birthday' and 'Horch was kommt von draußen rein'. She showed a fine musical sensitivity for the appropriate harmony, which was not always at her disposal to be played. In the playing of the drum her musical sensitivity in her reactions to the contrasting sound qualities of major and minor was reduced, but overall she had a pronounced perception of this harmonic realm of music. We see here, as in tests of language functioning, that the production, in this case of music, is impaired while perception remains.

Changes in the musical playing of the patient
In the rhythmical playing on drum and cymbal the therapist attempted to develop the patient's attention span through the use of short repeated musical patterns and changes in key, volume and tempo. She hoped to through changes in the sound to steer the patient to maintaining a stable musical form. This technique helped the patient to maintain a rhythmical pattern and brought her to the stage in which she could express her self, more strongly, musically. Beyond the emphasis on the basic beat in the music, the therapist searched for other ways to respond to, and develop a variety in, rhythmical pattern by moving away from the repetitive pattern played by the patient. In a quick tempo the patient was able to maintain a basic beat for a certain time. As soon as the tempo changed and became slower, or the music varied with the introduction of a semiquaver, the stable element of the music was disturbed and took on a superficial character.

A further change in the improvising was shown when the patient recognized, and could repeat rhythmical patterns which were frequently realized as a musical dialogue and brought into a musical context. In the last session of therapy the patient was able to change her playing in this way such that she could express herself more strongly by bringing her thoughtful and expressive playing into line (see Figure 9.1, Example 4).

A crucial point in the music came when she chose to play for a bar on the cymbal. Although after a while she trusted herself to play without help on two instruments, she could not get to grips with a new personal initiative on these instruments. This was also reflected in her continuing difficulty with what were initially strange instruments, like the temple blocks. She also expressed her insecurity as to how to proceed, and needed instructions about what to do next.

She displayed few changes in her dynamic playing. She reacted to dynamic contrasts and transitions, but powerful *forte* playing was only achieved in the last session. At times her playing had a uniform quality of attack which gave it a mechanistic and immovable character. For this patient it was not possible to build a freely improvised melody from a selection of tones. It was as if she was a prisoner of the search for melodies of known fixed songs; therefore she chose the free form of improvising on rhythm instruments.

INTENTIONAL PLAYING

From the first session of therapy the patient made quite clear her intent to sit at the piano, and play whatever melodies she chose and find the appropriate accompaniments. This wish and the corresponding will-power to achieve this end were shown in all the sessions. It was possible to use this impetus to play as a source for improvisation. In the sixth session Edith improvised a rhythmical piece in 4/4 time, which the therapist then transformed with a melodic phrase. At the end of the phrase the patient laughed with joy at the success of her playing and asked to play it again. The original lapses and slips in the form of the rhythmical playing could be carried by the intent and expression with which she played. While her overall intention to play was preserved, her attention to that playing, the concentration necessary for musical production and the perseverance required for completing a sequence of phrases progressively failed, and were dependent on the overall musical structure offered by the therapist.

Clinical changes

At the end of the treatment period, which also used homeopathic medicine, she was able to cook for herself and could find her own things about the house. The psychiatrist responsible for her therapeutic management reported an overall improvement in her interest in what was going on around her, and in particular that she maintained attention to visitors and conversations. The patient regained the ability to write her signature, although she could only write slowly. While wanting to speak, she still experienced difficulty in finding words.

It appears that music therapy has a beneficial effect on the quality of life of this patient, and that some of the therapeutic effect may have been brought about by treating the depression. While the patient came to the sessions with the intention of playing her ability to take initiatives was impaired, mirroring the state of her home life, where she wanted to look after herself yet was unable to take initiatives. The stimulus to take initiatives was seen as an important feature of the music therapy by the therapist, and appears to have a correlate in the way in which the patient began to take initiatives in her daily life. Active music making also promotes interaction between the persons involved, thereby promoting initiatives in communication which the patient also enjoyed, particularly when she accomplished a complete improvisation. Furthermore, the implications for the maintenance of memory by actively making music is significant. As Crystal *et al.* (1989) found in an 82-year-old musician with Alzheimer's disease, the ability to play previously learned piano compositions from memory was preserved, although the man was unable to identify the composer or titles of each work; and the ability to learn the new skill of mirror reading was also preserved while the man was unable to recall or recognize new information.

A contra-indication for music therapy with such patients, who are aware of their problems, is that the awareness of further deterioration in cognitive abilities (as this patient experienced in her piano playing) may exacerbate any underlying depression and demotivate the patient to continue. For Edith, not being able to find the appropriate harmonies to well-known tunes, that she could play when she was younger was yet another sign of her deteriorating status.

Music Therapy as a Sensitive Tool for Assessment
If we are unsure as to the normal process of cognitive loss in aging, we are even more in the dark as to the normal musical playing abilities of adults. The literature suggests that musical activities are preserved while other cognitive functions fail. Alzheimers patients, despite aphasia and memory loss, continue to sing old songs and to dance to past tunes when given the chance. Indeed, fun and entertainment are all part and parcel of daily living for the elderly living in special accommodation (Glassman 1983; Jonas 1991; Kartman 1990; Smith 1992). Quality of life expectations become paramount in any management strategy, and music therapy appears to play an important role in enhancing the ability to take part actively in daily life (Lipe 1991; Rosling and Kitchen 1992). However, the production and improvisation of music appear to fail in the same way in which language fails. Unfortunately no established guidelines as to the normal range of improvised music playing of adults is available.

Improvised music therapy appears to offer the opportunity to supplement mental state examinations in areas where those examinations are lacking (see

Tables 9.4 and 9.5). First, it is possible to ascertain the fluency of musical production. Second, intentionality, attention to, concentration on and perseverance with the task in hand are important features of producing musical improvisations and susceptible to being heard in the musical playing. Third, episodic memory can be tested in the ability to repeat short rhythmic and melodic phrases. The inability to build such phrases may be attributed to problems with memory or to an as yet unknown factor. This unknown factor is possibly involved with the organization of time structures. If rhythmic structure is an overall context for musical production, and the ground structure for perception, it can be hypothesized that it is this overarching structure which begins to fail in Alzheimer's patients. A loss of rhythmical context would explain why patients are able to produce and persevere with rhythmic and melodic playing when offered an overall structure by the therapist. Such a hypothesis would tie in with the musical hierarchy proposed by Swartz (Swartz et al. 1989, p.154), and would suggest a global failing in cognition while localized lower abilities are retained. However, the hierarchy of musical perceptual levels proposed by Swartz may need to be further sub-divided into classifications of music reception and music production.

Table 9.5 Musical elements of assessment and examples of improvised playing

Musical elements of assessment	Examples of improvised playing
testing of musical skills; rhythm, melody, harmony, dynamic, phrasing, articulation	improvisation using rhythmic instruments (drum and cymbal) singly or in combination
	improvisation using melodic instruments
	singing and playing folk songs with harmonic accompaniment
cortical disorder testing; visuo-spatial skills	playing tuned percussion (metallophone, xylophone, chime bars) demanding precise movements
cortical disorder testing; ability to perform complex motor tasks (including grip and right–left co-ordination	alternate playing of cymbal and drum using a beater in each hand
	co-ordinated playing of cymbal and drum using a beater in each hand
	co-ordinated playing of tuned percussion

Table 9.5 Musical elements of assessment
and examples of improvised playing (continued)

Musical elements of assessment	Examples of improvised playing
testing for progressive memory disintegration	the playing of short rhythmic and melodic phrases within the session, and in successive sessions
motivation to sustain playing improvised music, to achieve musical goals and preserve in maintaining musical form	the playing of a rhythmic pattern deteriorates when unaccompanied by the therapist as does the ability to complete a known melody, although tempo remains
'intention' a feature of improvised musical playing	the patient exhibits the intention to play the piano from the onset of therapy and maintains this intent throughout the course of treatment
concentration on the improvised playing and attention to the instruments	the patient loses concentration when playing, with qualitative loss in the musical playing and lack of precision in the beating of rhythmical instruments
flexibility in musical (including instrumental) changes	initially the musical playing is limited to a tempo of 120 Bp and a characteristic pattern but this is responsive to change
ability to play improvised music influenced by previous musical training	although the patient has a musical background this is only of help when she perceives the musical playing; it is little influence in the improvised playing
sensitive to small changes	musical changes in tempo, dynamic, timbre and articulation which at first are missing are gradually developed
ability to interpret musical context and relationship	the patient develops the ability to play in a musical dialogue with the therapist demanding both a refined musical perception and the ability of musical production

Music therapy appears to offer a sensitive assessment tool (see Table 9.5). It tests those prosodic elements of speech production which are not lexically dependent. Furthermore, it can be used to assess those areas of functioning, both receptive and productive, not covered adequately by other test instruments; i.e. fluency, perseverance in context, attention, concentration and intentionality. In addition it provides a form of therapy which may stimulate cognitive activities such that areas subject to progressive failure are maintained. Certainly the anecdotal evidence suggests that quality of life of Alzheimer's patients is significantly improved with music therapy (McCloskey 1985, 1990; Tyson 1989) accompanied by the overall social benefits of acceptance and sense of belonging gained by communicating with others (Morris 1986; Segal 1990).

Prinsley recommends music therapy for geriatric care as it reduces the individual prescription of tranquilizing medication, reduces the use of hypnotics on the hospital ward, and helps overall rehabilitation. He recommends that music therapy be based on treatment objectives: the social goals of interaction co-operation; psychological goals of mood improvement and self-expression; intellectual goals of the stimulation of speech and organization of mental processes; and the physical goals of sensory stimulation and motor integration (Prinsley 1986). Such goals as stimulation of the individual, promoting involvement in social activity, identifying specific individualized behavioural targets, and emphasizing the maintenance of specific memory functions are repeated throughout the music therapy literature (Prange 1990; Smith 1990; Summer 1981). Similarly, Smith (1990a) recommends behavioural interventions targeted at the more common behavioural problems (e.g., disorientation, age-related changes in social activity, sleep disturbances) of institutionalized elderly persons. In a matched control study of music therapy, or no music therapy, in two nursing homes, life satisfaction and self-esteem were significantly improved in the home where the residents participated in the musical activities (VanderArk, Newman and Bell 1983).

In terms of research, single-case within-subject designs with Alzheimer's appear to be a feasible way forward to assess individual responses to musical interventions in the clinical realm. Such studies would depend upon careful clinical examinations, mental state examinations and musical assessments. Unfortunately most of the literature concerning cognition and musical perception is based upon audition and not musical production. Like other authors we suggest that the production of music, as is the production of language, is a complex global phenomenon as yet poorly understood. The understanding of musical production may well offer a clue to the ground structure of language and communication in general. It is research in this realm of perception which is urgent not only for the understanding of Alzheimer's patients but in the general context of cognitive deficit and brain behaviour. It may be, as Berman (1981) suggests, that the non-dominant hemisphere is a reserve of functions in case of regional failure and this functionality can be stimulated to delay the progression of degenerative disease. Furthermore, it is important to point out that when the overall rhythmic pattern failed, the patient was able to maintain her beating in tempo. A similar situation applies in coma patients who cannot co-ordinate basic life pulses within a rhythmic context and thereby regain consciousness (Aldridge 1991b; Aldridge, Gustorff and Hannich 1990). We may need to address in future research the co-ordinating role of rhythm in human cognition and consciousness, whether it be in persons who are losing cognitive abilities, or in persons who are attempting to gain cognitive abilities.

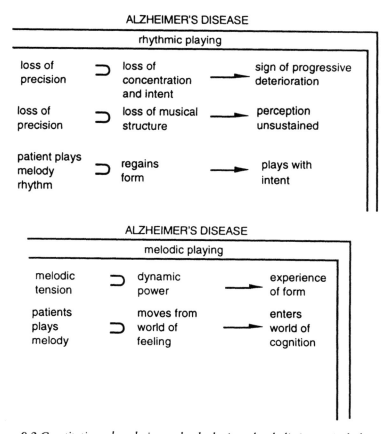

Figure 9.2 Constitutive rules relating to the rhythmic and melodic improvised playing of Alzheimer's patients

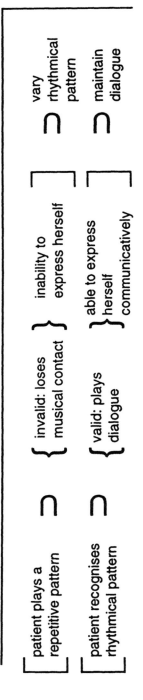

RHYTHMIC PLAYING OF A PATIENT WITH ALZHEIMER'S DISEASE

therapeutic assessment

loss of precision →

sign of progressive deterioration

Level 1 musical event

Level 2 description

Level 3 interpretation

Figure 9.3 Textual understandings of a musical phenomenon in therapeutic assessment

context of close friendship

patient plays a repetitive pattern ∩ invalid: loses musical contact } inability to express herself } ∩ vary rhythmical pattern

patient recognises rhythmical pattern ∩ valid: plays dialogue } able to express herself communicatively } ∩ maintain dialogue

Figure 9.4 Regulative rules relating to the rhythmic improvised playing of Alzheimer's patients and its meaning for dialogue in therapy

As a research point we can see how the use of texts relating to clinical practice can be used to build up a picture of clinical reasoning, as we also saw at the end of the last chapter. In this case we have constitutive rules (see Figure 9.2) relating to the rhythmical playing, where rhythmical precision is seen as a sign of progressive deterioration and evidence of a loss of concentration or loss of intent. Conversely, the maintenance of rhythm is construed as regaining form and evidence of playing with intent.

It is not only texts themselves that can be used to elicit meanings. We can see graphically in Figure 9.3 how a 'musical text' can be used as the basis for therapeutic assessment using a constitutive rules perspective. This assessment is based upon the same musical material as seen in Figure 9.1, Example 1 and the constitutive rule seen in Figure 9.2. By presenting material in this way we have a flexible means by which musical understandings can be constructed and demonstrated. That musical texts can be used is an important bridge between the experiences of the musician as therapist and the musician as researcher. This is a vertical understanding where level 1 is the musical experience itself, that is then 'neutrally' described at level 2, and interpreted at level 3.

Using these elements of rhythmical playing we can construct regulative, horizontal rules as they refer to the therapy process in time. In Figure 9.4 we see how when a repetitive pattern, which is interpreted as an inability on the part of the patient to express herself, is played, the therapist varies her own rhythmical pattern. If the patient recognizes such a change in rhythmical pattern, she is able to express herself communicatively and maintain the therapeutic dialogue. Having both a vertical form of analysis and a horizontal form of analysis allows us in some ways to display the element of performance that we have in a musical score. Vertically we have harmony and horizontally we have a substrate of time. In my method we have a vertical complexity of elicited understandings that are constructed horizontally as descriptions of therapeutic development. The benefit of this approach is that we can be clear about the material we are using as a basis for our description, and elucidate the stages of interpretation as they move away from the experience itself.

CHAPTER TEN

Hope, Meaning and Music Therapy in the Treatment of Life-Threatening Illness

> What strikes me is the fact that in our society, art has become something which is related only to objects and not to individuals, or to life. That art is something which is specialized or done by experts who are artists. But couldn't everyone's life become a work of art? Why should the lamp or the house be an art object, but not our life? (Michel Foucault quoted in Rabinow 1986, p.350)

In previous chapters I have tried to establish a foundation for working with music therapy in the treatment of intractable problems. In this chapter I turn to a problem facing modern society, the treatment of people with human immunodeficiency virus and AIDS, and women with cancer. I shall be returning to the theme of identity, which was raised earlier in the book, and the role that music plays in bringing hope for a future that may be drastically changed. As this future, like all our futures, is concerned with dying then I shall be introducing considerations of spirituality and the relevance that this has for clinical practice. For all three chronic diseases described in this book – chronic bowel disease, dementia in the elderly and chronic immunological challenge – hope is a mediating factor that will play a significant role in the maintenance of their daily lives.

The general proposal of this chapter is that the creative arts therapies have a significant role to play in the treatment of patients when their existence is threatened. Not only do they offer an existential form of therapy that accepts the person as they are, and offers them an opportunity to define themselves as they wish to be, they are primarily concerned with aesthetic issues of form and existential notions of potential, rather than concepts of pathology. That the person is infected with a virus recalcitrant to medical initiatives is given, and inarguable. What the person will become and how a personal future is defined, a future which is admittedly restricted and often tragically curtailed, are matters for joint therapeutic endeavour between therapist and patient and are not accessible to a normative medical science (Aldridge 1991a, 1992).

The end stage of our therapeutic endeavour is that the patient will die. This raises important questions about the nature and goals of therapy, with important implications for establishing the criteria for measuring or assessing the efficacy of our therapeutic endeavours. Many of the considerations we need to make, particularly with the dying, are not amenable to operational definition and thereby elusive to measurement (Feifel 1990). However, they are amenable to artistic expression in that they can be written as poetry, acted as drama, moved as dance, drawn, sculpted and painted as art, told as stories and played as music.

Creative arts therapies (music therapy, art therapy, dance therapy and drama therapy) have been developed for use in predominantly psychotherapy settings. Some creative arts therapists have developed the work with the dying in hospice settings (Dessloch *et al.* 1992; Frampton 1989), and Lee has developed the use of music therapy both with cancer patients in the hospice setting, and with AIDS patients (Lee 1991).

The following sets out some considerations which we may wish to incorporate into our treatment and research initiatives. As the treatment of AIDS patients occurs predominantly in medical settings it is necessary first to present some of the medical understandings of the problem. Those medical understandings, however, are partial. Medicine is a restricted set of practices from the repertoire of our possible healing strategies. What we also need are understandings gained from existential psychology and the creative arts themselves. Such understandings will be attempted in the latter part of the chapter.

The Chronically Immunologically Challenged

AIDS (Acquired Immunodeficiency Syndrome) is clinically complex. The process begins with infection through the bloodstream with the Human Immunodeficiency Virus (HIV). Initially there are no obvious symptoms. However, after about four weeks flu-like symptoms may occur, indicating an immune reaction. This reaction is the body's normal way of removing infections. What then occurs is the most dangerous part of the viral activity that makes HIV so intractable to treatment. The immune system is in part composed of 'helper cells'. It is these cells that act as a host to the virus, the structure of which the virus then changes. Every time an immune reaction occurs in the body the virus is replicated. What was formerly 'helping' is now 'infecting'. However, it must be stressed that not all HIV infected patients will undergo this process of seroconversion, i.e. changed immune status.

The stage is set for the development of AIDS; the development of which is variable from individual to individual. As the immune system deteriorates there are increasing possibilities of opportunistic infections. It is often these infections from which the patient eventually dies. As a condition AIDS was originally characterized by the following symptoms: (1) common infections, like pneumonia, to which the body has no immunity; (2) the development of malignancies like rare skin cancers; and (3) neurological disorders sometimes leading to dementia. However, a new AIDS definition has been proposed by The Centers for Disease Control in the United States regardless of symptomatic expression, to include those people who are seropositive for HIV and have a particular white blood cell count (CD4 T-lymphocyte) of less than $200/\mu l$ (Editorial 1992; Nelson 1992). The result of such a decision for research is that it will be easier to define cases. In practice such a decision means that the incidence of AIDS will rise sharply. Recently new AIDS indicator diseases have been recognized as pulmonary tuberculosis, recurrent bacterial pneumonia and invasive cervical cancer. The inclusion of pulmonary tuberculosis is 'more to do with efforts to control tuberculosis among HIV infected populations than its value as an indicator of severe immunodeficiency' (Editorial 1992; Nelson 1992). We see here that even in the apparently simple process of case definition, considerations of social control are raised, echoing the stigmatization of tuberculosis patients in the earlier part of this century.

Immunity, life events and social context

How the immune system reacts between viral infection and the development of AIDS is dependent upon the individual. However, the social and psychological conditions in which the infected persons live are also a contributory factor to the development of AIDS. As we are now becoming increasingly aware of the influence of lifestyle upon immune capabilities (Ader 1987; Darko 1986; Solomon 1987), it is in this arena of contact that we may be best able to offer therapeutic help. An already weakened system is further weakened by the threat of a lingering death, social isolation and condemnation. The contact between arts therapists and patient is the opposite of isolation, in that it offers the patient the chance to be a partner in a creative process that is without stigmatization.

There is a considerable body of work on the relationship between life events and psychological disorder, and this has been extended to working with AIDS patients (Atkins and Amenta 1991; Blaney *et al.* 1991; Dew, Ragni and Nimorwicz 1991; Ross 1990). In a study to determine the extent to which stigmatization influences mental health in 80 homosexual men there were significant associations between life events, and mental health and events related to AIDS had the highest correlations (Ross 1990). Ross suggests that the impact of life events may be amplified by stigmatization and that degree of life change is associated closely with psychological dysfunction. He concluded that life events, which are related to both stigmatization and related emotional distress, are significant predictors of psychological dysfunction.

For every patient living with the diagnosis of AIDS or a positive HIV test result, there is a turning point in his or her life. It is existential uncertainty and unpredictability that lie at the root of post-diagnostic problems. While the need for early treatment is evident, this also means a personal exposure to social scrutiny. AIDS is seen as threatening as no other current disease, which is in part exacerbated by information campaigns. Once the diagnosis is made the whole texture of social life and intimate relationships changes radically. Any future perspective on life is inhibited by the possibility of repetitive stays in hospital and deteriorating physical and mental status.

Physical problems go hand in hand with emotional problems, and these occur in a context of personal relationships. The consideration of physical, emotional and relational problems together is sometimes known as the biopsychosocial model (Engel 1977; Sadler and Hulgus 1990). Using such a model Wolf et al. (1991) evaluated 29 symptomatic and asymptomatic HIV-infected homosexual/bisexual men aged between 18 and 45 in the areas of psychiatric/psychosocial, neuropsychological, family, and immunological functioning. The outcome measures were mood disturbance, psychological distress, and white blood cell count (CD4). The most significant other family member, as selected by each subject, completed family measures. The subjects experienced psychological distress and neuropsychological problems. Coping was related to enhanced mood as was perceived social support, which was also related to lower psychological distress. Higher levels of neuropsychological functioning (verbal memory, visual memory, motor speed, and visual-motor sequencing) were associated with enhanced psychosocial functioning and/or immunological status. The authors conclude that it is then important to make longitudinal studies using a multi-dimensional approach in which HIV-infected persons and their most significant other family members are evaluated.

The suicide rate in persons with AIDS is significantly higher than in the general population (Cohen 1990; Grant and Hampton Atkinson 1990). Grant (Grant and Hampton Atkinson 1990) remarks that although some sub-groups of HIV positive individuals (e.g., military samples) may be at heightened risk of suicide, systematic studies showing an increased risk of suicide are lacking. Schneider considers suicidal ideation among relatively asymptomatic HIV positive gay men as a cognitive coping strategy which may alleviate emotional distress (Schneider *et al.* 1991). Certainly the picture is complex. Risk factors for suicide in the general population include hopelessness, impulsivity, substance abuse disorder, recent illness, recent hospitalization, depression, living alone and inexpressible grief. These factors are present in particular AIDS patients who are depressed, lonely and isolated and a high risk for suicide. Marital break-up, or a failing relationship which eventually ceases, is a significant feature leading to such loneliness. As Blaney remarks (Blaney *et al.* 1991), lack of social support is a strong predictor of psychological distress and implicated in the control of chronic disease. Suicidal behavior may be the end stage of a process of increasing psychological distress, related to both failing health status, in terms of increasing symptoms, and increasing isolation.

Help seeking

In a longitudinal survey of help-seeking and psychological distress among San Francisco gay men (Hays *et al.* 1990), those men reported high levels of anxiety, depression, and help-seeking from their social networks. High percentages of AIDS-diagnosed men sought help from all sources (peers, professionals, family), whereas non-diagnosed men were more likely to seek help from peers. Regardless of the men's HIV status, peers were perceived to be the most helpful source. Family members were less likely sought and perceived as least helpful.

However, in other studies family and friends appear to play an important, if sometimes ambiguous, role in caregiving. The psychological burden on the families and health workers involved in their treatment of AIDS patients is probably greater than in that of any other medical condition (Maj 1991).

In a study by Atkins and Amenta (1991) family adaptation to AIDS and to other terminal illnesses was compared by measuring the number of stressful events experienced by the family after diagnosis and role flexibility in response to medical stressors. Families of AIDS patients had significantly more stress, more rules prohibiting emotional expression, lower trust levels, and more illness anxiety than the other families.

In young children with AIDS, with the exception of transfusion-infected children, there is necessarily the presence of an infected adult, usually the mother. The problem in such a situation is not that of a child with a fatal illness but that of an entire family. In a study of 30 natural caregivers (mostly mothers but also fathers, aunts and grandmothers), most of the caregivers were economically disadvantaged and needed help in coping with stress and their life situation (Reidy, Taggart and Asselin 1991). Their need to confide in others was frequently not met, although they responded well to medical care, support and advice.

Social and ethical aspects

Few diseases since syphilis in the nineteenth century and tuberculosis in the early part of the twentieth century have raised the ethical, scientific and economic questions which AIDS has. The moral responsibility of the therapist to offer unconditional care for the patient has been threatened. The scientific principles of placebo trials and safe drug testing procedures have been consistently challenged by the community of AIDS activists (Faden and Kass 1990), and the cost of health care provision for European and American health care systems is potentially crippling. Furthermore, the disease has struck our modern society at its most vulnerable point in raising the issue of how we care for the sick, the poor and those whom we label as deviant (Ackerman 1989; Ribble 1989). Not only are patients infected with a recalcitrant virus, they are often infected by our attitudes of intolerance and condemnation (Johnston 1988).

As some of those persons contracting the AIDS virus are likely to belong to groups who are socially vulnerable (homosexual men and women, the urban poor of ethnic minorities and drug users), the challenge of offering treatment is one that reaches into the ethical resources of our healing communities.

It is precisely the source of contracting AIDS that causes many of the ethical problems. At a time when choice of sexual orientation was apparently becoming a matter of personal preference rather than one governed by genital endowment, and the tolerance of homosexual and lesbian activity was increasing, the AIDS virus served once more to condemn groups of people to a state of potential deviancy (Faden and Kass 1990).

Fear of contagion, coupled with prejudices about lifestyle, are undoubtedly strong factors influencing in the way that some caregivers treat their patients. A wide range of emotional reactions by the caregiver may occur, from refusal to provide care resulting in rejection, to a total immersion in the infected person's needs, leading to burnout. Since irrational fears and attitudes play an important role in conditioning these reactions, education alone for the caregivers may not be sufficient to change behaviour. Counselling sessions and mutual support groups are often the most appropriate contexts where fears and concerns can receive an individually tailored response, and where formal and informal caregivers can be helped to manage stress.

In contrast to other terminal illnesses, patients can often clearly say where, when and under which circumstances they contracted the disease. It is these circumstances that form the axis of judgement about the illness; they are either innocently infected victims or irresponsible deviants.

The conditions governing the attribution of the status sick (Parsons 1951) are that the sick (1) do not form groups, (2) recover within a prescribed time, and (3) are not causally responsible for their own demise. The last two of these conditions are violated by patients infected with the HIV virus. Furthermore, the AIDS activists who encourage sufferers to form groups and advocate changes in treatment and support on their own behalf are threatening a longstanding social requirement that the sick remain divided and powerless.

In addition, as a proportion of the AIDS infected population are drug users, the very virus is associated with an already socially stigmatized group. As Ribble (1989) points out, a nurse may feel a strong empathy for the sexually infected partner of an intravenous drug user, yet significantly less empathy for the infected drug user.

Maintaining integrity and hope

The immune system is the biochemical part of our identity. It is not only a system of reaction, but also a proactive system. Its actions are projected into the future to develop, restore and maintain our physiological identity based upon the experiences of today and yesterday. Immunological reactions are not only effects caused by aggressive stimuli; they are also meaningful memories of our physiological make-up. The immune system is the major integrative network within our bodies that facilitates our biological adaptation (Wiedermann and Wiedermann 1988).

For the HIV infected patient the task is one of maintaining an identity the source of which is partially, and perpetually, self-corrupted (in that the DNA material of some cells is changed). This itself calls for both an acceptance of self and the realization of a creative new self. It also calls for a massive new alignment of bodily immune regulation.

Positive emotions are known to be beneficial for the immune system. Yet it is possible to go further and say that the qualitative aspects of life; hope, joy, beauty and unconditional love are also vital and beneficial in therapy. This is precisely the ground in which the creative arts can have their own being. Patients can explore and express their being in the world which is creative and not limited by their infection. From such a perspective we would expect that although physical parameters may fluctuate or deteriorate, we would expect quality of life measures or existential indicators to show improvement.

A significant existential beneficial factor in enhancing the quality of life is hope. Hope has been identified as a multi-faceted phenomenon which is a valuable human response even in the face of a severe reduction in life expectancy. Herth's (1990) study explored the meaning of hope and identified strategies that were used to foster hope in a sample of 30 terminally ill adults. Cross-sectional data were collected on 20 of the subjects, and longitudinal data were collected on ten of the subjects in order to provide a clearer understanding of the hoping process during the dying trajectory. Hope was defined by Herth as an 'inner power directed toward enrichment of "being"'. With the exception of those diagnosed with AIDS, overall hope levels among subjects were high and were found to remain stable over time. Seven hope-fostering categories (interpersonal connectedness, attainable aims, spiritual base, personal attributes, light-heartedness, uplifting memories and affirmation of worth) and three hope-hindering categories (abandonment and isolation, uncontrollable pain and discomfort, devaluation of personhood) were identified.

Hope, like prayer (Saudia *et al.* 1991), is a coping strategy used by those confronted with a chronic illness which involves an expectation which goes beyond visible facts and which can be seen as a motivating force to achieve inner goals. These goals change. While a distant future of life expectancy no longer exists for AIDS patients, life aims can be redefined and refocused. With the progression of physical deterioration the future becomes less defined in terms of time but more defined in the meaning attributed to life events in relationships to others. In later stages there is a shift towards less concrete goals and a refocusing on the self to include the inner peace and serenity necessary for dying (Herth 1990). Music therapy, for example, with its ability to offer an experience of time which is qualitatively rich, and not chronologically determined, is a valuable intervention.

Music therapy can offer hope in situations of seeming hopelessness and is, therefore, a means of transcendence. This idea of transcendence, the ability to extend the self beyond the immediate context to achieve new perspectives, is seen as important in the last phases of life where dying patients are encouraged to maintain a sense of well-being in the face of imminent biological and social loss. As soon as I speak of prayer, transcendence and hope, I am entering into a discussion of spirituality to which I will later return.

Breast Cancer

I want now to turn to another life threatening disease and discuss the implications that music therapy has for its treatment. From the literature about breast cancer we know that it is important for patients to be able to express themselves. We know also that melody in our modern culture is an important form of expression. If expression is important for breast cancer patients, and melody is an important form of musical expression, then it makes sense to develop the melodic playing of patients in music therapy (Aldridge 1995). As we have previously seen in patients who are chronically immunologically challenged, the cancer sufferer often faces moral condemnation and psychological challenges that can exacerbate the course of the illness.

Breast cancer is the second leading cause of cancer incidence and mortality for women. Among approximately 200 different kinds of cancerous diseases, breast cancer is the most widespread among women and increasing in incidence (Carter 1994). Cancer is regarded in our society not only as an illness but also as a malicious enemy that can threaten life (Sontag 1990). The experience of breast cancer in our society, in which the breast of the woman is part of the cultural code for femininity and sexuality, is traumatic (Wear 1993). In facing a potentially fatal disease, a woman also faces the loss of a precious part of her body that is deeply embedded in her sexuality and femininity and a series of events that threaten her very existence.

Among the varying events that are most feared are: mutilation or amputation of one part of the body; the pain attached to that amputation; the uncertainty about the success of treatment; the possibility of the disease's recurrence; a deterioration of the women's current health condition; and death. To be faced with these possibilities causes deep and significant feelings 'that cannot be medicalized into neat stage theories or normalized by upbeat assurances' (Wear 1993, p.82).

At a time of increasing uncertainty, questions about guilt and one's own abnormal behaviour occur. Things one is afraid of, or which are felt as an insult or repulsive, may easily be identified with the disease. Susan Sontag (1990) sees cancer as being used by society as a metaphor for moralizing upon things that are seen as wrong. Similarly Wilkinson sees it as no coincidence that this disease is often viewed within a moral context (Wilkinson and Kitzinger 1993). A feature that has always been present in society is the attempt to combine the individual's point of view with a moral secular view, that reflects upon the existence of good and bad people. In applying this moral perspective to the body and health concerns, opinions are often expressed that describe 'inharmonious' individuals as susceptible to diseases. In this way the attribution of illness becomes a kind of moral judgement about the degree of control an individual has over her life.

As in the recognition of being HIV positive, the diagnosis of cancer can precipitate a state of profound anxiety that is associated with sensitivity, vulnerability, hopelessness, thoughts about death and uncertainty about the future (Wong and Bramwell 1992). This mental state may itself contribute to the progressive development of cancer. Spiegel (1991) also shows that the suppression of, and the inability to express, anger is in some ways associated with the appearance of cancer. Spiegel does not argue that cancer can be caused by this inability to express anger. In response to these psychological factors, there are indicators in the literature suggesting that survival and disease progression can be influenced by psychosocial interventions. Spiegel himself examined the effect of a psychosocial intervention on mood and pain, and discovered a positive effect on these variables. He found that there was not only reduced mood disturbance and less pain, but less phobic and better coping responses as well. For him the value and advantage of psychosocial intervention are in the fundamental improvement of the woman's quality of life.

Carter (1994) too points out that social stigma and discrimination lead to isolation, and both contribute to a negative view of the situation many working women are confronted with. The negative experience of going back to work may cause a problem of reconstructing a positive sense of self. Carter discusses the possibilities that facilitate a return to work and suggests recommendations for the further development of work re-entry programmes.

In determining the relationship between uncertainty and anxiety, Wong and Bramwell recommend supportive follow-up and the development of appropriate interventions, to assist breast cancer patients in dealing with their fears of recurrence and uncertainties regarding treatment effectiveness. Similar arguments are put forward by Carter (Carter and Carter 1993), who ascertained that women were not adequately prepared for their post-operative phase, since many of them continued to experience physical symptoms and depression four years after treatment. Patients described their post-operative experience as a survival process, of 'going through'. Each phase was experienced as a temporal context, having a past, a present, and an anticipated future, and as an experience of moving from something to something else. Each phase contained an element of pessimism. The integration of disease and illness makes sense within the context of the patient's life from the point of their lived experience, and it is this individual experiential voice of the woman that we must hear. Each woman has her own story to tell, and as Carter suggests, care might best be provided by understanding the context of each patient's life.

In the nursing literature, the claim for emotional support during the burdening phases of the course of the disease is a recurring theme where a number of risk factors for psychiatric morbidity are identified, and it is concluded that an increased awareness of such risk factors should lead to earlier detection and more appropriate treatment.

Meeting the relational and emotional needs of the patient

What we can take from the literature is also the fact that psychological and social factors are important aspects of patient care and have a crucial influence on the post-operative phase. Current medical treatment is a radical one (amputation, radiation/chemotherapy), yet it is not sufficient to provide the patients with the greatest possible healing chances. Medical treatment alone cannot be content with surgery and radiation but has to include, and offer, other psychosocial interventions that enable women to find a way of handling their disease and the consequences of medical intervention. Of these interventions, an emphasis can be made that enables women to find their own perspectives on the disease and encourage a new integration of understandings into their own biography.

Creative music therapy could be a valuable contribution to meet the patient's different needs. Fundamental questions emerge about how to deal with the body after amputation; how to deal with the emotional suffering that ensues; how to cope with the image that remains of an altered body; and how to handle the consequent social and professional problems (reorganizing life at home within the family, communicating with family, friends and acquaintances, dealing with possible financial difficulties). Furthermore, there is a problem of how to deal with the distance other people place between themselves and the sufferer, and the distance the sufferer may feel from her own body. By neglecting personal needs, feelings of isolation and distance from one's own body and illness can emerge. In becoming aware of her own intrinsic feelings during the actual musical playing, music therapy provides possibilities of promoting an intimacy with her own body for the woman, and creating an artistic dialogue to reinforce, and activate, interpersonal communication (Aldridge 1995).

Anxiety and depression are often cited as the predominant affective pattern in facing cancer. Patients are forced by their disease to know how to deal with their own emotional reactions. Some may succeed better than others, depending upon their nature. Music, while having everything to do with emotion, has nothing to do with the labels 'anxiety', 'depression' or 'aggression'. Music therapy has the effect of offering patients space and possibilities to express themselves directly out of their difficult situation, without normative expectations and without the fear of judgement, of doing everything wrong. It is presumed here that therapists are basing their reactions on acceptance and not moral judgements.

In having the ability to play as one feels in a creative way, there is a chance for women to achieve a sense of a new identity. To perform musically, as an active manifestation of self, may itself contribute to mood improvement and reduce negative feelings like despair, depression, loneliness and anxiety. As I have suggested earlier, in music therapy patients find their own way of expression that is creative and not limited by an illness. To start out from this way of looking, one could expect to find indicators that, in spite of a deterioration of physical parameters, point to an improvement of quality of life. This would be of special value for breast cancer patients and is related to the maintenance of hope.

Bailey (1983) also emphasizes the pervasive influence of music on mood improvement. In this respect music therapy should not only be used after a breast is removed surgically and during the post-operative phase, but also during different stages of the disease as a form of creative intervention. Music therapy as a receptive measure proves to be effective in that it not only provides patients with distraction but can reduce nausea and vomiting, promote relaxation and bring overall relief. Jacobsen (Jacobsen, Bovbjerg and Redd 1993) describes the relief of anticipated anxiety before a second treatment period of chemotherapy. Music therapy as a supportive action meets the needs of individual patients, fosters the expression of emotional problems, and stimulates creativity. Music therapy can promote a new personal integrity.

In being actively involved in the musical improvisation women can make decisions regarding that improvisation. The patient becomes an active partner in health care rather than putting her into the position of being a passive recipient of that care. This aspect of the woman's influence on her own fate is very important, and realizable in creative music therapy. She has the possibility of exerting influence on her own playing and taking respon-sibility for her actions.

The music therapeutic process, with its various demands and changes, is a joint effort. The function of the music therapist is that she is pointing the way towards new modes of expression and, in the context of the musical relationship, allowing a new identity to emerge. Within a context of musical communication, flexibility of expression may be encouraged within a sup-portive musical form. If music therapy is a powerful tool for promoting communication in terms of personal and interpersonal integration, isolation can be relieved. By the use of creative dialogues, interpersonal contact is maintained, and patients experience that they are not estranged within themselves, or estranged from others.

Expressivity

We know that cancer is a complex disease, demanding psychological, emotional and social consideration and moving away from a one-sided medical treatment of symptoms that reduces women to passive medical objects. A systemic model combines personal, social and cultural factors to achieve a deeper knowledge about the patient's adjustment to this disease.

Music therapy, as a receptive and active form of intervention, brings improvements by reducing anxiety, depression, fatigue and distraction. Not only is emotional suffering reduced, but a significant improvement in mood for the better can be achieved, as well as an improvement in communication with the family and loved ones.

Melodic improvisation promotes the important aspect of expressivity. Through melody the patient can find a way to put her feelings and musical intuition into her activity. Her creative energy is dynamically challenged and brought into an expressive form that makes sense to her. It may be that expressiveness, shown in this way, reflects the process of emotional recovery and points the way to a new identity. For breast cancer patients, faced with expressing overwhelming feelings, challenged with adjusting to a new, radically altered, future, the process of bringing their feelings into conscious form without any immediate verbal label may be a significant step on the road to recovery.

Simply exhorting women to express themselves, when that is the very problem itself, is futile. Encouraging the expression of anger may indeed be cathartic, but in the longer term may not be subtle enough, or positive enough, for prolonged recovery. Music therapy offers a means to expression that has no value labels of good or bad. Each woman is inspired to create her own expressions in her own time. She is given the opportunity to accept herself in a spontaneous, authentic way; she creates an identity that is aesthetic. In the therapeutic relationship this relationship is fostered as a form that is aesthetic, not moral. She performs, she is not judged. Her inner realities are experienced as beautiful.

Active, creative music therapy is an intervention that offers a chance for clients to use their own creativity and creative strength to cope with their crisis and maintain coherence on the way through the illness. In this sense music therapy can make a valuable contribution to the improvement in quality of life. In this way, it is possible to find a different musical form appropriate to the varying stages of the disease, whether they be towards recovery or through the accompaniment to dying. When we speak of accompanying the dying or promoting hope in the living, we are entering a realm of spiritual considerations.

Spirituality and Hope

> Our spirit is the real part of us, our body its garment. A man would not find peace at the tailor's because his coat comes from there: neither can the spirit obtain true happiness from the earth just because his body belongs to earth. (Khan 1979, p.76)

> Behind us all is one spirit and one life. How then can we be happy if our neighbour is not also happy? (Inayat Khan quoted in Khan 1979, p.123)

Terms like 'spirituality', 'hope', and 'creativity' are not commonly voiced in the world of medicine. However, palliative care has a tradition of breadth in its understanding of health care needs, and we find throughout the literature that the spiritual needs of patients are mentioned. It is this consideration of spirituality that I want to elaborate upon here, taking the link of hope with working creatively with music one step further.

What I am proposing is that in working with the dying and the chronically ill, we need to consider that which helps us to transcend our daily lives. Note that I am not separating practitioners and patients here, for we all surely face the great questions of life: 'What is the meaning of life, what is the nature of suffering, why me, what can I do?' Even though it is a fact that is often forgotten, we are all facing death, and in doing so we are all asked the question of how to live.

When we look at our lives from the perspective of how to live, we are faced with a crisis. I am using crisis here in a broad sense, to mean a judgement or discernment. Indeed, the difficulty faced in caring for dying patients is that while the problem appears to be that of chronic illness, in reality the challenges are acute and appear as a series of crises. Each crisis with a dying patient is a matter of identity: 'Who am I? What will become of me?'

We now have two questions, one concerned with existence and one with identity, and these questions have been the fundamental questions of all spiritual traditions. The practical ramifications of these questions are related to how we care for each other, and how we recognize each other's quality as a person? To answer these questions we need to be alive to a new consciousness.

The main emphasis of spirituality has always been that it will help us to achieve this new consciousness by transcending the moment. So too with the concept of hope; there is the expectation of a leap forward. In music therapy this transcending, expectant leap is made through the creative act.

Creativity occurs in the realization of an idea as created form. In the same way that the thoughts and ideas presented here have their own architecture realized in words; and as the architecture of the cathedral is realized in stone, so the architecture of music is realized in sounds. We can also be the architects of hope. By transcending the moment of suffering a new consciousness is created. This new consciousness is realized concretely in the performance of music. We play what we are. There is no precocious need to identify this as an emotional experience, rather to savour the experience in the moment itself.

As we saw in the first chapters, my assertion about the relationship between music and its benefit in clinical practice is that our human identity is a piece of symphonic music continually being composed in and of the moment. In contrast to a mechanistic metaphor of humanity that sees the body as an entity to be repaired, this view sees each being as vital and open to creation. We are improvised as a fresh identity according to every one of life's contingencies. Our very identities are created anew, although the theme may be repeated, and it is this repetition that gives us coherence as a 'personality'. Put another way, we are each a song that is continually being sung.

Music therapy is an activity which promotes the expression of this song. Each person is given the opportunity to define themselves creatively as they wish to be. What the person will become and how a personal future is defined, a future which is admittedly restricted and often tragically curtailed, are matters for joint therapeutic endeavour between therapist and patient (Aldridge 1991b). However, it is possible to realize ourselves in and of the moment not solely as a body restricted by infirmity, but transcended as a soul realizable in the music.

Even so, the end stage of our therapeutic endeavour is that the patient will die.

We know from clinical practice that the will to live is an important factor. Purpose and meaning in life are vital, and all too often are not questioned when we are in good health. But should we fall ill, then purpose and meaning become crucial to survival. Illness may be seen as a step on life's way which brings us in contact with who we really are. The positive aspect of suffering has been neglected in our modern scientific culture such that we, as practitioners and patients, often search for immediate relief. While the management of cancer pain has been a major contribution of the hospice movement, the understanding of suffering is still elusive in the literature. I am not suggesting that we actively seek out suffering, or deny that pain is debilitating, but want rather to remind us that part of the human condition is indeed to suffer. In seeking to relieve suffering we can value the opportunity it brings to learn. It may well be that the difficulties reported in effectively relieving pain are the result of the failure to identify suffering.

We are all asked the ultimate question of what meaning and purpose our lives would have had if we were to die now. Most of our activities cut us off from this brutal confrontation, except in the field in which you are working. While the management of pain is often a scientific and technical task, the relief of suffering is an existential task. In the major spiritual traditions suffering has always had the potential to transform the individual. As Tournier (1981) reminds us, it is love which has the power to change the sign of suffering from negative to positive.

What is spirituality?

The natural science base of modern medicine often ignores the spiritual factors associated with health. Health invariably becomes defined in anatomical or physiological, psychological or social terms. Rarely do we find diagnoses which include the relationship between the patient and their God. The descriptions we invoke have implications for the treatment strategies we suggest, and the way in which we understand how people can be encouraged to become healthy. Patience, grace, prayer, meditation, hope, forgiveness and fellowship are as important in many of our health initiatives as medication, hospitalization, incarceration or surgery. It is these spiritual elements of experience that help us to rise above the matters at hand such that in the face of suffering we can find purpose, meaning and hope.

Working as a psychiatrist, Hiatt (1986) offers an understanding of the spiritual in medicine which can also be worked with in psychological terms. 'Spirit refers to that noncorporeal and nonmental dimension of the person that is the source of unity and meaning, and "spirituality" refers to the concepts, attitudes, and behaviours that derive from one's experience of that dimension.' He suggests that by taking such a framework, we can discuss and use spiritual healing 'within a modified western framework [of medicine]' (p.742).

Table 10.1 Meanings of spirituality

author	description
Emblen, J. (1992)	'helping people to identify meaning and purpose in their lives, maintain personal relationships and transcend a given moment'
Kuhn, C. (1988)	'those capacities that enable a human being to rise above or transcend any experience at hand. They are characterized by the capacity to seek meaning and purpose, to have faith, to love, to forgive, to pray, to meditate, to worship, and to see beyond circumstances'
Hiatt, J. 91986)	'that aspect of the person concerned with meaning and the search for absolute reality that underlies the world of the senses and the mind and, as such, is distinct from adherence to a religious system'
Smyth, P. and Bellemare, D. (1988)	'that life has a purpose, to interpret personal illness in a way that makes sense of their world view'

Source: References in this book.

In recent years the word spiritual has appeared increasingly in the nursing literature where spiritual needs have been differentiated from religious needs (Boutell and Bozett 1990; Burkhardt 1989; Clark *et al.* 1991; Emblen 1992; Grasser and Craft 1984; Labun 1988; May 1992; Reed 1987; Stuart, Deckro and Mandle 1989). Within these approaches there is a core of opinion which accepts that suffering and pain are part of a larger life experience, and that they can have meaning for the patient, and for the carer(s) (Nagai Jacobson and Burkhardt 1989). The emphasis is placed upon the person's concept of God, sources of strength and hope, the significance of religious practices and rituals for the patient and their belief system (Soeken and Carson 1987). Spiritual well-being is also proposed as a hedge against suicide, providing some people with a reason for living (Ellis and Smith 1991) and as a mediator of depression (Fehring, Brennan and Keller 1987).

Spirituality, characterized by the idea of transcendence, has a broader perspective than religion. Religious care means helping people maintain their belief systems and worship practices. Spiritual care helps people to maintain personal relationships and relationship to a higher authority, God or life force (as defined by that individual); identify meaning and purpose in life; and transcend a given moment. This idea of transcendence, the ability to extend the self beyond the immediate context to achieve new perspectives, is seen as important in the last phases of life where dying patients are encouraged to maintain a sense of well-being in the face of imminent biological and social loss. Ross (1994) notes three necessary components to spirituality; the need to find meaning and purpose, the need for hope, and the need for faith in self, others and God.

Reed's study (1987) of spirituality and well-being in terminally ill hospitalized patients hypothesized that terminally ill patients would have a significantly greater spiritual perspective than non-terminally ill hospitalized adults with problems that were not typically life-threatening, and healthy non-hospitalized adults. For the terminally ill patients there was a shift towards greater spirituality, as indicated by a stronger faith and increased prayer.

Doctors, nurses and clergy have worked together to care for the dying (Conrad 1985; Reed 1987; Roche 1989), and a community approach which includes the family of the patient and his or her friends appears to be beneficial (Aldridge 1987). These benefits are a lessening of anxiety, general improvement in feelings of well-being and an increasing spiritual awareness for the dying person (Kaczorowski 1989). In addition, comprehensive treatment programmes for people with AIDS recommend that the spiritual welfare of the patient, and its influence on the well-being, is included (Belcher, Dettmore and Holzemer 1989; Flaskerud and Rush 1989; Gutterman 1990; Ribble 1989).

It is not only for the dying that spirituality plays a role. For the widow who must adapt to the loss of a partner, the ability to express her spirituality can, along with other criteria, play an important role in enhancing well-being. For young and old groups of widows attention to spiritual needs, physical exercise and a willingness to be self-indulgent all contributed to satisfy emotional and sexual needs.

Spirituality and religion, then, appear to be mediating factors for coping with an impending loss of life, and to be positive factors for maintaining well-being, particularly in older patients. When we consider patients in palliative care, then it is appropriate to consider what we can also do for their families and friends. Our patients rarely die alone, and surely the caregivers, familial, filial and professional, must be included for they too suffer, and it is they too who must transcend the moment.

Maintaining Integrity and Hope

> The true joy of every soul is in the realization of the divine spirit; the absence of realization keeps the soul in despair. (Inayat Khan 1979, p.105)

Positive emotions, which include the qualitative aspects of life – hope, joy, beauty and unconditional love – are known to be beneficial for the process of coping, both with the diagnosis of cancer, during the course of treatment and in post-operative recovery. This realm of positive emotion is precisely the ground in which the creative arts generally can have their own being. Patients can express themselves in a way which is creative and not limited by their disease. From such a perspective we would expect that although physical parameters may fluctuate or deteriorate, we would expect quality of life measures or existential indicators to show improvement.

Yates (1993) offers six dimensions of hope: the sensations and emotions of expectancy and confidence, a cognitive dimension that comprises positive perceptions and a belief that a desired outcome is realistically possible, a behavioural dimension where patients act on their positive beliefs to achieve their desires, a contextual dimension that links expectations with those of the family and friends, and a temporal dimension looking forwards or even backwards.

The true meaning of hope is that of an inclination towards something which we do not know. There is a longing for the unknown. We are all waiting for a change – even if it is a material change of circumstance – and this expectation is hope. Such hope cannot be touched, and often not understood; it is an attainment that may be described as beyond happiness, and above death.

Music therapy and the creative act

> Each individual composes the music of his own life. If he injures another he breaks the harmony, and there is discord in the melody of life. (Khan 1979, p.65)

Music therapy with its ability to offer an experience of time which is qualitatively rich, and not chronologically determined, is a valuable intervention. We are aware that music has soothing properties, and is used successfully as an anxiolytic (Aldridge 1993). Yet music can also be inspiring and uplifting (see Table 10.2). In its sacred use, music has been used to transport the listener to other realms of consciousness, and is used so in the final stages of dying (Schroeder-Sheker 1993). Indeed, the power of music is that it has the ability to calm us or to stir us in so many dimensions (Khan 1983) (see Table 10.3).

Table 10.2 Dimensions for fostering hope

Dimension of hope	Music therapy context
interpersonal context, relationship with others	therapeutic relationship
beliefs and cognition, identifying attainable aims	
spiritual base	uplifting music, the traditional role of sacred music, transcending the moment
personal attributes	being creative, being musical
light-heartedness	play in therapy
uplifting memories	listening to music, playing and singing remembered songs
affirmation of worth	activity of mutual music making

Table 10.3 Different dimensions of music

Dimension	Influence
popular	inducing motions of the body
technical	satisfying the intellect
artistic	that which has a tendency to beauty and grace
appealing	that which pierces the heart
uplifting	that in which the soul hears the harmony of the spheres

Music therapy, with the potential for bringing form out of chaos, should offer hope in situations of seeming hopelessness, and therefore a means of transcendence. This idea of transcendence, the ability to extend the self beyond the immediate context to achieve new perspectives, is seen as important in the last phases of life where dying patients are encouraged to maintain a sense of well-being in the face of imminent biological and social loss. Even in the midst of suffering it is possible to create something that is beautiful. This aesthetic expectation of self-in-relationship is positive – it is hope made manifest.

Significantly for many AIDS patients, personal relationships are deteriorating. Either friends die of the same illness, or social pressures urge an increasing isolation. Spontaneous contacts are frowned upon, and the intimacy of contact is likely to be that of the clinician rather than the friend. Music therapy offers an opportunity for intimacy within a creative relationship. This relationship is both non-judgemental and equal. The patient is encouraged to creatively form a new identity that is aesthetic, even in the face of disfigurement.

Working together in a creative way to enhance the quality of living can help patients make sense of dying (Aldridge 1987a). It is important for the dying, or those with terminal illness, that approaches are used which integrate the physical, psychological, social and spiritual dimensions of their being (Feifel 1990; Gary 1992; Herth 1990) (see Table 10.4). In addition, how we care for the sick and dying, no matter how they contracted their disease, is both a matter of our own personal responsibility and a collective measure of our humanity (Aldridge 1991a, 1991c).

Table 10.4 Coping requirements and changes associated with terminal illness

Coping with physical changes	Anticipation of pain
	Management of pain
	Management of the physical consequences of illness (nausea, incontinence) and change in physical appearance
	Management of the physical consequences of treatment
Coping with personal changes	Loss of hope, fitness and identity
	Anxiety and depression about the future
	Loss of role in family and in employment
	Frustration and helplessness
Coping with relationship changes	Resolution of conflict
	Change in parental roles
	Anxiety about future welfare (emotional and financial)
	Anticipated hospital contacts and treatment
	Anticipated loss of a family member or partner
	Planning the future
	Social isolation

Table 10.4 Coping requirements and changes
associated with terminal illness (continued)

	Changes in family boundary, and of family and marital emotional distance
	Negotiation of dependence/independence
	Saying, 'goodbye' and talking about dying
	Handling the above personal and physical changes within the context of an intimate relationship
	Changes in, and loss of, sexual activity
Coping with spiritual changes	Feelings of loss, alienation and abandonment
	Understanding suffering
	Accepting dependency
	Handling anger and frustration
	Forgiving others
	Discovering peace
	Discussing death
	Grieving
	Planning the funeral
	Discovering hope and the value of living

Note: It must be emphasized that these changes have ramifications at differing levels. Personal changes have implications for an intimate relationship, within the family and throughout the social environment.

In music therapy, the patient is required to be an active self-defining agent. The requirement is that the patient is moral, i.e. actively partaking and self-defining, when he or she is sick and suffering, not that they be subjected to our morality and definition.

Music therapy, with its emphases on personal contact and the value of the patient as a creative productive human being, has a significant role to play in the fostering of hope in the individual. Hope involves feelings, thoughts and necessitates action; i.e. like music it is dynamic and susceptible to human influence. Stimulating the awareness of living, in the face of dying, is a feature of the hospice movement where being becomes more important than having. The opportunity, offered by music therapy, for the patient to be remade anew in the moment, to assert an identity which is aesthetic, in the context of another person, separate yet not abandoned, is an activity invested with that vital quality of hope. Hope, when submitted to the scrutiny of the psychologist and not conforming to an established reality, can easily be interpreted as denial. For the therapist, hope is a replacement for therapeutic nihilism, enabling us to offer constructive effort and sound expectations (Menninger 1959).

Any therapeutic tasks must concentrate on the restoration of hope, accommodating feelings of loss, isolation and abandonment, understanding suffering, forgiving others, accepting dependency while remaining independent and making sense of dying. Music therapy can be a powerful tool in this process of change. Change can be accommodated within the overall rubric 'quality of life'. While the elusive life qualities inherent in creative activities, joy, release, satisfaction, simply being, are not readily susceptible to rating scales, we can hear them when they are played and feel them when they are expressed.

Music therapy appears to open up a unique possibility to take an initiative in coping with disease, or to find a level to cope with being close to death. It is this opening up of the possibilities which is at the core of existential therapies (Dreyfus 1987). Rather than the patient living in the realm of pathology alone, they are encouraged to find the realm of their own creative being, and that is in the music.

The Therapeutic Relationship

If the progress of disease is an increasing personal isolation, then the musico-therapeutic relationship is an important one for maintaining interpersonal contact. A contact that is morally non-judgemental, where the ground of that contact is aesthetic. For the sick, maimed, disfigured and stigmatized, the opportunity to partake in a greater beauty is important. Furthermore, the therapeutic question is not 'What am I?', a question which lies in the realm of categorization and cognition; but 'How am I?', which is one of being.

It is necessary to emphasize how important it is to keep our idea of creativity broad. A patient, when asked about the values of the various arts therapies he had recently had, commented, 'I did not want to be so intensely creative [as in the art therapy], but I did enjoy the music therapy where I could sing'. If being creative is used as a metaphor for new growth, and understood solely in its material implications, then no wonder that it will be rejected by some patients for whom new growth is a sign of a deterioration in health. Creativity can be used in the non-material sense, as in making music, as transcending the moment. In this transcendence, the essence of spirituality, we take a leap, which is hope, into a new consciousness. That this new consciousness is not bound up with our bodies, our instincts, our motor impulses, nor our emotions, awakens our awareness to another purpose within us.

Finally in our treatment initiatives, and research projects, it appears prudent to include the patient's caregivers. While this may be alien to some individual therapeutic directions, the overwhelming burden of care and suffering of daily living lies outside the clinic. If we consider the course of life, which includes dying, as a developmental process, that process will have a personal ecology. This ecology is relationship.

When we work over a long period of time, then we must include our selves and colleagues too in that ecology as we accompany our patients, in faith and hope, on that long journey which awaits us all.

Implications for Treatment

The intensification of the inner life through artistic activity helps provide a refuge from the emptiness of existence in a threatened future, but also provides a platform from which the next existential spring can be made. Having AIDS changes the experience of time. Many of those who have the disease are young. Suddenly they are faced with a provisional and uncertain existence. Without a goal, it is difficult to live for the future. To do something positive, to create, to play, is to take life seriously. The creative act then is to take the opportunity to live.

The creative act gives us the possibility of realizing something of value in the world. While passive appreciation of art and beauty enhance our aesthetic appreciation, the act of creation offers a way forward into the future. For those who are suffering, the creative act, no matter how small, offers the chance to achieve something concretely (Frankl 1963). By painting, singing, dancing, acting, or making music together we can bring the emotion of suffering into the world into a concrete form. Suffering made external as expression, and brought into form by art, gives the individual the chance to grapple with the meaning of that suffering and thereby bring about change. To quote Frankl (1963):

> Whenever one is confronted with an inescapable, unavoidable situation, whenever one has to face a fate that cannot be changed, such as an inoperable cancer, just then is one given a last chance to activate the highest value, to fulfil the deepest meaning, the meaning of suffering. For what matters above all is the attitude we take toward suffering, the attitude in which we take our suffering upon ourselves. (p.178)

The meaning of life is discovered, then, in concrete acts of creation which are aesthetic. What is internal is expressed externally as form. By bringing onto paper, or forming as sound, by moving the body in a sequence of dance or creating a narrative with dramatic intent, the individual takes responsibility for answering the questions which life asks. The answer to these questions of meaning are answered in what we do; that is, concrete activities performed out of individual destinies. Thus, the creative act retains its individuality and cannot be prescriptive. Furthermore, such an act is aesthetic, it brings into form, making coherent and manifest what is unintelligible and hidden (Arnheim 1992). As Langer (1953) writes, 'The function of art is to acquaint the beholder with something he has not known before' (p.22). Each situation is unique and needs a creative response. In this sense the creative act is one similar to play, which lies between the most personal, intimate and subjective sphere and the external world of objects (Winnicott 1951), in that it bridges the internal world of the individual and the external world of the therapeutic relationship (Robbins 1992).

The art form presents the whole intelligible form as an intuitive recognition of inner knowledge projected as outer form: subjective is made objective but in the terms of the subject and thereby unconventional. In artistic expression we have the possibility of making perceptible an inner experience. Music, drama and visual art are concerned not with the stimulation of feeling, but the expression of feeling. It may be more accurate to say here that feelings are not necessarily emotional state, more an expression of what the person knows as inner life (Aldridge 1989).

Our treatment initiatives should also be made early in the patient's illness career, soon after diagnosis, such that a relationship is made with the patient, and with the carers (see Table 10.5). The therapeutic relationship offers intimacy at a time when the individual is often threatened with isolation and rejection. We can help our patients discover their own sense of meaning by living out their lives in individual creative acts within the context of the therapeutic relationship. (Robbins (1992, p.178) refers to such situations as 'creative holding environments'). What we need is time, and the opportunity, to maintain long-term stability in the relationship, although the physical consequences of the disease continually remind us of the precariousness of corporeal existence. It is this very balance between the temporal aspects of the body and the existential act of living in that body which is at the crux of the therapeutic act.

Table 10.5 Treatment recommendations

Start early after diagnosis

Consider creative arts therapies as diagnostic tool

Develop a stable team, encourage long-term stability

Include the caregivers or partner in the therapy plan

Establish a support group for the professional caregiving team

Promote teamwork and identify common aims

Be ready for changes in physical status of the patient

Integrate the physical, psychological, social and spiritual

Be aware of the existential anxiety of working with AIDS patients; death, contagion, sexuality and disempowerment

Research Suggestions

Because of the nature of the disease and its individual progression it will be necessary to formulate research designs which follow individual patients over time (see Table 10.6). Such designs are longitudinal. There have been calls elsewhere for such longitudinal designs, combining scientific and artistic intellectual rigour, which follow the individual patient as they chart their course through the depths and shallows of their illness (Aldridge 1991a).

In any such study it is also necessary to consider various a recurring theme which is heard from varying perspectives. This theme concerns the necessity to include the views of the partners, or immediate family, of patients in any long-term therapeutic initiatives (Wolf et al. 1991).

To carry out such long-term research, which follows the course of an illness, it is necessary to develop a core team of practitioners and researchers who will remain with a project for its duration. The establishment of such a team is dependent upon adequate research funding, sufficient academic support and personal supervision for the personnel involved to sustain interest in a field of work which is notorious in the toll which it takes on the professionals involved. As research interviews and therapeutic practice can be emotionally demanding it is imperative to implement adequate supervision; a feature which is accepted in therapy but often neglected in research.

Table 10.6 Research recommendations

Promote prospective longitudinal studies

Develop a stable core research team, academic and clinical

Establish ethical guidelines for the use of collected information

Install procedure for continuing current literature review

Gather data from patients and their partners/families

Consider creative arts therapies as diagnostic tool

Identify appropriate health measures; life quality scales, hope index, diary recordings

Establish art and music archive of patient creations

Distinguish parameters for discerning treatment costs

Propose specific hypotheses for doctoral studies

As the field of practice is changing so rapidly, it is important to maintain a review of the current literature. There are a number of databases that provide background information about the field of AIDS research and will furnish the research team with valuable insights from other practitioners.

As neurological problems are a feature of HIV infection it should be possible to explore the contribution which the arts therapies can make to the detection of behavioural and functional changes. Creative arts therapies appear to offer sensitive assessment tools. They can be used to assess those areas of functioning, both receptive and productive, not covered adequately by other test instruments, i.e. fine motor behaviour, perseverance in context, attention, concentration and intentionality. In addition they provide forms of therapy which may stimulate cognitive activities such that behaviours subject to progressive failure are maintained (Aldridge and Aldridge 1992).

Buckwalter (Buckwalter et al. 1991) describes the outcomes of a study involving family members of communication-impaired long-term care residents in a collaborative nursing/speech language pathology intervention designed to increase the residents' communication ability. Family members provided memorabilia and artefacts or produced audio or videotapes, for use in conjunction with a speech therapy programme. Findings revealed that, despite a minimal improvement in speech ability, there was a dramatic increase in family members' satisfaction. As peers, partners or family play an important role in the process of therapy, and are susceptible to considerable distress too, then we must include assessments of their perceptions of therapeutic change.

Quality of life has become accepted in the assessment of cancer treatment programmes. If the HIV virus is endemic to populations and there is no cure for AIDS, our research endeavours must include some appraisal of quality of life (Catalan 1990). To this end, the use of established quality of life scales alongside individual assessment protocols will provide the therapist with feedback about the impact of their work on the ever-changing life of the patient.

There are varying quality of life scales in existence which have been tested for reliability and validity (Aaronson 1989; Bowling 1991; Clark and Fallowfield 1986; Gold 1986; Oleske, Heinze and Otte 1990; Porter 1986; Spitzer 1987).

The Hospital Anxiety and Depression scale was developed, from clinical experience, as a brief rating instrument to detect the extent of mood disorders as distinguished from the physical illness of the patient. Zigmond and Snaith (1983) purposefully excluded all items relating to physical disorder retaining only items relating to psychic symptoms, which is valuable with AIDS patients whose physical condition may deteriorate but psychological condition improve. As a scale in daily use it has proved to be reliable, easily understood by patients and easy to administer and evaluate by clinicians (Clark and Fallowfield 1986). Because the Hospital Anxiety and Depression scale is a self-report questionnaire, the patient gives an account of his or her own perception of quality of life. The generally accepted, but cruder, Karnofsky Performance Scale (Karnofsky, Abelmann and Craver 1948), while weighted towards the physical dimensions of quality of life, is physician-rated and considered to be flawed in that there are discrepancies between what doctors perceive and what patients perceive.

It is important to understand when using such scales that 'quality of life' has a multiplicity of meanings and, therefore, to some therapists the scales may seem naive and limited. Those researchers who have developed the scales know themselves that such limitations exist. Rather than develop an unwieldy global package, some researchers have concentrated on specific items gleaned from a factor analysis of many previously posed questions with an eye to developing a refined clinical instrument.

In addition to quality of life, the fostering of hope is seen as a valuable activity in patient care (Herth 1990, 1991). Herth's Hope Index is a useful screening tool that assesses hope over time and validates nursing diagnoses of hopefulness and hopelessness. Hope is a complex concept with many dimensions, yet it is possible using such a scale to assess the way in which patients view their future.

The message from all of this is to select the required test from a number of suggestions according to the particular research question being asked which is appropriate to clinical practice. Clinical scales are generally designed as a guide for practice and are easy to administer. Research instruments are often comprehensive in scope, time-consuming to administer (occasionally requiring training) and time-consuming to evaluate, and rich in material. Using previously validated questionnaires builds bridges between small initiatives and a greater body of knowledge helping the researcher to see the value of his or her work.

The above measures are concerned with the health status of the patient from a particular medical orientation, albeit broad in its incorporation of psychical, emotional, psychological, relational and social dimensions. What is clearly missing is the collection of material from the creative arts activities.

A standard method for active music therapy is to make an audio, or video, recording of the therapy session and then index this recording after the session. Such material is then available for assessment according to given criteria, and for evaluation for validation by peers. Similarly, graphic (Niederreiter 1990; Oliveri 1991) and plastic material produced in the studio can be saved to show a progression during the course of the therapy. This work can also be photographed when each item is completed, or at stages during the course of creation. With new advances in computer technology it is possible to develop photographs as prints, and to commit the same images for archiving electronically on a compact disc. Such images then can be saved in a database, displayed later on a monitor screen and incorporated into research documents. By saving images over time it is possible to gain an overview of recurring elements, variations, and changes in composition and form.

Although it is difficult enough for music therapists to agree on an established language for research, there are grounds to believe that active co-operation is possible between creative arts therapeutic disciplines (Aldridge, Brandt and Wohler 1990). It is important that a research structure is established such that creative arts therapists regularly meet to discuss their work, and in doing so develop a common language. Our experience is that changes in form whether sculpted, painted, drawn or played occur concurrently. The task we face is to correlate such changes in the creative therapies with changes according to other measures of health outcome. Furthermore, we need to establish what are our expectations of patients in their first therapy sessions. We know little about how adults spontaneously create in various media, i.e. sing, move, draw or paint, particularly when they are previously untutored and unpractised.

With the extended costs of health care for the AIDS patient playing a significant role in health care delivery; when medical insurance support is likely to be exhausted; or for the poor, non-existent (Faden and Kass 1990); the financial burden of health care is going to fall on to the shoulders of the wider community. Any new initiatives will need to establish the cost of treatment over time. While the creative arts therapies are labour-intensive and time-consuming, the potential savings in terms of the use of fewer expensive pharmaceutical products, less long-term use of medical facilities, and possible extended survival rates, are valuable (Krupnick and Pincus 1992). The estimation of such costs will depend upon developing methodologies which include clinical outcome measures (e.g. the above-mentioned quality of life scales), functional outcome measures (e.g. the ability to care for the family, number of days lost from work) and the costs of health care utilization. To do this we need to establish the routine inclusion of cost data in our studies and establish clinical outcome criteria which make sense for the patients, clinicians and therapists involved and the policymakers responsible for third party methods of reimbursement (Aldridge 1990a).

McCormick et al. (McCormick et al. 1991) observe that AIDS has become a chronic disease, and the demand for long-term care has increased. The authors studied a cohort of hospitalized persons with AIDS to determine the proportion and characteristics of 120 AIDS patients who could appropriately be cared for in long-term care facilities with skilled nursing on the medical wards of five Seattle tertiary care hospitals. The appropriateness for long-term care was determined by the patients' physicians, nurses, and social workers according to four admission criteria: impaired activities of daily living, diagnosis of central nervous system illness or poor cognition, living alone, and weight loss. One-third of hospitalized persons with AIDS were considered to be appropriate for care in long-term care settings, accounting for one-third of the days AIDS patients currently spend in hospitals. These patients could be identified early in hospital stays using a simple clinical index based on the criteria above.

In formulating such a research proposal it is apparent that the suggestions are general. We must develop specific research studies, but as yet we have limited experience. The research tradition in the creative arts therapies is limited. Music therapy, in particular, has no established research methodology although there is a body of research material in the music therapy and medical press (Aldridge 1993, 1993c). There are, however, research methods and clinical outcomes measures which can be utilized from other spheres of practice. A priority must be to get started doing research as a series of longitudinal pilot studies.

Cautions about practice and research

Music therapy can be used as an adjuvant therapy complementary to medical initiatives in palliative care. In modern scientific medicine people are transformed into the objects of research. They are classified into disease groupings. This objectification, and the conditional requirement that they remain passive to keep the status 'sick' not 'deviant', is challenged by AIDS patients. In contrast, the creative therapies expect the patient to be an active self-defining agent. The requirement is that the patient is moral, i.e. actively partaking and self-defining, when he or she is sick and suffering, not that they be subjected to our morality and definition, i.e. passive and judged.

Foucault challenges us to find a new truth which is creative and performed free from the politics of medical authority (Rawlinson 1987). It is this freedom of truth and practice which we must encourage with our AIDS patients. The therapist and the patient can challenge the notions that we must always be able to do something and that everything which is humanly significant is subject to measurement.

At the centre of the AIDS debate is a massive existential anxiety which patients, and we as therapists, face. This anxiety is based upon the confrontation with death, the fear of contagion, the challenge to our sexual orientation, the exercise of power over another, and the reality of poverty in a material world.

Death, the inevitable end process of living which is so often ignored, comes into the foreground, and thereby the normal expectation of medical endeavour, that the patient will recover to a state of normative health, is challenged.

Contagion, the fear of being invaded, is ever-present. Despite our knowledge of the transmission of the virus, our fears of contagion have little to do with such rationality. For example, in talking with general practitioners and oncologists about working with cancer patients the difficulty for the doctors was the fear of 'catching cancer'; an irrational fear in a purportedly rational scientific enterprise (Aldridge 1987c).

Sexuality, which we learn to express, and which we take for granted as part of our identity, is seen as a matter of choice and preference, not as solely dictated by our genetic make-up. The notion of 'sex' makes it possible to group together in an artificial unity anatomical elements, biological functions, conducts, sensations and pleasures suitable to the scrutiny of modern scientific medicine (Dreyfus 1987).

Foucault (1988, 1989) describes such a tendency, to normalize all aspects of human behaviour and bring them under medical control, as bio-power. The effect of this power on the patient is that he responds in the same way to every situation as if his possible responses had become reduced to one form. For Foucault the therapeutic act is to bring about a change in such structuring, to give the life of the patient the stability and the uniqueness of a work of art as we saw in the epigraph that opens this chapter.

We know too that patients are socially vulnerable, and that their caregivers, particularly in the face of children with AIDS, are disadvantaged. Poverty is a challenge to us all in that no matter what therapeutic skills we bring to bear, and no matter how we strive for our own empowerment, we are continually faced with the blight of material neglect. How we care for the poor, the sick and the dying, no matter how they contracted their disease, is both a matter of our own personal responsibility and a collective measure of our humanity (Aldridge 1991b).

Fostering Hope and the Quality of Life

Music therapy, with its emphasis on personal contact and the value of the patient as a creative productive human being, has a significant role to play in the fostering of hope in the individual. Hope involves feelings and thoughts and necessitates action; that is, it is dynamic and susceptible to human influence. Stimulating the awareness of living, in the face of dying, is a feature of the hospice movement where being becomes more important than having. The opportunity offered by the creative arts activities, for the patient to be remade anew in the moment, to assert an identity which is aesthetic in the context of another person, separate yet not abandoned, is an activity invested with that vital quality of hope and also true to the epigraph at the beginning of this chapter. For the therapist, hope is a replacement for therapeutic nihilism, enabling us to offer constructive effort and sound expectations (Menninger 1959).

Any therapeutic tasks must concentrate on the restoration of hope, accommodating feelings of loss, isolation and abandonment, understanding suffering, forgiving others, accepting dependency while remaining independent and making sense of dying. Creative arts therapies can be powerful tools in the this process of change. These changes can be accommodated within an overall rubric of quality of life. While quality of life scales exist for the general clinical assessment of cancer patients, they fall short of meeting the requirements for individual patients. Expectations of quality of life differ. Furthermore, the elusive life qualities inherent in creative activities, joy, release, satisfaction, simply being, are not readily susceptible to rating scales. We can, however, hear them when they are played, see them when they are painted or danced, and feel them when they are expressed drama-turgically.

In the next chapter, we shall also see that providing hope for children who are deemed to be developmentally delayed is also a significant factor in promoting their potential as children, but plays an important role for the well-being of the caregivers to those children too. Creative music therapy as described in these chapters is concerned with individual treatment. However, the ramifications of that treatment are not solely for the individual. Knowing that something can be done to relieve discomfort and pain, to lighten the burden of daily living, is an important understanding. When a cure cannot be found, or is not immediately in sight, then our therapeutic responsibilities do not cease. Indeed, for the patients who are presented within these pages, there is no immediate cure in sight. The children in the following chapter are irretrievably handicapped. However, the implications of a handicap should not be restricted through our desire for heroic treatment endeavours or an idealized picture of the perfect human form. We are all in some ways damaged, and all have the opportunity to present ourselves as works of art, and thus perfect in our very being.

CHAPTER ELEVEN

Creative Music Therapy in the Treatment of Children with Developmental Delay

This chapter attempts to demonstrate that creative music therapy is a viable therapeutic form for developmentally delayed children, and in doing so elucidate what it is in the therapy that is valuable. For referring parents, paediatricians, and payers (potential funding agencies and third party medical insurers) alike, we need to present evidence that the work that we are engaged in has a value that makes sense to them. This book has been about my conviction that music therapy is a valuable enterprise within the field of health care. While I am convinced of the value of this work according to my criteria, the overall endeavour of this book has been to convince readers that music therapy is effective, or at least that it is worthy of serious consideration. In the following pages I am going to turn my gaze to working with children with developmental delay and suggest ways in which I believe that music therapy helps them. This means that the wheel of understanding presented in this book has turned full circle. I started with my observations of music therapy with a woman with disabilities, moving through various considerations of working with patients in hospital, older patients and, in the last chapter, those who are dying. Now I return to the theme of disability again, this time in children. In the bigger scheme of things, it is also a return to the roots of this form of music therapy as it was developed out of work with autistic and severely disabled children by Paul Nordoff and Clive Robbins (1971, 1975, 1977).

I shall be using an integrated approach to music therapy research that combines both a quantitative approach, as shown by the measurement of changes, and a qualitative approach, as argued from the interpretation of empirical data. While this first purpose may seem rather paradoxical, given the arguments proposed in previous chapters, the underlying reason is that I hope to show that in music therapy research we can creatively adapt techniques and forms of argumentation to suit our needs. We do not have to take a polarized stance, either for or against qualitative or quantitative methods. Indeed, the danger of my previous arguments has been to maintain an ideological position, either falling into the trap of methodolatry on one hand, or scientism on the other. By emphasizing one approach we are in danger of prematurely restricting our research possibilities. However, I stand behind the arguments that music therapy needs methods related to the music itself and that quantities and scales cannot adequately reflect personal meanings. What is emerging is that no single approach can meet all the needs of music therapy research. We have to find methods appropriate to the task in hand, and to the audience for whom the research is intended. Our knowledge gleaned here from practice is for real people; this is not a disembodied academic debate. Indeed, as mentioned above, the purpose of the research throughout this book has been to convince a variety of readers. This diversity in the audience will inevitably mean a variety of forms of evidence, collected by various activities. Rather than rebutting one approach in favour of another, I am seeking a tolerance of variety that seeks varying indications for demonstrating the efficacy of music therapy. In a field where we have few research findings, then our primary purpose is to gather together what we have to serve the purpose of helping our patients.

Research methods are simply tools for structuring our thinking, and gathering the evidence that we will use to support our arguments. In some ways I am rehearsing a debate that has already been comprehensively argued in both the fields of nursing (Dzurec and Abraham 1986, 1993) and social psychology (Shadish and Fuller 1994). By relating both sets of information, qualitative and quantitative, it may be possible to generate insights not available from the two types of information separately (Heyink and Tymstra 1993).

The overall aim here is to present music therapy with children suffering from a variety of developmental challenges, and propose that by using a particular form of assessment available to other music therapists we can see that a beneficial change occurs quantitatively. The reason for that change, I shall argue, is attributable to specific qualities of creative music therapy. Some of the benefits of music therapy we will see, while not being quantifiable, are significant to the parents of the children involved.

The music therapy approach taken here is based upon Nordoff and Robbins' improvised music therapy, which has its origins in working with children with developmental delay. However, while there is a wealth of case study material in the music therapy literature concerning music therapy with such children (Bang 1986; Bean 1995; Bunt 1994; Howat 1995; Oldfield

1995; Warwick 1995; Wigram 1995; and see Bruscia 1991 and Decker-Voigt, Eschen and Mahns 1993 for collected works), and a considerable literature suggesting the value of music therapy for child development (Wilson and Roehmann 1987), there have been few controlled studies of Nordoff–Robbins music therapy with children with disabilities.

An important feature of childhood development is the acquisition of speech and the ability to communicate meaningfully with another person. Music therapy encourages children without language to communicate and has developed a significant place in the treatment of developmental delay in children. How such communication is achieved, and how in some instances it leads to speech, are as yet unknown. Indeed, the very ability to develop and achieve speech in normal children is a miracle of daily living which continues to baffle linguists and psychologists. While this chapter makes no attempt to solve the riddle of how speech is brought about, I will attempt to demonstrate how music therapy helps the developmentally/challenged child progress towards a richer communicative life.

Developmental delay can be the consequence of various difficulties, physical, mental or social (Lewis and Volkmar 1990). Children who are developmentally challenged experience the same emotional conflicts and difficulties as normal children; however, they are also more likely to experience rejection when they fail to meet standards of expectation associated with their chronological age. This rejection can lead to behavioural disturbances. The successful social integration of children with developmental delay relies upon a sensitive and adaptable social environment, as does the sequence of development itself. If the environment is both modified to meet the needs of the children and to enhance communication possibilities according to the child's potential, then we might expect fewer behavioural problems. Children who are developmentally delayed face the same developmental tasks and challenges, and have the same needs to be loved, stimulated and educated, as any child. What they face is a progression that may be slower and which may perhaps limit their future capabilities. Our therapeutic task is to respond to abilities and potentials such that those limitations themselves are minimized. If both environment and the individual are important for developmental change, the therapist provides, albeit temporarily, an environment in which individual change can occur. It is this ecological understanding of child, or infant, in interaction that is at the heart of music therapy and many current speculations about the development of communication (Cohen and Levesque 1994; Elias and Broerse 1995; Reed 1995).

Child Development and Challenges to Theory

Child development itself is subject to various theories and is a continuing source of active academic debate. All children are now conceived of as very active constructive thinkers and learners, rather than passive copiers of what is given to them (Case 1993; Lewis 1993). Children select and transform what is meaningful for them from the context within which they find themselves. What is selected and transformed is in part in accordance with their cognitive abilities, yet these abilities are not separate from other related developmental processes. Each child may differ in his or her development. Furthermore, children not only take from the environment, they too give out signals which modify their environment. Infants give clues to their mothers about how they expect them to react. Improvised creative music therapy, then, with its emphasis on activity within a dynamic personal relationship, may play a role in encouraging development, particularly when it focuses on communicative abilities.

The idea that children change in regular stages that are governed by their biology, and that they become progressively better in a linear evolutionary development, is being challenged (Florian 1994; Macnamara 1993; Morss 1992; Ross, Friman and Christophersen 1993; Siegel 1993; Sipiora 1993; Spieker and Bensley 1994; Wagner, Torgesen and Rashotte 1994). Morss (1992) calls for an interpretative, as opposed to a causal-explanatory, approach to human experience and proposes that studies of infancy are often studies of scientists studying infancy, and, like Sipiora (1993), finds that the infant under study is often absent. Sipiora criticizes Piaget for skewing the natural choice of questions answerable only by a child to those of an adult consciousness. Pure observation cannot always distinguish the child from his or her beliefs, and it is the inner life of the child, what he or she wishes to communicate, which should be the focus of our attention. Siegel (1993) reminds us that this debate is not entirely new and, interestingly for the creative arts therapies, that non-verbal tasks are the best means of representing the thinking of the very young child. She also emphasizes that Piagetian developmental stages are not supported empirically and what may seem to be an orderly sequence of acquisition may indeed be an artefact of the way in which tasks are structured. The outcome of this debate is that in understanding children we are encouraged to study processes rather than products, and that those processes when related to assessment will always occur in a dialogue between child and therapist.

If we return briefly to the research purpose of this chapter, we can propose that a qualitative method of research will be necessary to look at this process of developmental change as it occurs between therapist and child, and a quantitative method can help us to identify specific changes.

The above challenge to Piagetian orthodoxy is based partly on a questioning of the orthodoxy of the spoken word as being primary (Ross, Friman and Christophersen 1993). Some authors are concentrating on how children perform in the world, which is a 'world-of-others', as the principal focus for attention. Play is seen as a mental act including unconscious fantasies and wishes, a physical act which is observable and a necessary awareness that what is being enacted is 'play'. Play, when defined by its functions, facilitates the libidinization of the body and is an area of importance bridging the realms of the personal and the social (Lewis 1993). For Vygotsky (1978) this intermediary realm, the distance between what children can do on their own and what they can do with the help of an adult, is referred to as the proximal zone. It is such a 'zone' which we find in creative music therapy. Musical activity is based upon what the child can do in musical play, but the potential of what the child can do further is based upon what child and therapist are capable of together. Furthermore, with an emphasis on the activity of musical playing within the context of a personal relationship, the libidinization of the body is achieved as a communicative act.

In our work we emphasize the role of the therapist as encouraging and providing the context in which musical communication take place. The therapeutic relationship is a relationship that mirrors the primary relationship of learning to communicate in which development emerges. Vandenberg (1991) reminds us that looking, hearing, smelling, sucking and grasping are some of the early reflexes for assimilating objects and the basis from which cognitive development emerges. At birth, children are most responsive to the human voice through hearing. It is this orientation to the social world of others which is of such importance. The special relationship with others is something that is 'elaborated from those primitive forms of attunement' (p.1282). This is a reflection of the position taken by Stern (1985) that the infant has a core self which is in a relationship with the core self of the other, and this relationship forms a crucial axis of development. The symbolic world of the child is imbued with the relationship with the caregiver and others of significance. My proposal is that such a relationship is essentially 'musical'.

In Chapter Three I emphasized the importance of rhythmic interaction for the development of language and socialization in the infant. From birth the infant has the genetic basis of an individually entrained physiology, that is, a self-synchronicity. The infant has its own time, yet the process of socialization and the use of language depend upon entraining those rhythms with those of another. Biorhythms are considered to be a basic of life in terms of co-ordinating oxygen requirements, gastric reflux, the pattern of melatonin and serotonin secretion (which is linked to colic and crying) the sleep–wake cycle and respiratory rhythms (Thomas 1995). Cycles of rhythmic interaction between infants and mothers reflect an increasing ability by the infant to organize cognitive and affective experience within the rhythmic structure provided by the parent. This organization, however, is not a one-sided phenomenon. Infants produce forms of expression and gesture that are not imitations of maternal behaviour. Both baby and mother learn each other's rhythmic structure and modify their own behaviour to fit that structure. Arousal, affect and attention are learned within the rhythm of a relationship.

The competence of infants is not solely a quality inherent within the individual. Individuals are located in particular environments, those of their significant relationships. Gaussen (1985) criticizes maturational models of child assessment in that they do not take into account the variability and individual differences of the developmental processes. Assessment methods rely on how the child responds and moves; they tell little about what the child knows and responds to. Such a criticism echoes that of the authors above, who wish to know more of the inner life of the child, a life which is not solely dependent upon intact motor responses.

Nevertheless, communication is dependent upon motor co-ordination, and motor responses, as we shall read below, are important indicators that a child is developing. For the parent, rather than the theoretician and psychologist, the pragmatics of understanding the child is based upon what that child can do. Furthermore, communication is also dependent upon doing. What that 'doing' means is important, but achieving that 'doing' and co-ordinating with another person, is primary. Hence the value of non-verbal therapies, and the establishment of a communicative relationship before the complexities of lexical meaning are necessary.

Motor Development, Gesture and Communication

The development of the child demands many integrated skills. One important skill is to control motor activity, that is, to be able to draw, and write, handle a knife and fork, play with a ball and run. Children who do not master such activities are often labelled as clumsy, whereupon they meet with disapproval from their peers and often from family members. On reaching play-school or school age these children find themselves facing ridicule. Such ridicule may then lead to a lack of self-esteem and confidence which is further exacerbated by social withdrawal (Laszlo and Sainsbury 1993). Once such children find they cannot perform 'properly' they give up trying. The consequences of such personal and social handicap as clumsiness, or perceptual-motor dysfunction, remain in adult life.

Three main processes are assumed to be necessary for the performance of motor skills: kinaesthesis, muscle control and timing (Laszlo and Sainsbury 1993). Kinaesthesia is 'the conscious ability to discriminate the position of body parts and the amplitude, direction, timing and force of movement without visual or auditory cues' (Willoughby and Polatajko 1995, p.790). This sixth sense, referred to by Sacks as 'proprioception', is a sense which we have in our bodies and is 'that continuous but unconscious sensory flow from the movable parts of our body (muscles, tendons, joints), by which their position and tone and motion is continually monitored and adjusted, but in a way which is hidden from us because it is automatic and unconscious' (Sacks 1986, p.42).

Proprioception is indispensable for our sense of self, in that we experience our bodies as our own. Muscle control refers to the way in which movement is directed and controlled spatially. These movements must also be co-ordinated, and this involves timing. Laszlo and Sainsbury (1993), however, argue that kinaesthesis is the overarching factor which unites both direction and timing in the control of posture, in error detection and in memorizing movements. Indeed, the co-ordinating of action involves the whole body and von Hofsten (1993) asserts that it can only be understood as a purposive dynamic future-oriented interaction between the organism and the external world. Actions originate not from reflexes, but from spontaneously produced, purposeful controlled movements; in other words, actions develop through action. Yet this action must be structured, and this structure is that of time. Active music therapy would seem to be an ideal medium for encouraging purposeful controlled movement in a time structure that is formed yet flexible.

Gestures also help us understand what a child means, and what stage of understanding a child is in (Alibali and Goldin-Meadow 1993; Goldin-Meadow, Alibali and Church 1993). Gesture is spontaneous and often idiosyncratic, whereas speech conforms to an established form. Some expressive events may be better encoded in communications as gestures for some children at their stage of understanding, in that gesture maps the phenomena closely. Indeed gestures in a communication dialogue are pre-verbal and do not need the extra abstract and lexical dimension of speech (Braake and Savage-Rumbaugh 1995). It is gestural activities that are actively utilized in the repertoire of play songs used in the Nordoff–Robbins approach, and that I am suggesting are significant precursors in the promotion of speech using music therapy interventions.

Active music therapy then would seem to be a relevant therapy form as it concentrates on, and fosters, the use of purposive co-ordinated movements which occur in a context of time and relationship, i.e. music, offering a form for communication without words. It is important to emphasize the concept of dialogue as a joint activity (Cohen and Levesque 1994). Both parties to a music therapy improvisation are responsible for that activity, and must have a joint commitment to its continuing. Such joint commitment must take into account the intentionality of the children themselves to join in the musical playing. Vedeler (1994) describes intentionality as being a dynamic relationship that appears at first as a social-communicative intentionality and then as a thing-oriented intentionality.

Developing Children and Music Therapy

Twelve patients were assessed, selected and randomly allocated into two groups of six children (see Figure 11.1). Each child was to receive individual music therapy. This formed a treatment group, and an initial non-treatment

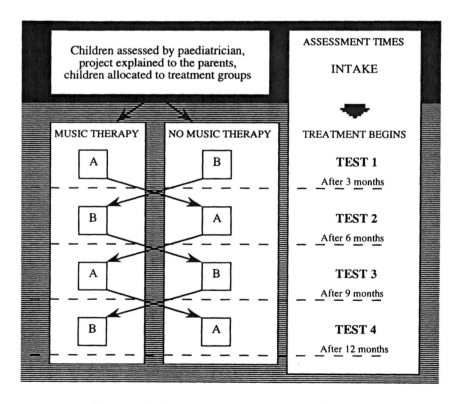

Figure 11.1 Allocation of children to treatment groups and study design

group to serve as a waiting-list control. The non-treatment group received music therapy after waiting for three months, while the previously treated children had a break from therapy. Our intention was to stay as close to the clinical practice of music therapy as possible. This intention influenced the timing of the treatment stages in that a course of music therapy treatment takes about three months followed by a three-month pause. Similarly, we could only ever take on six new patients in one treatment period. All the subjects of this study would receive music therapy, and the maximum treatment delay after intake would be for three months.

Entrance criteria were that the children should be 4 to 6.5 years old in chronological age, with a developmental age of 1.5 to 3.5 years; and that the selected children had no previous experience of music therapy. Children were excluded from the study if they had a physical problem which was degenerative, if the child was currently receiving psychopharmaceutical treatment, or if the child was currently attending another form of creative art therapy. Play-school or kindergarten attendance was not interrupted.

The use of a waiting-list control and alternating treatment periods met our ethical demands for the treatment of children in terms of clinical research, in that both procedures mirrored our normal practice. Furthermore, the study was clearly explained to all the participating parents and caregivers of the children, who were assured that refusal to take part in the study would not disqualify their children from treatment. Similarly, all participants were asked to give permission for the use of the data as part of a research project and for possible publication.

Referrals were from a local paediatrician who assessed the children before treatment began (at intake). We had previously set the criteria for the clinical assessment of developmental change (see below). A medical student, trained in the assessment of children, saw the children and their caregivers every three months to assess any clinical changes according to the medical criteria (Tests 1, 2, 3 and 4 after intake). She was initially 'blind' as to whether the children were in the treatment or non-treatment group.

The main assessments were *developmental* according to psychological and functional criteria (the Griffiths' test; see Table 11.1), and *musical* according to the Nordoff–Robbins rating scales (see Figures 11.2 and 11.3). Music therapy sessions were recorded on audiotape and later indexed according to music therapy criteria.

Table 11.1 Contents of the Griffiths Scales of Assessment

Griffiths' Subscales

A: Locomotor Development

pushes with feet, lifts head, kicks vigorously, begins to crawl, climbs, can walk on tiptoe, catches a ball, hops and skips

B: Personal-Social Scale

responds to being held, smiles, resists adult taking a toy away, anticipatory movements, plays 'pat-a-cake', plays with other children, has a special friend

C: Hearing and Speech

most intellectual of the scales, indicative of hearing problems; startled by sounds, vocalization other than crying, searches for sound visually, listens to music,[1] listens to conversations, rings bell, likes rhymes and jingles, enjoys story-books, develops words and speech, names objects, defines by use, comprehends sentences

D: Hand and Eye Co-ordination

by observing the hands of the child, follows visually moving objects, uses hands for exploration, points with fingers, likes holding toys, plays with bricks, scribbles freely, builds a tower, folds paper, copies shapes, draws recognizable figures and objects

E: Performance Tests

measures skill in manipulation, speed of working and precision with an awareness of the child's eagerness and persistence; searches for toy under a cup, manipulates cubes and boxes, opens screw-topped jars, makes patterns[2]

F: Practical Reasoning

recognition of differences in size and categorizing as 'bigger', this scale measures the ability to reason in 'embryo'. Any child before he or she can express ideas verbally can look, listen, think and learn the foundations of knowledge and the way in which the mind works in apprehension of the environment

Note:
[1] there is an overall neglect of musical ability.
[2] there is, however, no mention of musical patterns.
Source: after Griffiths (1954).

Rating Sheet

Child: **Date:**   **Session:**
                                               Therapist: **Rater:**

Level of participation	*Qualities of resistiveness*	*Ratings*
(10) Establishment of functional independence in group work		
(9) Stability and confidence in musical relationships. Constructive participation in group activities	Through identification with the therapist's expectation resists own regressive tendencies	
(8) Mutuality in the expressive mobility of the music	(a) crisis-towards resolution (b) no resistiveness	
(7) Assertive co-activity. Working relationship	Perseverative compulsiveness and/or assertive inflexibility. Contest. Rebelliousness	
(6) Activity relationship developing	Perversity and/or manipulativeness	
(5) Limited response activity	Evasive defensiveness	
(4) Wary ambivalence. Tentative acceptance	Anxious uncertainty. Tendency toward rejection	
(3) Awareness but not acceptance	Continuous negativism	
(2) Fleeting signs of awareness	Withdrawal to the autistic state	
(1) Total obliviousness	Imperviousness. Rage reaction when pressed	

Source: Nordoff and Robbins (1977, p.182)

Figure 11.2 Scale 1: Child–Therapist Relationship in Musical Activity

Rating Sheet

Child: **Date:**   **Session:**
                                              Therapist: **Rater:**

	Modes of activity			
Levels of communicativeness	*Instru-mental*	*Vocal*	*Body movements*	*Rating totals*

(10) Commitment to musical
     objectives in group work

(9) Musical intelligence and
     skills freely functioning
     and communicable

(8) Enthusiasm for musical
     creativity. Musical
     competence

(7) Attentive mobile
     responsiveness. Self-
     expressive musical
     confidence

(6) Participating communicative
     response-ability established.
     Involvement in indiv-
     idualized forms of activity

(5) Sustaining of directed
     response-impulses setting
     up musical communication

(4) Momentary musical
     perception and directedness

(3) Evoked responses (ii): more
     sustained and musically formed

(2) Evoked responses (i): fragmentary

(1) No communicative responsiveness

Source: Nordoff and Robbins (1977, p.196)
Figure 11.3 Scale 2: Musical communicativeness

Our main hypothesis was that there would be greater developmental changes in the music therapy treatment group, in the first session of the treatment period, compared with the non-treatment group. Our secondary hypothesis was that by the end of the two treatment sessions both groups would have changed equally.

The Griffiths Scale and the Nordoff–Robbins Rating Scale

Ruth Griffiths, as a psychologist, spent a great deal of time observing babies and small children. From these observations she developed a series of scales which could be used to gain insight into areas of learning in young children. The function of these scales was not to say categorically what the reason might be for a child's slowness to learn, rather to diagnose those areas of a child's capability and to provide a profile of capabilities from which the child might respond to treatment. This emphasis on the positive potential of the scales was initially attractive for our work as it reflected, and had features complementary with, the approach of Nordoff–Robbins music therapy in focusing on the inherent potentials of the child rather than concentrating on the known pathologies. Reading her book (Griffiths 1954), which was written over 40 years ago, is a fascinating insight into the rigour of a scientist who clearly has a love for children, and how that rigour can be applied in the assessment of behaviour. Sometimes creative arts therapists criticize science for seemingly leaving out the individual and thereby losing any relevance for treatment. With Griffiths, however, there is a constant reminder that these scales were crafted from a devotion to the lot of those children who were in need such that we, as carers of those children, could better our own observations to meet their needs.

There are six sub-scales with equal degrees of difficulty. Each sub-scale tests a different avenue of learning with the intention of discovering true potentialities in the child with disabilities (Griffiths 1954, pp.171–172). Once such potentials are recognized, help can be brought as early as possible when needed. Indeed, the tests are intended to educate the carers and the educators about the needs of the child. While the central plank of the assessment work is to provide a differential diagnosis of mental status (see Figure 11.4), that diagnosis is clearly linked with potentials for treatment.

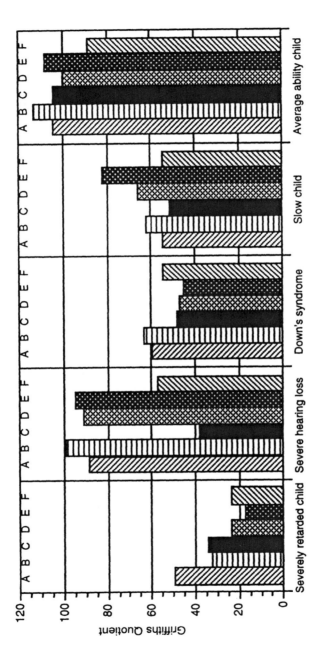

A = locomotor development
B = personal-social relationship
C = hearing and speech

D = hand and eye co-ordination
E = performance tests
F = practical reasoning

Figure 11.4 Examples of Griffiths' profiles for varying groups of children

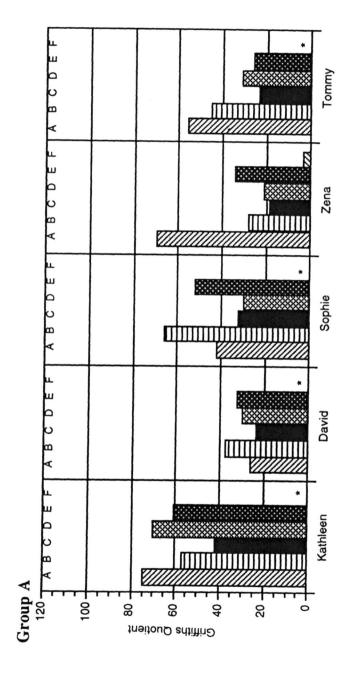

Figure 11.5 Griffiths quotient intake profiles

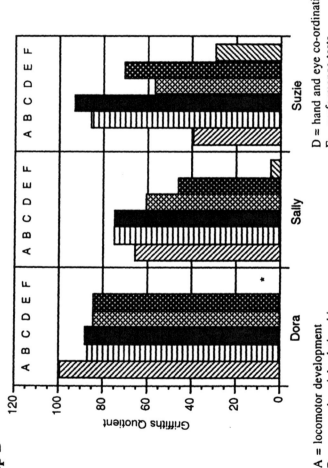

A = locomotor development   D = hand and eye co-ordination
B = personal-social relationship   E = performance tests
C = hearing and speech   F = practical reasoning
Note that four of the children in Group A, and one child in Group B, do not score on the practical reasoning
scale.

Figure 11.5 Griffiths quotient intake profiles (continued)

Attempts were made by Nordoff and Robbins as early as 1964 to develop rating scales for individual music therapy (Nordoff and Robbins 1977). However, these evaluative scales proved to be difficult to compose so as adequately to meet the complexity of musical responses. Two years later, scales for evaluating autistic children in a day centre were adapted for music therapy use, and evolved as 'Scale 1: Child–Therapist Relationship in Musical Activity' (Figure 11.2) and 'Scale 2: Musical Communicativeness' (Figure 11.3).

Scale 1 evaluates the relationship between child and therapist as it develops from what may be total obliviousness, through limited response, to a stability and confidence in the mutuality of playing music together. It must be stressed that it is in the musical activity that the relationship is developed, and the vocabulary used to evaluate the performance of the child is mainly musical. While Nordoff and Robbins stress that the evaluation is of the relationship itself, the language itself places emphasis on evaluating the child, that is, we would not expect the therapist to be totally oblivious to the child.

Scale 2 attempts to evaluate both the state of musical communication in the session, and 'provides an index to the personality development of a child through assessing the character and consistency of the musical communicativeness he manifests' (Nordoff and Robbins 1977, p.193). The scale includes three modes of activity: instrumental, vocal and body movement, which provide an aggregate rating on ten levels of communication ranging from 'no communicative response', through active participation, to an intelligent musical commitment. Both scales are rather rough-and-ready and have never really been validated in clinical practice as research instruments, although the scales do provide a valuable guide to clinical practice and evaluation for assessing individual change. A comprehensive third scale exists but is demanding in use, and has similarly not been subjected to validation.

Results

A clinical trial, even with limited numbers, is an exercise in good will, good planning and good fortune. Although planning to treat twelve children, we 'lost' four children in the study – lost in the sense that four children could not be included in the end results for a variety of reasons. One boy during the first sessions of music therapy was discovered to be profoundly deaf rather than mentally handicapped and developmentally delayed, which meant that he had to be fitted with a hearing aid. This finding seems to point to music therapy assessment as a valuable diagnostic method for developmentally delayed children simply because it brings attention to active hearing in an almost naturalized setting. One other child had been abused by a

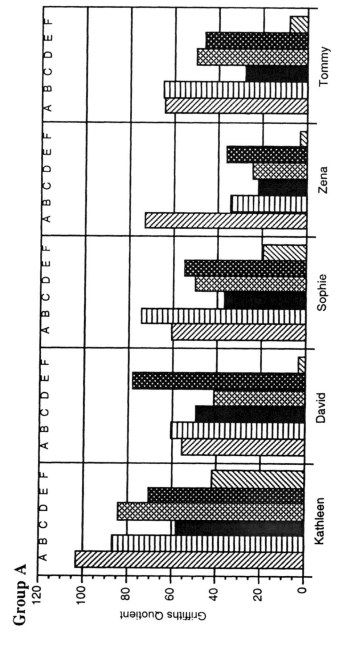

Figure 11.6 Griffiths quotient final assessment profiles

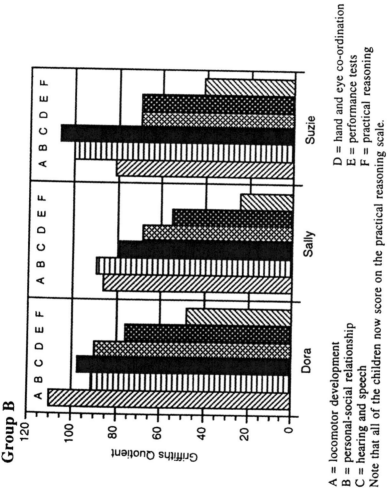

A = locomotor development
B = personal-social relationship
C = hearing and speech
D = hand and eye co-ordination
E = performance tests
F = practical reasoning
Note that all of the children now score on the practical reasoning scale.

Figure 11.6 Griffiths quotient final assessment profiles (continued)

member of her family and it was not possible to continue the full programme of treatment and assessment. Two children came from families of ethnic minorities and it was both difficult to get them to music therapy sessions, and to maintain the continuity of follow-up.

By the end of the study there were two unbalanced groups, similar in chronological age, but different in mental age despite the random allocation. We see in Figure 11.5, which illustrates the Griffiths sub-scale scores for the children in both groups, in comparison with Figure 11.4, that the children range from what is considered to be severely delayed to the 'slow' child. Five out of the eight children failed to score on the practical reasoning scale (Sub-scale F). Sub-scale F is heavily dependent upon speech and represents the general language deficits in these children. However, we see by the final assessment sessions, Figure 11.6, that all the children have developed some capacity for practical reasoning. Indeed all the children improve, as would be expected. Children develop with or without music therapy. But the rate at which they develop, and how it is possibly influenced by music therapy, is the subject of this study.

We see in Figure 11.7 that the changes in the Griffiths scores do indeed differ according to which group the children are in. During the same period of time from intake, the first treatment group (A) changes more than the children on the waiting list (measured at Test 1). When the waiting-list group are treated and then tested (at Test 2), and the children who were treated take a rest, the newly treated children start to catch up in their development. Such differences can be demonstrated at a level of statistical significance and support our initial hypothesis that music therapy will bring about an initial change. While it appears clear that music therapy does make a difference to the development of these children, it does not immediately tell us why music therapy helps, or what indeed is changing specifically.

There are significant differences between the groups. First, there is a continuing significant difference on the hearing and speech sub-scale and a significantly changing ability to listen and communicate. The personal-social interaction sub-scale (B) also proves to be the significant differentiator at Tests 1 and Tests 3. After Test 3, the children in Group A have received two treatment periods of music therapy. It must be noted here that Tests 2, 3 and 4 are all made after children have been treated at least once with music therapy. Music therapy seems to have an effect on personal relationship, emphasizing the positive benefits of active listening and performing, and this in turn sets the context for developmental change. However, the groups also differ initially on hand–eye co-ordination (sub-scale D), and this is not

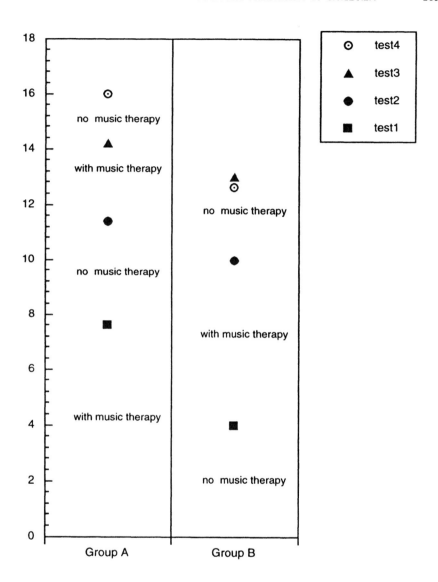

These changes are the mean changes from when the children were measured at intake; that is, the intake is the baseline, zero. The test scores, 1, 2, 3 and 4 are the mean changes in the Griffiths quotients for each group at three months, six months, nine months and one year following the initial measurement at intake. Note at test 4 in Group B there appears to be a regression in the changes.

Figure 11.7 Group differences in Griffiths' test score mean changes from intake

surprising given that the playing of musical instruments demands such manipulative and perceptive skill.

While focused listening in a personal–social relationship sets the scene for music therapy, and provides the context in which change can occur, a further investigation of the data reveals an important variable related to hand–eye co-ordination that is correlated with significant clinical changes when the children are tested. Sub-scale D, which measures hand and eye co-ordination, and is taken to be demonstrative of non-verbal communication (Muenzenmaier, Meyer and Ferber 1993), is significantly correlated with change throughout the series of test times. At Test 1 (Pearson r 0.915, Bonferroni p 0.001), and Test 2 (Pearson r 0.903, Bonferroni p 0.002), hand–eye co-ordination is correlated with the hearing and speech scale change, Sub-scale C. A change occurs on both scales of non-verbal communication and potential verbal communication. Furthermore, at Test 3, hand–eye co-ordination is correlated with changes in the performance tests, Scale E (Pearson r 0.902, Bonferroni p 0.033); and later at test 4, hand–eye co-ordination is correlated with changes in practical reasoning (Pearson r 0.933, Bonferroni p 0.010). The active element of musical playing, which demands the skills of hand and eye co-ordination and listening, appears to play a significant role in developmental changes.

Case Vignettes

In these two examples we see that while clear developmental changes accessible to assessment take place, it is the qualitative subtleties of personal meaning that play an important role for the parents. In the first child presented here, Dora, a clear quantitative change takes place in the Griffiths test score. In the second example, while no clear objective change occurs in the test scores over time, the parents see important qualitative changes that they perceive as improvements.

Dora

Dora, the child of a developmentally disabled mother and a socially disturbed father, was adopted at birth. While experiencing feeding difficulties she put on weight. She was developmentally delayed, hyperactive and often uncontrollable. As a baby she received physiotherapy because she started to walk late, and, at the time therapy began, was still in nappies. Her major problem was presented as episodes of agitation and restlessness after which she appeared to have lost much of what she had previously learnt. After such episodes she said that she would fall, or her head would fall off. An electroencephalogram showed no obvious signs of pathology. Socially she was distant from other children and adults, was extremely anxious in the presence of others, and protected her eyes with her arms clamped to the sides of her head. She would not listen to others or make eye contact. Sometimes her voice, according to her caregivers, had a strange 'fairy-tale' character and she had been seen by a child psychiatrist.

At the beginning of the music therapy Dora cried a lot and had to be held in the arms of the co-therapist throughout the session. When he tried to put her down she cried even louder. Eventually she responded to the musical structure that was offered to her, and although making no eye contact with the therapist at the piano, rang a small bell with her finger. Gaining in confidence, while remaining in the arms of the co-therapist, she played the cymbal continuously. When asked if she had finished playing, she replied clearly that she had. Eventually, in the fourth session, she had confidence to play a drum alone. Now there was no crying and she looked confidently at the therapist. The therapist had composed her a special 'goodbye song' and she sang too! By the tenth session, her musical playing was formed and she played a crescendo alone.

At first Dora told her adopted mother that she would not come to music therapy, but, after the first few sessions, appeared to come gladly. At home she displayed both sympathy for others, and sadness. That she could express herself emotionally was an important experience for her mother. In addition, Dora made it clear she was happy to see her adopted mother and said that she loved her. While previously distant, she now cuddled others and was happy to be cuddled. After two music therapy sessions Dora began to sleep well, and sleep alone, which was a great benefit for the parents. When she had an episode of agitation she said that she no longer needed to be held and could manage alone. Instead of using single words, she combined words together as phrases and could say 'I', 'we' and 'you' in the proper context.

After the second treatment block, she became dry during the day. The table in her bedroom, once used for changing her nappies, became a desk. Although not particularly comfortable at the kindergarten, she started to make friends.

Sophie

Sophie was a much-wanted child, as her mother had previously miscarried twice. While being able to sit alone at four months, she failed to crawl and failed to pull herself up to stand. There appeared to be no organic cause for such a delay. The physiotherapist found that Sophie had difficulties with both her fine and coarse motor control. Although able to hear normally, she failed to speak. Sophie also played alone and was not interested in distractions. After a virus infection, and a fever of up to 42°C when she was unconscious for a short time, her mother became very anxious. An electroencephalogram showed no obvious signs of irregularity.

In the first session Sophie clung to her mother and was carried into the therapy room by the co-therapist, on whose arm she remained. Her hands shook, she whimpered and was very anxious. She played a small bell and a chime bar so quietly that they could hardly be heard.

In the second session she was also very withdrawn and came crying into the room. However, with the support of the co-therapist she played single tones on the piano, sat on the co-therapist's lap and separately played both drum and cymbal.

By the fourth session she was able to come into the therapy room alone, and, after a while, came to the piano where she played single unrelated tones which, at times, accidentally met the music played for her by the therapist. Sophie was very insecure in the musical pauses and immediately retreated from rhythmical impulses. However, in the fifth session she played more often in relationship to the music, using both hands to beat the drum in parallel and alternately. She was surer in the therapeutic relationship and made considerably more effort to play, even when it was manually difficult for her.

After this treatment period Sophie's mother described her as being much freer in daily life. For example, she investigated the family's newly acquired caravan alone. When travelling on the local bus, she greeted the child by whom she sat. When the door bell rang, she opened the door. When she wanted to play with her mother she would find the toys herself, a reverse of the previous situation. She showed more initiative. Furthermore, although speaking in a general babble, she could remember words and situations. If misunderstood, she would become annoyed and show it.

In the next treatment period her playing on drum and cymbal remained at first impulsive. But, by the seventh session she came happy and expectant directly to the piano, where she played with more security.

A significant change came about in the eighth session where she was constantly active and the musical aspects of her playing were more recognizable. She could accompany, and play, changing tempi; decide between loud and soft playing; repeat musical motifs; she brought some continuity to her playing, which was no longer spoilt by small distractions. Her accidental changes were supported in the music such that they became parts of the musical whole, and she worked hard to maintain the musical relationship.

In the following, ninth session Sophie's playing sounded ambivalent and not so related as in the previous week. She seemed withdrawn and unsure in what she did. However, by the next session she was restored to her previous level of progress and was able to express herself in diverse musical activities. With help, she was able to play the drum with parallel and alternative arm movements, and by the final session had many developed musical improvisational possibilities at her disposal.

Sophie's mother described her daughter as being much more capable of playing with her brother, and able both to dress herself and put on her shoes. Although she was defiant when asked to repeat a word, for instance, she babbled more and often repeated the first syllable of a word that she had heard. Sophie was more independent. On visiting a friend of her mother's, Sophie had gone to the refrigerator to fetch a drink when no one had understood that she was thirsty. She had become much more aware, and appeared to be surprised by her own capabilities. The consequences were that she became braver and more energetic in taking new things on, would play with others and sit next to her brother or her parents. On going to bed, she took her teddy bear with her along with other cuddly toys. For her mother it was a personal breakthrough when Sophie allowed her hair to be cut and styled, and agreed to wear a slide in her hair.

It is important to emphasize here the role of parental observation. When therapeutic change occurs, the primary arena for expression of that change is not solely in the therapy room. What parents are expecting is that children will be different at home. These changes are often subtle and too varied for a standardized questionnaire. Therefore, the personal interview with the parents is of equal importance for understanding changes in children. I have chosen to weave subjective observations and objective results together as part of the creative nature of this inquiry, and this can be done once the criteria for the way in which our data are collected are established. Here I have used a quantitative assessment procedure from a paediatrician 'blind' to the treatment allocation of the children. In addition, there is qualitative data collected from interviews with the parents and therapists following the music therapy sessions. Neither assessor was aware of the assessments of the other.

The Co-Ordination of Senses in a Relational Context

Children will develop. Some develop more slowly than others, and for an even smaller minority that development is delayed through a variety of causes. We argue, like others before us, that music therapy can facilitate development, and enhance the rate of development in those children whose development is in some way impaired. When we speak of developmental change we are in the main speaking about the ability to communicate either non-verbally or verbally. Indeed, the parents of the children treated in this study had an expectation that what they and their children did together would make some sense to them, that their children could communicate needs, desires and emotions, and that they too, the parents and caregivers, could communicate their feelings to the children. That Sophie could show both sadness and happiness was considered to be important for her mother. That she could also cuddle was a significant milestone in the emotional relationship of child and mother.

In this study we have gone some way to fulfilling our first purpose in demonstrating that developmental change can be perceived according to standardized testing in the context of clinical research. The Griffiths test is acceptable to us and to referrers, in that it is based upon a broad base of clinical observations and makes sense when applied to the lives of the children being assessed. Like music therapy itself, the emphasis is on eliciting the potential of the children.

We can say that children, when they partake in improvised creative music therapy, achieve significant developmental milestones in comparison to those children who are not treated. Later, when a comparison group of children are treated, they too rapidly achieve developmental goals. It must be mentioned here that at no stage in the study was music therapy targeted to specific developmental achievements, or aimed at particular behavioural activities. What we were interested in was what developmental changes took place, rather than trying to manipulate children such that targeted changes occurred. The reason for not specifying behavioural goals is that creative music therapy is not based on a behavioural plan of identifying specific clinical aims, as that would detract from the essential aim of making music together. As all the children were so completely different, as is the nature of developmental delay, the same target variable could not apply to all the children. Furthermore, as this was a preliminary study, we could not know what we were to focus on before we had done the study. However, there is a paradox inherent in creative music therapy research in that we emphasize the musical activity as paramount in therapy, yet it is the behavioural changes that we champion as therapeutic success.

My initial purpose was also to discover what it is in the activity of making music that is important. Clearly the activity of listening, in a structured musical improvisational context, without the lexical demands of language, is a platform for communicational improvement. The building blocks of language – rhythm, articulation, sequencing (Jusczyk, Cutler and Redanz 1993), pitch, timbre (Weinert 1992) and turn-taking (Bechtel 1993) – are musical in nature. Focused listening to another person is a prerequisite of effective mutual communication and dialogue. In addition, musical dialogue in the music therapy relationship seems to bring about an improvement in the ability to form and maintain personal social relationships in other contexts.

Hand and eye co-ordination, which is dependent on a wider body awareness, appears to be the third vital component in developmental change. That hand movement plays such an important role is also supported by the literature emphasizing the role of non-verbal communication and gesture in the subtle aspects of emotional expression (Barrett, Zahnwaxler and Cole 1993), the acquisition of language (Merlin 1993), and in cognitive development (Alibali and Goldin-Meadow 1993; Goldin-Meadow, Alibali and Church 1993). The active playing of a drum demands that the child listens to the therapist who in turn is listening to, and playing for, her. This act entails the physical co-ordination of a musical intention within the context of a relationship. We would argue that this unity of the cognitive, gestural, emotional and relational is the strength of active music therapy for developmentally challenged children.

In addition, the importance of the visual system in generating speech is important to bear in mind. Shuren, Geldmacher and Heilman (1993) propose that there is a visual semantic system storing codes for concrete words and picture names, and a verbal system for conceptual knowledge of a more abstract type. Both systems work together, yet the second is more dependent upon internal stimuli or self-generated dialogues. The activation of hand and eye together in this study, visual-semantic and gestural, may have had an influence on the speech-related practical reasoning Sub-scale F which all children exhibited by the end of the study.

The proximal zone, where child and therapist play together, awakening a potential, and extending the possibilities for the child, appears to be an important concept for music therapy and is critical in achieving new creative possibilities in the therapeutic relationship. While the musical therapeutic relationship is the domain of this zone, the means of achieving this relationship is in the encouragement of active listening. Yet, such listening is also related to performing. The intention to communicate is brought into a structure such that communication can be achieved as performance. In this case the structure is musical, and has the advantage of flexibility, and is built upon the capabilities of the individual child. His or her own capabilities, no matter how limited, are brought into the mutual realm of musical relationship with the therapist, and therefore are open to variety, and thereby, development.

The caregivers of the children in this study said that a benefit of music therapy was that they could enjoy their children and what the children did began to make more sense. If through this 'making sense' a child achieves independence by the expression of needs, desires and wishes, and the ability to act accordingly, then we have gone some small way in our study to demonstrate a benefit of creative music therapy. Listening and performing in the musical relationship, that is, action and purposeful movement in a relational context, appear to be the building blocks of developmental change and of relevance for cognitive change. That these factors are pre-verbal, and not language-dependent, would argue for the importance of music therapy in the treatment of developmentally delayed infants.

A secondary purpose was to find a suitable research approach integrating quantitative and qualitative methods. Empirical data have been used that can be analysed statistically, but as in all statistical methods, the analysis must be applied and interpreted. By using multi-variate techniques I have chosen to investigate the relationship between variables as shown by the data. We saw the same process of interpretation earlier when I used a principal components analysis of the repertory grid data. The relationship between variables, while being suggested as significant by the analysis, must be interpreted as clinically significant by the researcher and further validated by the clinicians. As Dzurec and Abraham (1986) remark,

> For the researcher using multivariate analysis, as for the researcher using phenomenology, meaning is not inherent in data as they are analysed, but is implied by the researcher's view of reality and the construction of reality to be conveyed in a given situation. Hence attribution of meaning to objective data collected using either multivariate analysis or phenomenology is a subjective task. (p.61)

The above work needs to be validated with a larger population of children, and is best considered as a pointer in a general direction rather than as a conclusive statement. The clinical controlled trial is a rather clumsy approach for music therapy purposes. Even a small number of children are radically different in their capabilities. The treatment approach could not, in practice, be blinded from the assessor in the first phase as parents would ask her when their child would eventually get to music therapy. What did emerge was the importance of a reliable assessment instrument such as the Griffiths profile that could be systematically applied over longer treatment periods. Longitudinal single case designs would appear to be appropriate for further studies. Ideally, we would also have used a child musical development instrument if one had been available. The Nordoff–Robbins scales are not reliable instruments for comparative research, but they do provide a guide to individual assessment. For future researchers, it is important to repeat that the interview with the parents or caregivers is of equal value, in that subtle individual and relational changes are reported which would otherwise escape the attention of a questionnaire or formal assessment instrument. A qualitative study would emphasize in the future the relationship between the musical processes of change and the various changes as they occur in the life of the child at home. What is important to discover is that patterns of communication occurring in the music therapy sessions can be transferred to other situations with siblings, caregivers or other therapists.

While generalizations can be made from the above work, it is important for music therapists as researchers to stay in contact with the individual child. This does not invalidate group research methods. As we see here, the comparison of groups alerted me to significant changes. Hopefully, future research will reflect the creative tensions between generalizability and specificity; that is, what we can say about music therapy with children in general and what happens to the individual child in the process of therapy. Quantitatively, we have assessed changes through the collection of data according to a particular instrument, the Griffiths test. Qualitatively, we have interpreted those data to develop inferences from what is observed. At the end of the day when the paediatrician sees an appreciable change in the child that she has referred to music therapy using a method of assessment that makes sense to her, and the parents of that child say that they can appreciate that child a little more, then we have evidence enough. When a child shows that he knows we are there, when our infants begin to get a good night's rest (and we do too), when the first few words emerge after years of waiting, then no scale will be refined enough to express the significance of such events. While I will continue to argue for a broad spectrum of research methods appropriate to the task in hand, we must not exclude from that research endeavour the comments of those whom we serve. To do so is to deny the validity of simple everyday human expression, and that would be to deny the very task in which we are engaged in music therapy.

CHAPTER TWELVE

The Credible Practitioner
in the Community of Inquiry

The current state of the music therapy world is one in which bridges are being built between understandings; between medical practitioners and music therapists; between music therapists and therapists from differing therapeutic backgrounds; between patients and therapists; and between differing groupings of music therapists. There are often differing values and beliefs, but a common purpose can be sought, and that is to provide the best possible service for those who come to us for help. Indirectly this will be reflected in our teaching initiatives and our research endeavours.

I hope that in these pages some of those understandings have been elucidated such that values can be reconciled. What I have been aiming for is to establish a community of inquiry whereby we can share experiences as 'credible practitioners' (Bayley 1995). In building this community we often come across the problem of which language to use. There are the varying languages of medicine, psychology, anthropology, sociology and musicology. Within the arts therapies there are varying languages, and even within music therapy itself the dialects are such that one tribe may not understand another. By turning to particular contexts and particular situations it is possible to focus upon the therapeutic intention rather than the diversity of potential misunderstandings.

The metaphor of building a bridge is deliberate. Although we may differ, we have to agree upon what it is that will be connected; that someone on one side, your side, will want to meet with someone on the other side, my side. There is a divide that has to be crossed. We suppose then a common purpose of joining two opposing, or separate, positions for mutual benefit. In this case, it is for the constituency of patients that we serve.

In the 1980s I worked on a project in London that was jointly led by two visionary men. One had a vision of converting his church into a healing centre that would include the very best of modern medicine. Secular activities and spiritual interventions would work side by side. The other man had a similar vision. Health would be delivered to a local community and incorporate the whole of the patient, including his or her spiritual needs. Yet, although these two men had similar visions, the source of those visions had not made it clear exactly whose vision was to predominate. Indeed, in the realization of those visions the bridge that could have been built to unite them failed to be built. Certainly the project was, and remains, successful in meeting the needs of the local community. Both groups, however, work in tandem. They go their parallel ways. A real merging of minds never really took place.

To build a bridge there must be a firm foundation on both sides of the divide that is to be crossed. Medicine has this, and I hope that this book demonstrates that music therapy has a secure basis to its claims too. Upon those platforms, a bridge can be built. This building will require an architect to understand the purpose of the bridge, and that is often the task of the researcher who attempts to meet the mutual needs of the parties involved.

A bridge is built for traffic, for achieving exchanges. Although the bridge itself is important, and depends upon an appropriate architecture to support the loads that pass over it, we have really to concentrate on the processes of exchange and what it is that is being carried. We need to know from whom the exchanges come and to whom we are making our exchanges.

Having a bridge will bring the potential for change. Nobody is being forced to cross that bridge. The implications of this book do not have to be acted upon. However, once the potential of movement from one position to the other is established, then we have a choice. Choices can have their negative sides too. Bridges can divert business away from a locality and starve the population. As in complementary medical research, we have deprived many creative arts therapists of research funding and thereby ghettoized them. Condemning music therapists as lacking research support ignores the ways in which that support has been denied them.

Some bridges can bring too much activity and overload the inhabitants. My music therapy colleagues have been so successful in their work with post-comatose patients in neurological rehabilitation that they simply cannot provide enough music therapists for the hospital positions. Similarly, the needs of handicapped children, and the possibilities that music therapy offers, cannot be met in that we do not have enough capacity in our clinics to treat them. Need has outstripped our training capabilities since the bridge of credibility has been constructed.

We speak too of the information super-highway and the massive bridges that can be built to span continents. This does not mean that we all have to travel through such international landscapes. The danger of a super-highway is that it can transport more information than we can handle. More data does not necessarily lead to more understanding. It may be that our task is simply to perform the equivalent of spanning a stream with a plank. Although there are magnificent motorways throughout the whole of Europe delivering people and goods to their multifarious destinations, there are still bridges over, and tunnels under, these massive highways for shepherds and cowswains. We may have to be engaged in constructing lots of little bridges at first to serve the needs of our colleagues. We have partial knowledge that may not be in the mainstream of understanding.

This book was being written at a time when the historic bridge at Mostar had been destroyed. The bridge had become an icon of civilization in a nationalist war at the heart of Europe, where brutality appeared to be triumphing over enlightenment. While bridges undoubtedly have a function and historic purpose that may be forgotten, they also have an aesthetic. We must contemplate the landscape in which a bridge is built before we reflect upon its architecture and construction. A bridge provides an important function in the ecology of social life. Finally, building a bridge is symbolic. Building is intentional and requires prior co-operation from both sides. It is a symbolic act of a mutual agreement. Destruction, however, can be one-sided.

In each of the previous chapters I have tried to place small planks across the divides of understanding. Even a review of the literature has as its subtext the intention of bringing two worlds together. In the research approaches I have tried to suggest possible ways forward such that we can discern how various clinical understandings are elicited. The danger is always that the world of understanding is related to texts. Before the text there is the experience, and the value of music, like all fundamental human activities, is that we can participate without words. It is the use of words that provokes misunderstandings. No more so than in the world of music therapy research where there appears to be a move towards 'conceptual cleansing' where factions identifying themselves as creative or receptive, qualitative or quantitative are claiming a universal knowledge that is misplaced and unsupported. If we have escaped in music therapy from the hegemony of medicine and psychology, there is no need to replace it with the tyranny of partial knowledge that claims to be ubiquitous.

Talking About Music and Music Therapy

In the aesthetics of music there is a debate about the autonomy of music. Music is claimed to be neither a language of emotion nor of anything else

(Shibles 1995, p.73). In music therapy we have the same debate taking place. The difficulty is that music therapists are not solely musicians but have entered an arena of therapy whereby they undertake a social contract to help another person. At some point they will be called upon to describe or explain what they have been doing and what benefits this may bring for the patient or client with whom they have worked. In terms of research, and the distribution of the results of that research, then the use of verbal descriptions is demanded.

Throughout the chapters of this book I have tried to weave a thread of research understanding within the fabric of clinical practice. Such a sequential development is deliberate. Research develops slowly. What I have tried to establish is that at one level we have the experience of the music itself as it is performed, and recognizing that, we can then understand that any other verbal understandings or attempts to describe those phenomena are descriptive, at another level, and interpretative, at yet another level. Thus we have a system for understanding how meanings are gleaned and constructed from performance and the way in which those meanings are woven together, regulated, in practice. Knowing what we are describing, and from which system of understandings we are interpreting, is a vital step forward. Such understandings are meant to be particular, referring to restricted contexts. In this way I am following a path that is currently being trod in the movement of qualitative research methods. However, while qualitative methods are my method of choice, I do not want to suggest that only qualitative methods are appropriate for music therapy research. We have a broad spectrum of methods available to us in clinical practice, and we should be able to choose the method that suits the practice itself, the abilities and resources of the practitioner and researcher and the target audience for that research. As we saw in the chapter about working with developmentally delayed children, quantitative and qualitative methodologies need not be exclusive. We can utilize a variety of differing explanations from the same phenomena.

Towards the Development of a European Research Culture in Music Therapy

Over the past ten years we have seen an emerging demand for music therapy research in Europe. A number of individual researchers based in different countries have attempted to promote music therapy research. Music therapy itself, like nursing, psychotherapy and other helping professions, is also being challenged to produce research results.

The source of that challenge is coming both from within the profession itself, and from without. From within the profession, a new generation of music therapists is demanding academic credibility, and this need is linked to the establishment of postgraduate music therapy courses leading to masters qualifications. Music therapists are also demanding within their own career trajectories that they can deepen their understanding of what they are doing and gain academic credentials by further study. Combined with this internal demand, we are seeing throughout the European Union a demand for outcomes research related to varying therapeutic initiatives both from third party funders and from employing health institutions. With Government cutbacks in health and education, enhanced scrutiny in university spending, and fiscal demands for efficiency and productivity, music therapy departments are having either to justify their existence by producing material evidence of their efficacy or produce research papers to improve their academic points rating. This means that a relatively new profession is being forced to develop research results without having had the chance to establish research training, without a satisfactory background of research material and without the opportunity to negotiate an acceptable way of doing research that is related to therapeutic outcome. Indeed, we are not alone in this; rehabilitation medicine and general medical practice in the Western world stand under the same spotlight of scrutiny.

In addition, we are faced with a relative lack of research expertise. Some of us have a research career that has experience of various forms of research projects. However, few of our colleagues have had the opportunity to do post-graduate research and are being expected to teach research methods and supervise research projects. While this may be a necessity, driven by need, I suggest that in some cases we will find that colleagues are being prepared for an over-idealized world of academic research that perhaps reflects the lack of experience within the profession, rather than research that is focused upon clinical practice. It is vital that we develop a sound basis of research-oriented clinical practitioners.

There are also differences in the purposes of research. At the moment, in a junior profession we have researchers preparing masters material and doctoral studies. These studies are often of a different nature from postgraduate research studies and research contracted to outside agencies. Doctoral studies are focused on the development of the doctoral candidate. They are there for the sole process of developing someone who will later be able to carry out research. Therefore the work itself will often be of an intensely deep and inward-looking nature. The research that is carried out by experienced researchers will be more outward-looking and often at the request of some external agency wanting to see some material benefit from their investment. Therefore, the purposes and the methods used will differ. I am arguing that we need both these forms of research. Only to foster an inward-looking research will restrict the nature of music therapy research, and thereby practice, in the future. As a rational step forward the single case research designs proposed in Chapter Six are a positive way forward, fostering both process-oriented work and the assessment of clinical outcomes.

As we have seen in earlier chapters, what kind of research we do, and the methods we use to go about researching, will be influenced by the philosophy of science that we have. My main proposal has been that science is a process, an activity, not a set of commandments set in stone for all time as the basis for a dogma. In a post-modern world, where all the major themes are challenged and deconstructed, it is our responsibility to construct themes that are appropriate to the knowledge that we need. While this debate is often set out as differences in truth claims – that is, 'Is truth relative?', or 'Is there one truth?' – my argument is that such a position belongs to a previous era of debate. Claims about truth have already been discussed in other scientific disciplines. What we are really making claims about are objectivity and subjectivity and local knowledge. This debate can currently be found in the nursing literature, in the world of psychology, in journals dedicated to social science and, particularly over the last ten years, in the field of complementary medicine.

Science for music therapists

First, let me make an observation about science in a broad sense. The word science itself in its English usage springs from the Latin *scire*, 'to know', originally meaning 'to cut', and thereby 'to decide', and has a relationship with the Latin adjective *scius*, which means 'knowing'. So, on the one hand we have a derivation of science that appears to be about making decisions, cutting and separating. Or we can follow another route, and look at the adjective *scius* as it refers to knowing, and as it occurs in the Latin word *conscius* (literally *con* = together *scius* = knowing). Perhaps this is what we are searching for in our scientific activity; how we can share knowledge, or how can we bring knowledge into consciousness.

Yet another perspective would take us to the German word for science, 'Wissenschaft'. *Wissen* is 'to know' or 'to know about', and is related to knowledge and judgement, and *schaffen* is 'to make' or 'create', or 'to manage' or 'accomplish'. So, from another European perspective we can see science as the activity of creating knowledge, and perhaps it is this creative activity that may appeal to many of us today; and perhaps some of us feel it has become lost to the scientific activity. Knowledge is something that can be done, it is a creative activity, a process not a fixed product. Indeed the word knowledge in English is distantly derived from a root that means 'I can' (Middle English *Ic can*, German *können* and *kennen*) and is perhaps best described as the statement, 'I can know'. Once we take such a position of knowledge being actively acquired, then we can speculate upon the various arts of doing science. This is a move away from the Cartesian position that consciousness of the word derives from the mind – 'cogito ergo sum' (I think therefore I am) towards 'ago ergo sum' (I perform therefore I am).

What remains to be added to these descriptions from the Latin and the German roots is the notion of decision or judgement, therefore doing science – or the activity of sciencing – is a matter of deciding. It is therefore a moral activity.

How do we create knowledge, then? This question lies at the centre of many modern scientific debates, and is a question of methodology. One of our critiques of modern science-doing is that the argument rarely concentrates on the subject matter of our inquiry that leads to a new creative discovery for the person who wants to know. The activity of science seems more like the pressure for us to conform, in our knowing, to a set of prescriptions that are applied to a given body of knowledge, that is, methodolatry not methodology. It is this struggle with an appropriate methodology that we find in the current creative arts therapy literature, and one that has been hotly debated during the last decade within other fields of applied therapeutic practice.

We see this breaking out in the debate about quantitative or qualitative research, where one is proposed as the only form of research inquiry. While music therapists in the United States, partly because of their education structure, have a tradition of music therapy research, that tradition has often been polarized into two opposing camps: qualitative research versus quantitative research. The grounds for this polarization appear to be historically based in the establishment of a political professional identity within the field of practice. What I have tried to do is to avoid such polarization and foster a climate of tolerance that allows a music therapy research strategy to develop that suits music therapists and their various purposes. All too often this methodological debate has been at the foreground of research initiatives and has masked the underlying political debate about which group should hold political sway within the profession. We could just as easily translate this debate into the intolerance of varying music therapy schools for one another. Such arguments really are superfluous at a time when the profession itself is ripe to develop, and in its maturity should be ready to extend the tolerance necessary for knowing together.

What I am arguing is that if science is a creative doing of knowledge, then the way that we can do knowledge about being human is not restricted to instrumentation through machines; rather, knowledge is something that can be sung, or played, or danced or acted. Underlying this approach is a philosophy of the world presented in Chapter Two that moves away from a solely materialistic perspective to a perspective that sees the world as a living organism improvised in the moment in which we are all taking part.

Teaching and individualism

A new generation of music therapists is being trained that demands a choice of learning approaches which suits its approach to music and to therapy. The pioneer approach of the teacher–pupil relationship no longer holds sway, and while the restriction of the relationship may be lost, so too is the security. Furthermore, as there is no established tradition of music therapy research, we have the luxury of deciding what methods are appropriate to use in our scientific endeavour. While some of us will research alone, others will decide to work together in groups. What we need to avoid is one group making an exclusive claim to determine the doing of knowledge according to their own principles. To establish tolerance we need to understand each other and our varying purposes.

The activity of doing research, or sciencing as knowing, is concerned not with restricting us to a one-dimensional sense of being according to an accepted orthodox world-view, but with the possibility of interpretation of the self as new. What we choose to know, and how we know, is a matter of judgement, and therefore one of moral agency. How each one of us decides to know in the future, with whom we share that knowledge, and how we tolerate and incorporate what others know, will determine the scientific culture of music therapy.

While a benefit of music therapy training is that it promotes individualism and allows for the unique expression of clinical expertise, the danger is that groups then form that are so convinced of their own unique value that they believe that all others should work in their superior way and that they have the right to dictate the standards of individuals. This is tribalism and is the ultimate danger in a post-modern society. We form groups when our identity is threatened. Indeed, music therapists have struggled for years to find a voice that will be heard in the community of practitioners. However, in their searches for modern identities some have resorted to falling back on a traditional background. While this is undoubtedly expedient, and resurrects a heritage that itself may provide innumerable riches, it is also in danger of resurrecting identities that are no longer viable in current practice. Where such individual identities are isolated from the practice of others, and make unique claims for knowledge that is superior, we have the triumph of insecurity and its babbling cliques over a set of particularized understandings that may lead us to realizing our community of practitioners.

A Way Forward

It is important that international connections for the discussion of research methods and clinical practice are maintained and fostered. One way to accomplish this will be by exchanging teaching staff interested in research, or providing the opportunity for extended visits. Promoting research placements for higher-level students, or junior members of staff, is also a possibility that would benefit the institutions. For example, we have had visiting music therapists who have sat in on the teaching sessions, experienced a series of therapy sessions and undertaken a review of literature on a theme that has interested them. There are a number of institutions throughout Europe that have areas of special interest for music therapists, and an extended working visit is a good way of getting to know other institutions.

We need to encourage a standard of music therapy writing that will bring the exciting clinical work that is being done throughout Europe to the attention of other clinicians. In our various training schemes we often fail to promote the skill of writing and the communication of clinical results. While accepting that music therapy must be learned as a set of skills, so too must the skills of writing be learned and presentation be learned. Furthermore, we need to encourage the possibility of academic writing and theoretical discussion. This can only be achieved by a journal that will act as a forum for such debate. As our chosen medium is music, and non-verbal, then the challenge of developing new media possibilities arises in these times of modern technology. We do not need a new *printed* publication. I suggest that we investigate the publication of music therapy material on CD-Rom. Material published in this way could be both text, musical scores, musical extracts as recorded sounds, video clips, photographs and database items.

We certainly need to collaborate on providing a research infrastructure. By this I mean that we have to share our various resources for offering methodological advice and teaching research methods. There is enough expertise, the problem remains of how to utilize it and co-ordinate it. We have access to databases and literature archives. What we do not have, as yet, is a means of giving a broad access to such material. Setting up co-operating centres within the differing countries would establish nodes of expertise, but that would mean that they would have to communicate with each other!

One important way forward would be to promote a 'single case' agency where we could co-ordinate single case methods teaching, offer a suitable research format, and collect research examples. By doing this we could develop a set of clinical studies as a clinical studies database. A clinical studies database would necessitate translating the clinical studies into a common set of European languages and offer clinical researchers a pool of comparative data.

Within the music therapy programme at the University Witten Herdecke, a literature support service has been initiated that is also being shared currently with Denmark, Holland and other Nordic and Scandinavian countries. This literature support service has been based on our recognition of a need for research support within Germany to meet the needs of students who have trained with us and who are now colleagues in practice. In addition, there are other colleagues who do not have the benefit of institutional support, and it is our responsibility to support them at least in whatever way they can should they wish to begin clinical research.

Music and Living: A Spontaneous Activity

Improvisation demands the maintenance of a theme that must change to gain liveliness. So are our lives improvised, from the cellular to the cerebral, to maintain our identities intact. In all such processes, listening to one other is a central method for gaining information, negotiating relationship and maintaining credibility whether it is the cell communicating with the cell, person with person, or community with community.

However, we must return once more to the central role of the body in modern society. The relationship with the self is with the body; it is here that we have the interface of internal and external. How we experience the unfolding of our experience is reflected in our bodies. The body tells us how language works; the meta-communication, as it were. The reason that the expressive arts as therapies are so powerful is that they emphasize the lived body as being sensed, not only as being said. So expressing ourselves as a musical identity, or as a danced piece, even as a dramatic event, may stay closer to the reality of symptoms as they are expressed. Expressive culture is the projection of the body into an expressive medium. Manipulation of that medium is expressiveness, and culture is dedicated to understanding how to use that medium. Form is given to feelings and cognitions. Symptoms too are bodily expressions involving feelings and cognitions, sometimes conforming to a medical interpretation, but also demanding an existential interpretation that cannot be spoken. From this perspective, we can perhaps understand that some seemingly chronic diseases, and predominantly those seen as psychosomatic, are problems that are being dynamically expressed upon the stage of the body and failing to be interpreted adequately in the context of treatment. While symptoms are the embodiment of distress, it is in the arena of their performance that we are engaged as practitioners and researchers. The means we use to understand that drama is being questioned by those who claim an identity other than that of the stigmatized sick. Patients perform their lives before us. How we come to realize that potential as enhancing, as aesthetic, is the task of the music therapist. Demonstrating the benefit that that performance may have for people in their daily lives is the task of music therapy research.

If the big narratives of modernism are now being replaced by our own personal sets of meaning made locally with those whom we seek to live (Warde 1994), we need to understand more about the person that comes to us for therapy. How that person creates an identity will be indicative of how that person will resolve his or her problems. How that person plays will be the foundation of their recovery. We are challenged to participate in the aesthetics of health in terms of becoming whole. Many non-medical appraisals of health care activity seem be based upon holistic considerations that include feelings of mood and vitality (Andersen and Lobel 1995). If changes of mood are ignored, or assessed as potentially pathological by health care practitioners, and the philosophy of vitality is generally regarded as invalid in modern scientific medicine, we should not wonder that people come to music therapists for help. If, as in traditional Chinese medicine, for example, health seeking becomes a pleasure, that sequesters 'a body that can not only taste sweetness but be sweet, not only report painful symptoms, but also dwell on and cultivate the quiet comforts of health' (Farquhar 1994, p.493) then maybe we can understand that the seeking of a positive identity in a post-modern world is an activity that can be enjoyed. We may indeed have to learn to seek out those personal and local truths that our patients are themselves choosing to embody.

We have to understand how people 'do' their lives, not simply what they think and say about their lives. It is in the body that individual identity is expressed, and the body is the interface between the individual and society. It is what people do together that binds them together with the groups with whom they perform their lives. This performance will be bound up with lifestyle, leisure activities, exercise, dieting and dress. In this sense, 'lifestyle' is not something that can be read about in books, it is an activity. Making sense of the world is an activity achieved through the body. Swimming cannot be learned about by reading about it, or by gathering together a band of expert swimmers together to tell you about their experiences, nor by attending a conference of hydro-physicists. At some time we have to jump into the water and, through experience, swim. The body grasps what it needs to do. Having a teacher in the water certainly helps.

So too with health and a change in 'lifestyle'. If we wish to encourage people to do something differently, we have to understand that it will be intimately connected with their identity as a person and with those with whom that identity is validated. Change is brought about by influencing small groups and understanding their way of being in the world. Music therapy offers the chance to do something differently. A new identity can be created. However, the patient is not left alone to find their own way; the music therapist accompanies them. Rather than describe the way forward for someone, we accompany them along part of the way, reviving the old notion of the therapist as one who attends to the needs of a fellow traveller as well as the musical accompanist who provides a basis from which the other can perform.

One factor that we must take into account is that the serious business of living can also be fun. While we know a lot about health care activities and their impact, we know little about the importance of leisure activities and their ramifications for health. Positive emotions, according to new thinking, influence our health status for the better. Optimism and a sensual pleasure in everyday activities and situations are valuable for promoting personal health. The absence of symptoms and a sense of enjoyment, coupled with a zest for living, appear to play a significant role in the subjective assessment of health (Wenglert and Rosén 1995). Once more, health may be described as an activity with sensual ramifications concerned with pleasurable activities that are themselves integrated with an overall sense of 'lifestyle'. This may be more appealing than our current unilateral exhortations to follow expert health care prescriptions based on warnings and denial. Music has a vast potential for pleasure. Music is to be played. Play can be a serious business, as any child will remind us. Perhaps as adults too, we can be reminded that play is not a trivial activity, and a little bit of fun is a powerful medicine. As I said at the beginning of this book, having fun is not disputed as an activity that is beneficial; my task has been to demonstrate that music therapy is more than simply having fun. How our lives are performed is a serious activity, and music therapy is an important healing activity through which our futures can be orchestrated.

References

Aaronson, N. (1989) 'Quality of life assessment in clinical trials: methodologic issues.' *Controlled Clinical Trials 10 (4 Supplement)*, 195S–208S.

Ackerman, F. (1989) 'Family-systems therapy with a man with AIDS-Related Complex.' *Family Systems Medicine 7*, 3, 292–304.

Adams, L. (1988) 'Apollo and Marsyas: a metaphor of creative conflict.' *Psychoanalytic Review 75*, 2, 319–38.

Ader, R. (1987) 'Brain, behavior and immunity.' *Brain, Behavior and Immunity 1*, 1–6.

Aizenberg, D., Schwartz, B. and Modai, I. (1986) 'Musical hallucinations, acquired deafness, and depression.' *Journal of Nervous and Mental Disorders 174*, 5, 309–311.

Aldridge, D. (1984) 'Suicidal behaviour and family interaction: a brief review.' *Journal of Family Therapy 6*, 309–322.

Aldridge, D. (1987) 'A team approach to terminal care: personal implications for patients and practitioners.' *Journal of the Royal College of General Practitioners 37*, 364.

Aldridge, D. (1987a) *One Body: A Guide to Healing in the Church.* London: SPCK.

Aldridge, D. (1987b) 'Families, cancer and dying.' *Family Practice 4*, 212–218.

Aldridge, D. (1987c) 'A team approach to terminal care: personal implications for patients and practitioners.' *Journal of the Royal College of General Practitioners 37*, 364.

Aldridge, D. (1988) 'Treating self-mutilatory behavior: a social strategy.' *Family Systems Medicine 6*, 1, 5–19.

Aldridge, D. (1989) 'A phenomenological comparison of the organization of music and the self.' *The Arts in Psychotherapy 16*, 91–97.

Aldridge, D. (1989a) 'Music, communication and medicine: discussion paper.' *Journal of the Royal Society of Medicine 82*, 12, 743–746.

Aldridge, D. (1990) 'Making and taking health care decisions.' *Journal of the Royal Society of Medicine 83*, 720–723.

Aldridge, D. (1990a) 'The delivery of health care alternatives.' *Journal of the Royal Society of Medicine 83*, 179–182.

Aldridge, D. (1991) 'Single case research designs for the clinician.' *Journal of the Royal Society of Medicine 84*, 249–252.

Aldridge, D. (1991a) 'Aesthetics and the individual in the practice of medical research: a discussion paper.' *Journal of the Royal Society of Medicine 84*, 147–150.

Aldridge, D. (1991b) 'Creativity and consciousness: music therapy in intensive care.' *The Arts in Psychotherapy 18*, 359–362.

Aldridge, D. (1991c) 'Spirituality, healing and medicine.' *Journal of British General Practice 41*, 425–427.

Aldridge, D. (1991d) 'Physiological change, communication, and the playing of improvised music: some proposals for research.' *The Arts in Psychotherapy 18*, 59–64.

Aldridge, D. (1992) 'The needs of individual patients in clinical research.' *Advances 8*, 4, 58–65.

Aldridge, D. (1993) 'Music therapy research: I. A review of the medical research literature within a general context of music therapy research. [Special Issue: Research in the creative arts therapies].' *The Arts in Psychotherapy 20*, 1, 11–35.

Aldridge, D. (1993a) 'Observational methods: a search for methods in an ecosystemic research paradigm.' In G. Lewith and D. Aldridge (eds) *Clinical Research Methodology for Complementary Therapies.* London: Hodder and Stoughton.

Aldridge, D. (1993b) 'Single case research designs.' In G. Lewith and D. Aldridge (eds) *Clinical Research Methodology for Complementary Therapies.* London: Hodder and Stoughton.

Aldridge, D. (1993c) 'Music therapy research II: Research methods suitable for music therapy.' [Special Issue: Research in the creative arts therapies.] *The Arts in Psychotherapy 20*, 2, 117–131.

Aldridge, D. (1994) 'Unconventional medicine in Europe.' *Advances 10*, 2, 52–60.

Aldridge, D. and Aldridge, G. (1992) 'Two epistemologies: music therapy and medicine in the treatment of dementia.' *The Arts in Psychotherapy 19*, 243–255.

Aldridge, D. and Brandt, G. (1991) 'Music therapy and inflammatory bowel disease.' *The Arts in Psychotherapy 18*, 113–121.

Aldridge, D. and Dallos, R. (1986) 'Distinguishing families where suicidal behaviour is present from families where suicidal behaviour is absent.' *Journal of Family Therapy 8*, 243–252.

Aldridge, D. and Pietroni, P. (1987) 'Research trials in general practice: towards a focus on clinical practice.' *Family Practice 4*, 311–315.

Aldridge, D. and Rossiter, J. (1984) 'A strategic assessment of deliberate self harm.' *Journal of Family Therapy 6*, 119–132.

Aldridge, D. and Rossiter, J. (1985) 'Difficult patients, intractable symptoms and spontaneous recovery in suicidal behaviour.' *Journal of Systemic and Strategic Therapies 4*, 66–76.

Aldridge, D., Brandt, G. and Wohler, D. (1990) 'Towards a common language in the arts therapies.' *The Arts in Psychotherapy 17*, 189–195.

Aldridge, D., Gustorff, D. and Hannich, H. (1990) 'Where am I? Music therapy applied to coma patients [editorial].' *Journal of the Royal Society of Medicine 83*, 6, 345–346.

Aldridge, G. (1995) 'A walk through Paris: the development of melodic expression in music therapy with a breast-cancer patient.' (Submitted for publication).

Alibali, M. and Goldin-Meadow, S. (1993) 'Gesture–speech mismatch and mechanisms of learning: what the hands reveal about a child's state of mind.' *Cognitive Psychology 25*, 468–523.

Allen, K.D., Barone, V.J. and Kuhn, B.R. (1993) 'A behavioral prescription for promoting applied behavior analysis within pediatrics.' *Journal of Applied Behavior Analysis 26*, 4, 493–502.

Altenmüller, E. (1986) 'Brain correlates of cerebral music processing.' *European Archives of Psychiatry 235*, 342–354.

Altshuler, I. (1948) 'A psychiatrist's experience with music as a therapeutic agent.' In D. Schullian and M. Schoen (eds) *Music and Medicine.* New York: Henry Schuman.

Alzheimer, A. (1907) 'Über eine einartige Erkrankung der Hirnrinde.' *Allgemeine Zeitschrift für Psychiatrie und Psychisch-Gerichtliche Medizin 64*, 146–148.

Andersen, M. and Lobel, M. (1995) 'Predictors of health self-appraisal: what's involved in feeling healthy?' *Basic and Applied Social Psychology 16*, 1 and 2, 121–136.

Ansdell, G. (1995) *Music for Life: Aspects of Creative Music Therapy with Adults.* London: Jessica Kingsley Publishers.

Armstrong, D. (1987) 'Theoretical tensions in biopsychosocial medicine.' *Social Science and Medicine 25*, 11, 1213–1218.

Arnheim, R. (1992) 'Why aesthetics is needed.' *The Arts in Psychotherapy 19*, 149–151.

Atkins, R. and Amenta, M. (1991) 'Family adaptation to AIDS: a comparative study.' *Hospital Journal 7*, 1–2, 71–83.

Ayer, A. (1982) *Philosophy in the Twentieth Century.* London: Weidenfeld and Nicolson.

Ba, G. (1988) 'Strategies of rehabilitation in the Day Hospital.' *Psychotherapie und Psychosomatik 50*, 3, 151–6.

Babikian, V., Wolfe, N., Linn, R., Knoefel, J. and Albert, M. (1990) 'Cognitive changes in patients with multiple cerebral infarcts.' *Stroke 21*, 7, 1013–1018.

Baer, D.M. (1993) 'A brief, selective history of the department of human development and family life at the University of Kansas – the early years.' *Journal of Applied Behavior Analysis 26*, 4, 569–572.

Bailey, L. (1983) 'The effects of live music versus tape-recorded music on hospitalised cancer patients.' *Music Therapy 3*, 1, 17–28.

Bailey, L. (1984) 'The use of songs with cancer patients and their families.' *Music Therapy 4*, 1, 5–17.

Bailey, L. (1985) 'Music's soothing charms.' *American Journal of Nursing 85*, 11, 1280.

Baker, G.H. (1987) 'Invited review: Psychological factors and immunity.' *Journal of Psychosomatic Research 31*, 1–10.

Bang, C. (1986) 'A world of sound and music: music therapy and musical speech therapy with hearing-impaired and multiple-handicapped children.' In E. Ruud (ed) *Music and Health.* Oslo: Norsk Musikforlag.

Barfield, O. (1978) *The Case for Anthroposophy.* London: Rudolf Steiner Press.

Barison, F., Pradetto, A. and Valer, T. (1984) 'The musical productions of autistic children [letter].' *Journal of Autism and Developmental Disorders 14*, 4, 453–454.

Barlow, D. and Hersen, M. (1984) *Single Case Experimental Designs: Strategies for Studying Behavior Change.* New York: Pergamon Press.

Barlow, D., Hersen, M. and Jackson, M. (1973) 'Single-case experimental designs.' *Archives of General Psychiatry 23*, 319–325.

Barnason, S., Zimmerman, L. and Nieveen, J. (1995) 'The effects of music interventions on anxiety in the patient after coronary artery bypass grafting.' *Heart and Lung 24*, 2, 124–132.

Barrett, K.C., Zahnwaxler, C. and Cole, P.M. (1993) 'Avoiders vs amenders – implications for the investigation of guilt and shame during toddlerhood.' *Cognition Emotion 7*, 6, 481–505.

Bason, B.T. and Celler, B.G. (1972) 'Control of the heart rate by external stimuli.' *Nature 4*, 279–280.

Bateson, G. (1941) 'Experiments in thinking about observed ethnological material.' *Philosophy of Science 8*, 53–68.

Bateson, G. (1972) *Steps to an Ecology of Mind.* New York: Ballantine.

Bateson, G. (1978) *Mind and Nature.* Glasgow: Fontana.

Bateson, G. (1991) *A Sacred Unity.* New York: HarperCollins.

Bayles, K.A., Boone, D.R. and Tomoeda, C.K.(1989) 'Differentiating Alzheimer's patients from the normal elderly and stroke patients with aphasia.' *Journal of Hearing and Speech Disorders 54*, 74–87.

Bayley, C. (1995) 'Our world views (may be) incommensurable: now what?' *The Journal of Medicine and Philosophy 20*, 271–284.

Bean, J. (1995) 'Music therapy and the child with cerebral palsy: directive and non-directive attention.' In T. Wigram, B. Saperston and R. West (eds) *The Art and Science of Music Therapy: A Handbook.* Chur, Switzerland: Harwood Academic Publishers.

Beatty, W. and Goodkin, D. (1990) 'Screening for cognitive impairment in multiple sclerosis: An evaluation of the Mini-Mental State Examination.' *Archives of Neurology 47*, 3, 297–301.

Beatty, W.W., Zavadil, K.D. and Bailly, R.C. (1988) 'Preserved musical skills in a severely demented patient.' *International Journal of Clinical Neuropschology 10*, 158–164.

Bechtel, W. (1993) 'Decomposing intentionality: perspectives of intentionality drawn from language research with two species of chimpanzee.' *Biology and Philosophy 8*, 1–32.

Behrends, L. (1983) 'Erfahrungen mit einer kombinierten Gruppenpsychotherapie bei Adolescenten.' *Psychiatrie, Neurologie, Medizin und Psychologie, Leipzig 35*, 3, 154–157.

Belcher, A., Dettmore, D. and Holzemer, S. (1989) 'Spirituality and sense of well-being in persons with AIDS.' *Holistic Nursing Practice 3*, 4, 16–25.

Benjamin, B. (1983) 'The singing hospital – integrated group therapy in the Black mentally ill.' *South African Medical Journal 63*, 23, 897–899.

Beresford, S., Walker, J., Banks, M. and Wale, C. (1977) 'Why do women consult doctors? Social factors and the use of the general practitioner.' *British Journal of Social and Preventive Medicine 31*, 220–226.

Berman, I. (1981) 'Musical functioning, speech lateralization and the amusias.' *South African Medical Journal 59*, 78–81.

Bernard-Opitz, V., Roos, K. and Blesch, G. (1989) '[Using computers with autistic handicapped children].' *Zeitschrift für Kinder und Jugendpsychiatrie 17*, 3, 125–130.

Berrios, G. (1990) 'Musical hallucinations: a historical and clinical study.' *British Journal of Psychiatry 156*, 188–194.

Blalock, J.E. and Smith, E.M. (1985) 'The immune system: our mobile brain?' *Immunology Today 6*, 115–117.

Blampied, N.M. and France, K.G. (1993) 'A behavioral model of infant sleep disturbance.' *Journal of Applied Behavior Analysis 26*, 4, 477–492.

Blaney, N., Goodkin, K., Morgan, R., Feaster, D., Millon, C., Szapocznik, J. and Eisdorfer, C. (1991) 'A stress-moderator model of distress in early HIV-1 infection: concurrent analysis of life events, hardiness and social support.' *Journal of Psychosomatic Research 35*, 2–3, 297–305.

Bloch, D. (1987) 'Family "disease" treatment systems: a co-evolutionary model.' *Family Systems Medicine 5*, 277–292.

Bolton, A. and Adams, M. (1983) 'An investigation of the effects of music therapy on a group of profoundly mentally handicapped adults [news].' *International Journal of Rehabilitation Research 6*, 4, 511–512.

Bolwerk, C. (1990) 'Effects of relaxing music on state anxiety in myocardial infarction patients.' *Critical Care Nursing Quarterly 13*, 2, 63–72.

Bonny, H. (1975) 'Music and consciousness.' *Journal of Music Therapy 12*, 3, 121–135.

Bonny, H. (1978) *GIM Monograph No.2. The Role of Taped Music Programs in the GIM Process.* Baltimore: ICM Press.

Bonny, H. (1983) 'Music listening for intensive coronary care units: a pilot project.' *Music Therapy 3*, 1, 4–16.

Bonny, H. (1986) 'Music and healing.' *Music Therapy 6a*, 1, 3–12.

Bonny, H. (1989) 'Sound as symbol: Guided imagery and music in clinical practice. National Association for Music Therapy California Symposium on Clinical Practices (1987, Costa Mesa, California).' *Music Therapy Perspectives 6*, 7–10.

Bonny, H. and McCarron, N. (1984) 'Music as an adjunct to anesthesia in operative procedures.' *Journal of the American Association of Nurse Anesthetists* Feb., 55–57.

Bortoft, H. (1986) *Goethe's Scientific Consciousness. Monograph Series No.22.* Tunbridge Wells, England: Institute for Cultural Research.

Boutell, K. and Bozett, F. (1990) 'Nurses' assessment of patients' spirituality: continuing education implications.' *Journal of Continued Education in Nursing 21*, 4, 172–6.

Bowling, A. (1991) *Measuring Health: A Review of the Quality of Life Assessment Scales.* Buckingham: Open University Press.

Braake, K. and Savage-Rumbaugh, E. (1995) 'The development of language skills in Bonobo and chimpanzee. I. Comprehension.' *Language and Communication 15*, 2, 121–148.

Brett-Jones, J., Garety, P. and Hemsley, D. (1987) 'Measuring delusional experiences: a method and its application.' *British Journal of Clinical Psychology 26*, Pt 4, 257–65.

Brewster Smith, M. (1994) 'Selfhood at risk: postmodern perils and the perils of postmodernism.' *American Psychologist 49*, 5, 405–411.

Brody, R. (1988) 'Which music helps your muscles?' *American Health 7*, 80–84.

Brown, S. and Fenwick, P. (1989) 'Evoked and psychogenic epileptic seizures: II. Inhibition.' *Acta Neurologica Scandanavia 80*, 6, 541–547.

Bruce, T. (1986) 'Emotional sequelae of chronic inflammatory bowel disease in children and adolescents.' *Clinical Gastroenterology 15*, 89–104.

Bruscia, K. (1987) *Improvisational Models of Music Therapy.* Springfield, IL: Charles Thomas.

Bruscia, K. (1988) 'Standards for clinical assessment in the arts therapies.' *The Arts in Psychotherapy 15*, 5–10.

Bruscia, K. (ed) (1991) *Case Studies in Music Therapy.* Phoenixville, PA: Barcelona.

Bruscia, K. (1995) 'The process of doing qualitative research: Part 1: Introduction.' In B. Wheeler (ed) *Music Therapy Research: Quantitative and Qualitative Perspectives.* Phoenixville, PA: Barcelona.

Bruscia, K. (1995a) 'The process of doing qualitative research: Part 3: The human side.' In B. Wheeler (ed) *Music Therapy Research: Quantitative and Qualitative Perspectives.* Phoenixville, PA: Barcelona.

Brust, J. (1980) 'Music and language: musical alexia and agraphia.' *Brain 103*, 367–392.

Bryant, G. (1989) 'Myofacial pain dysfunction and viola playing.' *British Dental Journal 166*, 9, 335–336.

Bryant, W. (1991) 'Creative group work with confused elderly people: A development of sensory integration therapy.' *British Journal of Occupational Therapy 54*, 5, 187–192.

Buckwalter, K.C., Cusack, D., Kruckeberg, T. and Shoemaker, A. (1991) 'Family involvement with communication-impaired residents in long-term care settings.' *Applied Nursing Research 4*, 2, 77–84.

Budde, E. (1989) 'Musik–Klang–Farbe.' *Musik und Bildung 2*, 68–75.

Bunt, L. (1994) *Music Therapy: An Art Beyond Words.* London: Routledge.

Burgin, V. (1989) *The End of Art Theory: Criticism and Postmodernity.* London: Macmillan.

Burkhardt, M. (1989) 'Spirituality: an analysis of the concept.' *Holistic Nursing Practice 3,* 3, 69–77.

Burkhardt, R. and Kienle, G. (1980) 'Controlled clinical trials and drug regulations.' *Controlled Clinical Trials 1,* 151–164.

Burkhardt, R. and Kienle, G. (1983) 'Basic problems in controlled trials.' *Journal of Medical Ethics 9,* 80–84.

Butcher, P. (1984) 'Existential-behaviour therapy: a possible paradigm?' *British Journal of Medical Psychology 57,* 3, 265–274.

Calkins, B.M. and Mendeloff, A.I. (1986) 'Epidemiology of inflammatory bowel disease.' *Epidemiological Reviews 8,* 60–91.

Caramazza, A. (1986) 'On drawing inferences about the structure of normal cognitive systems from the analysis of patterns of impaired performance: the case for single-patient studies.' *Brain and Cognition 5,* 1, 41–66.

Carter, B.J. (1994) 'Surviving breast cancer: a problematic work re-entry.' *Cancer Practice 2,* 2, 135–140.

Carter, R.E. and Carter, C.A. (1993) 'Individual and marital adjustment in spouse pairs subsequent to mastectomy.' *American Journal of Family Therapy 21,* 4, 291–300.

Casby, J.A. and Holm, M.B. (1994) 'The effect of music on repetitive disruptive vocalizations of persons with dementia.' *American Journal of Occupational Therapy 48,* 10, 883–889.

Case, R. (1993) 'Theories of learning and theories of development.' *Educational Psychologist 28,* 3, 219–233.

Cassem, N. and Hackett, T. (1971) 'Psychiatric consultation in a coronary care unit.' *Annals of Internal Medicine 75,* 9.

Catalan, J. (1990) 'Psychosocial and neuropsychiatric aspects of HIV infection: review of their extent and implications for psychiatry.' *Journal of Psychosomatic Research 22,* 3, 237–248.

Chetta, H. (1981) 'The effect of music and desensitization on preoperative anxiety in children.' *Journal of Music Therapy 18,* 2, 74–87.

Christie, M.E. (1992) 'Music therapy applications in a skilled and intermediate care nursing home facility: A clinical study.' *Activities, Adaptation and Aging 16,* 4, 69–87.

Clair, A. (1990) 'The need for supervision to manage behavior in the elderly care home resident and the implications for music therapy practice.' *Music Therapy Perspectives 8,* 72–75.

Clair, A. (1991) 'Music therapy for a severely regressed person with a probable diagnosis of Alzheimer's Disease.' In K. Bruscia (ed) *Case Studies in Music Therapy.* Phoenixville, PA: Barcelona.

Clair, A. (1992) 'Music therapy for a severely regressed person with a probable diagnosis of Alzheimer's Disease.' In K. Bruscia (ed) *Case Studies in Music Therapy.* Phoenixville, PA: Barcellona Publishers.

Clair, A. and Bernstein, B. (1990) 'A comparison of singing, vibrotactile and nonvibrotactile instrumental playing responses in severely regressed persons with dementia of the Alzheimer's type.' *Journal of Music Therapy 27,* 3, 119–125.

Clair, A.A. and Bernstein, B. (1990a) 'A preliminary study of music therapy programming for severely regressed persons with Alzheimer's-type dementia.' *Journal of Applied Gerontology 9*, 3, 299–311.

Clark, A. and Fallowfield, L. (1986) 'Quality of life measurements in patients with malignant disease: a review.' *Journal of the Royal Society of Medicine 79*, 165–169.

Clark, C.C., Cross, J.R., Deane, D.M. and Lowry, L.W. (1991) 'Spirituality: integral to quality care.' *Holistic Nursing Practice 5*, 3, 67–76.

Clark, M.L. (1986) 'The role of nutrition in inflammatory bowel disease: an overview.' *Gut 72*, S1, 72–75.

Clouse, R. (1986) 'The relationship of psychiatric disorder to gastrointestinal illness.' *Annual Review of Medicine 37*, 283–295.

Cohen, M. (1990) 'Biopsychosocial approach to the human immunodeficiency virus epidemic: a clinician's primer.' *General Hospital Psychiatry 12*, 2, 98–123.

Cohen, P. and Levesque, H. (1994) 'Preliminaries to a collaborative model of dialogue.' *Speech Communication 15*, 265–274.

Colletti, V., Fiorino, F., Carner, M. and Rizzi, R. (1988) 'Investigation of the long-term effects of unilateral hearing loss in adults.' *British Journal of Audiology 22*, 2, 113–118.

Condon, W. (1975) 'Multiple response to sound in dysfunctional children.' *Journal of Autism and Childhood Schizophrenia 5*, 37–56.

Condon, W. (1980) 'The relation of interactional synchrony to cognitive and emotional processes.' In M. Key (ed) *The Relationship of Verbal and Non-verbal Communication.* The Hague: Mouton.

Condon, W. and Ogston, W. (1966) 'Sound film analysis of normal and pathological behavior patterns.' *Journal of Nervous and Mental Disorders 14*, 338–347.

Conrad, N. (1985) 'Spiritual support for the dying.' *Nursing Clinics of North America 20*, 2, 415–426.

Cook, D.J., Guyatt, G.H., Adachi, J.D., Clifton, J., Griffith, L.E., Epstein, R.S. and Juniper, E.F. (1993) 'A diagnostic and therapeutic N-of-1 randomized trial.' *Canadian Journal of Psychiatry 38*, 251–254.

Cook, J. (1981) 'The therapeutic use of music.' *Nursing Forum 20*, 3, 252–266.

Cook, J. (1986) 'Music as an intervention in the oncology setting.' *Cancer Nurse 9*, 1, 23–28.

Coons, P. (1986) 'Treatment progress in 20 patients with multiple personality disorder.' *Journal of Nervous and Mental Disorders 174*, 12, 715–721.

Cooper, J., Mungas, D. and Weiler, P. (1990) 'Relation of cognitive status and abnormal behaviors in Alzheimer's disease.' *Journal of the American Geriatric Society 38*, 8, 867–870.

Corr, C. (1993) 'Coping with dying: Lessons that we should and should not learn from the work of Elisabeth Kübler-Ross.' *Death Studies 17*, 69–83.

Cottraux, J. (1984) 'Agoraphobia and panic attacks: biological and behavioral approaches.' *Encephale 10*, 1, 13–9.

Courtright, P., Johnson, S., Baumgartner, M., Jordan, M. and Webster, J. (1990) 'Dinner music: does it affect the behavior of psychiatric inpatients?' *Journal of Psychosocial Nursing and mental Health Services 28*, 3, 37–40.

Coyle, N. (1987) 'A model of continuity of care for cancer patients with chronic pain.' *Medical Clinics of North America 71*, 2, 259–270.

Crick, N.R. and Dodge, K.A. (1994) 'A review and reformulation of social information-processing mechanisms in children's social adjustment.' *Psychological Bulletin 115*, 1, 74–101.

Crossley, N. (1995) 'Body techniques, agency and intercorporeality: on Goffman's relations in public.' *Sociology 29*, 1, 133–149.

Crystal, H., Grober, E. and Masur, D. (1989) 'Preservation of musical memory in Alzheimer's disease.' *Journal of Neurology, Neurosurgery and Psychiatry 52*, 12, 1415–1416.

Cuddy, L., Cohen, A. and Miner, J. (1979) 'Melody recognition: the experimental application of musical rules.' *Canadian Journal of Psychology 33*, 148–157.

Dalessio, D. (1984) 'Maurice Ravel and Alzheimer's disease.' *Journal of the American Medical Association 252*, 24, 3412–3413.

Dallos, R. and Aldridge, D. (1986) 'Change: how do we recognise it?' *Journal of Family Therapy 8*, 45–59.

Darko, D. (1986) 'A brief tour of psychoneuroimmunology.' *Annals of Allergy 57*, 4, 233–238.

Daub, D. and Kirschner-Hermanns, R. (1988) 'Reduction of preoperative anxiety: a study comparing music, Thalamonal and no premedication.' *Anaesthesist 37*, 9, 594–597.

Davis-Rollans, C. and Cunningham, S. (1987) 'Physiologic responses of coronary care patients to selected music.' *Heart and Lung 16*, 4, 370–378.

Decker-Voigt, H.-H., Eschen, J. and Mahns, W. (1993) *Kindermusiktherapie.* Lilienthal/Bremen: Eres.

Declaration of Helsinki (1975) *Recommendations Guiding Doctors in Biomedical Research.* Twenty-ninth World Medical Assembly Conference Proceedings. Tokyo.

Dellmann-Jenkins, M., Papalia Finlay, D. and Hennon, C. (1984) 'Continuing education in later adulthood: implications for program development for elderly guest students.' *International Journal of Aging and Human Development 20*, 2, 93–102.

Denzin, N. and Lincoln, Y. (1994) *Handbook of Qualitative Research.* London: Sage.

Dessloch, A., Maiworm, M., Florin, I. and Schulze, C. (1992) 'Hospital care versus home-bound hospice care – quality of life in patients with terminal cancer.' *Psychotherapie, Psychosomatik, Medizin und Psychologie 42*, 12, 424–429.

Devisch, R. and Vervaeck, B. (1986) 'Doors and thresholds: Jeddi's approach to psychiatric disorders.' *Social Science and Medicine 22*, 5, 541–551.

Dew, M., Ragni, M. and Nimorwicz, P. (1991) 'Correlates of psychiatric distress among wives of hemophilic men with and without HIV infection.' *American Journal of Psychiatry 148*, 8, 1016–1022.

Dielman, T., Butchart, A., Moss, G., Harrison, R., Harlan, W., and Horvarth, W. (1987) 'Psychometric properties of component and global measures of structured interview assessed Type A behavior in a population sample.' *Psychosomatic Medicine 49*, 458–469.

Dillon, K.M. and Baker, K.H. (1985) 'Positive emotional states and enhancement of the immune system.' *International Journal of Psychiatry 15*, 13–17.

Dimsdale, J. and Stern, M.E. (1988) 'The stress interview as a tool for examining psychologic reactivity.' *Psychosomatic Medicine 50*, 64–71.

Diserens, C.M. (1920) 'Reaction to musical stimuli.' *Psychological Bulletin 20*, 173–199.

Dossey, L. (1982) *Space, Time and Medicine.* Boulder, CO: Shambala.

Drachman, D., O'Donnell, B., Lew, R. and Swearer, J. (1990) 'The prognosis in Alzheimer's disease.' *Archives of Neurology 47*, 851–856.

Dreyfus, H. (1987) 'Foucault's critique of psychiatric medicine.' *The Journal of Medicine and Philosophy 12*, 311–333.

Dudley, H. (1983) 'The controlled clinical trial and the advance of reliable knowledge: an outsider looks in.' *British Medical Journal 287*, 957–960.

Dunnell, K. and Cartwright, A. (1972) *Medicine-takers, Prescribers and Hoarders.* London: Routledge and Kegan Paul.

Dzurec, L. (1989) 'The necessity for and evolution of multiple paradigms for nursing research: a poststructuralist perspective.' *Advanced Nursing Science 11*, 4, 69–77.

Dzurec, L. and Abraham, I. (1986) 'Analogy between phenomenology and multivariate statistical analysis.' In P. Chinn (ed) *Nursing Research Methodology: Issues and Implementation.* Gaithersburg, MD: Aspen.

Dzurec, L. and Abraham, I. (1993) 'The nature of inquiry: Linking quantitative and qualitative research.' *Advanced Nursing Science 16*, 1, 73–79.

Editorial (1992) 'Changing case-definition for AIDS.' *The Lancet 340*, 1199–1200.

Edmans, J. and Lincoln, N. (1989) 'Treatment of visual perceptual deficits after stroke: four single case studies.' *International Disability Studies 11*, 1, 25–33.

Edwards, K.J. and Christophersen, E.R. (1993) 'Automated data acquisition through time-lapse videotape recording.' *Journal of Applied Behavior Analysis 26*, 4, 503–504.

Elias, G. and Broerse, J. (1995) 'Temporal patterning of vocal behaviour in mother–infant engagements: infant-initiated "encounters" as units of analysis.' *Australian Journal of Psychology 47*, 1, 1–7.

Elliott, D. (1994) 'The effects of music and muscle relaxation on patient anxiety in a coronary care unit.' *Heart and Lung 23*, 1, 27–35.

Ellis, J.B. and Smith, P.C. (1991) 'Spiritual well-being, social desirability and reasons for living: is there a connection?' *International Journal of Psychiatry 37*, 1, 57–63.

Emblen, J.D. (1992) 'Religion and spirituality defined according to current use in nursing literature.' *Journal of Professional Nursing 8*, 1, 41–47.

Engel, G. (1977) 'The need for a new medical model: a challenge for biomedicine.' *Science 196*, 129–136.

Engelmann, I. (1995) 'Musiktherapie in psychiatrischen kliniken.' *Nervenarzt 66*, 217–224.

Eustache, F., Cox, C., Brandt, J., Lechevaliet, B. and Pnos, L. (1990) 'Word-association responses and severity of dementia in Alzheimer disease.' *Psychological Reports 66*, 3 Pt 2, 1315–1322.

Evers, S. (1990) '[Music for rheumatism – a historical overview] Musik gegen Rheuma – Ein historischer überblick.' *Zeitschrift für Rheumatologie 49*, 3, 119–124.

Faden, R. and Kass, N. (1990) 'AIDS will pose moral dilemmas well into 1990s.' *Kennedy Institute of Ethics Newsletter 4*, 3, 1–2.

Fagen, T.S. (1982) 'Music therapy in the treatment of anxiety and fear in terminal pediatric patients.' *Music Therapy 2*, 1, 13–23.

Fais, L. (1994) 'Conversation as collaboration: some syntactic evidence.' *Speech Communication 15*, 231–242.

Farquhar, J. (1994) 'Eating Chinese medicine.' *Cultural Anthropology 9*, 4, 471–497.

Faustman, W., Moses, J.J. and Csernansky, J. (1990) 'Limitations of the Mini-Mental State Examination in predicting neuropsychological functioning in a psychiatric sample.' *Acta Psychiatra Scandanavia 81*, 2, 126–131.

Fehring, R., Brennan, P. and Keller, M. (1987) 'Psychological and spiritual well-being in college students.' *Research Nursing and Health 10*, 6, 391–398.

Feifel, H. (1990) 'Psychology and death: meaningful rediscovery.' *American Psychologist 45*, 4, 537–543.

Feinstein, A. (1966) 'Symptoms as an index of biological behavior in human cancer.' *Nature 209*, 241–245.

Fenton, G. and McRae, D. (1989) 'Musical hallucinations in a deaf elderly woman.' *British Journal of Psychiatry 155*, 401–403.

Finney, J.W., Miller, K.M. and Adler, S.P. (1993) 'Changing protective and risky behaviors to prevent child-to-parent transmission of cytomegalovirus.' *Journal of Applied Behavior Analysis 26*, 4, 471–472.

Fitzgerald Cloutier, M.L. (1993) 'The use of music therapy to decrease wandering: An alternative to restraints.' *Music Therapy Perspectives 11*, 1, 32–36.

Flaskerud, J. and Rush, C. (1989) 'AIDS and traditional health beliefs and practices of black women.' *Nursing Research 38*, 4, 210–215.

Fletcher, V. (1986) 'The mobile accident team: when the music stopped.' *Nursing Times 82*, 18, 30–32.

Florian, J.E. (1994) 'Stripes do not a zebra make, or do they? Conceptual and perceptual information in inductive inference.' *Developmental Psychology 30*, 1, 88–101.

Foley, K. (1986) 'The treatment of pain in the patient with cancer.' *Cancer Archives 36*, 4, 194–215.

Folstein, M.F., Folstein, S.E. and McHugh, P. (1975) 'Mini-Mental State: a practical guide for grading the cognitive state of patients for the clinician.' *Journal of Psychiatric Research 12*, 189–198.

Formby, C., Thomas, R., Brown, W.J. and Halsey, J.J. (1987) 'The effects of continuous phonation on 133xenon-inhalation air curves (of the kind used in deriving regional cerebral blood flow).' *Brain and Language 31*, 2, 346–363.

Foucault, M. (1988) *The Use of Pleasure: The History of Sexuality.* London: Peregrine.

Foucault, M. (1989) *The Birth of the Clinic.* London: Routledge.

Frampton, D. (1986) 'Restoring creativity to the dying patient.' *British Medical Journal of Clinical Research 293*, 6562, 1593–1595.

Frampton, D. (1989) 'Arts activities in United Kingdom hospices: a report.' *Journal of Palliative Care 5*, 4, 25–32.

Frandsen, J. (1989) 'Nursing approaches in local anesthesia for ophthalmic surgery.' *Journal of Opthalmic Nursing Technology 8*, 4, 135–138.

Frank, J. (1985) 'The effects of music therapy and guided visual imagery on chemotherapy induced nausea and vomiting.' *Oncology Nursing Forum 12*, 5, 47–52.

Frankl, V. (1963) *Man's Search for Meaning.* New York: Washington Square Press.

Fraser, W., King, K., Thomas, P. and Kendell, R. (1986) 'The diagnosis of schizophrenia by language analysis.' *British Journal of Psychiatry 148*, 275–278.

Freeling, P. (1985) 'Health outcomes in primary care: An approach to problems.' *Family Practice 2*, 177–181.

Freeman, L. (1986) 'Emotion, heart rate and hyperventilation.' *Journal of Psychosomatic Research 30*, 4, 429–436.

Freer, C. (1980) 'Self care: a health diary study.' *Medical Care 18*, 853–861.

Freyberger, H., Künsbeck, H.J., Lempa, W., Wellmann, W. and Avenarius, H.J. (1985) 'Psychotherapeutic interventions in alexithymic patients with special regard to ulcerative colitis and Crohn patients.' *Psychotherapeutic Psychosomatics 44*, 72–81.

Fried, R. (1990) 'Integrating music in breathing training and relaxation: I. Background, rationale, and relevant elements.' *Biofeedback and Self-Regulation 15*, 2, 161–169.

Friedman, A. and Glickman, N. (1986) 'Program characteristics for successful treatment of adolescent drug abuse.' *Journal of Nervous and Mental Disorders 174*, 11, 669–679.

Friedmann, E., Thomas, S., Kulick-Ciuffo, D., Lynch, J. and Suginohala, M. (1982) 'The effects of normal and rapid speech on blood pressure.' *Psychosomatic Medicine 44*, 545–553.

Froehlich, M. (1984) 'A comparison of the effect of music therapy and medical play therapy on the verbalization behavior of pediatric patients.' *Journal of Music Therapy 21*, 1, 2–15.

Fry, D. (1971) *Some Effects of Music. Monograph Series No.9.* Tunbridge Wells, England: Institute for Cultural Research.

Fulder, S. (1988) *The Handbook of Complementary Medicine.* London: Coronet.

Furnham, A. (1994) 'Explaining health and illness: lay perceptions on current and future health, the causes of illness and the nature of recovery.' *Social Science and Medicine 39*, 5, 715–725.

Gagnon, M., Letenneur, L., Dartigues, J., Commenges, D., Orgogozo, J., Barberger Gateau, P., Alperovitch, A., Decamps, A. and Salamon, R. (1990) 'Validity of the Mini-Mental State examination as a screening instrument for cognitive impairment and dementia in French elderly community residents.' *Neuroepidemiology 9*, 3, 143–150.

Galasko, D., Klauber, M., Hofstetter, C., Salmon, D., Lasker, B. and Thal, L. (1990) 'The Mini-Mental State Examination in the early diagnosis of Alzheimer's disease.' *Archives of Neurology 47*, 1, 49–52.

Gary, G. (1992) 'Facing terminal illness in children with AIDS: developing a philosophy of care for patients, families, and caregivers.' *Home Health Nurse 10*, 2, 40–43.

Gates, A. and Bradshaw, J. (1977) 'The role of the cerebral hemispheres in music.' *Brain and Language 4*, 403–431.

Gaussen, T. (1985) 'Beyond the milestone model – a systems framework of infant assessment procedures.' *Child Care, Health and Development 11*, 131–150.

Gerdner, L.A. and Swanson, E.A. (1993) 'Effects of individualized music on confused and agitated elderly patients.' *Archives of Psychiatric Nursing 7*, 5, 284–291.

Gergen, K. (1991) *The Saturated Self: Dilemmas of Identity in Contemporary Life.* New York: Basic Books.

Gerstner, G. and Goldberg, L. (1994) 'Evidence of a time constant associated with movement patterns in six mammalian species.' *Ethology and Sociobiology 15*, 181–205.

Gilbert, J. (1977) 'Music therapy perspectives on death and dying.' *Journal of Music Therapy 14*, 4, 165–171.

Gilchrist, P. and Kalucy, R. (1983) 'Musical hallucinations in the elderly: a variation on the theme.' *Australia and New Zealand Journal of Psychiatry 17*, 3, 286–287.

Gillberg, C., Winnergard, I. and Wahlstrom, J. (1984) 'The sex chromosomes– one key to autism? An XYY case of infantile autism.' *Applied Research in Mental Retardation 5*, 3, 353–360.

Gillon, R. (1986) 'On sickness and health.' *British Medical Journal 292*, 318–320.

Giorgio, A. (1994) 'A phenomenological perspective on certain qualitative research methods.' *Journal of Phenomenological Psychology 25*, 2, 190–220.

Glassman, L.A. (1983) 'The talent show: meeting the needs of the healthy elderly.' *Music Therapy 3*, 1, 82–93.

Glenn, S. and Cunningham, C. (1984) 'Nursery rhymes and early language acquisition by mentally handicapped children.' *Exceptional Children 51*, 1, 72–74.

Glynn, N. (1986) 'The therapy of music.' *Journal of Gerontological Nursing 12*, 1, 6–10.

Godley, C. (1987) 'The use of music therapy in pain clinics.' *Music Therapy Perspectives 4*, 24–27.

Gold, J. (1986) 'Quality of life measurements in patients with malignant disease.' *Journal of the Royal Society of Medicine 79*, 622.

Goldin-Meadow, S., Alibali, M.W. and Church, R.B. (1993) 'Transitions in concept acquisition – using the hand to read the mind.' *Psychology Review 100*, 2, 279–297.

Gollek, R. (1989) *Brennpunkt der Moderne: Der blaue Reiter in München*. Munich: Piper.

Goloff, M. (1981) 'The responses of hospitalised medical patients to music therapy.' *Music Therapy 1*, 1, 51–56.

Grant, I. and Hampton Atkinson, J. (1990) 'Neurogenic and psychogenic behavioral correlates of HIV infection.' In B. Wakeman (ed) *Immunologic Mechanisms in Neurologic and Psychiatric Disease*. New York: Raven Press.

Grasser, C. and Craft, B. (1984) 'The patient's approach to wellness.' *Nursing Clinics of North America 19*, 2, 207–218.

Gray, J. and Robertson, I. (1989) 'Remediation of attentional difficulties following brain injury: three experimental single case studies.' *Brain Injury 3*, 2, 163–170.

Green, E. (1986) 'Chord perception in schizophrenia.' *British Journal of Clinical Psychology 25*, Pt 1, 69–70.

Gregg, I. (1985) 'The quality of asthma in general practice – a challenge for the future.' *Family Practice 2*, 94–100.

Griffiths, R. (1954) *The Abilities of Babies*. London: University of London Press.

Grimm, D. and Pefley, P. (1990) 'Opening doors for the child "inside".' *Pediatric Nursing 16*, 4, 368–369.

Groene, R.W. (1993) 'Effectiveness of music therapy 1:1 intervention with individuals having Senile Dementia of the Alzheimer's Type.' *Journal of Music Therapy 30*, 3, 138–157.

Grohmann, W. (1987) *Paul Klee*. London: Thames and Hudson.

Gross, J.-L. and Swartz, R. (1982) 'The effects of music therapy on anxiety in chronically ill patients.' *Music Therapy 2*, 1, 43–52.

Guba, E. and Lincoln, Y. (1989) *Fourth Generation Evaluation*. London: Sage.

Gustorff, D. (1990) 'Lieder ohne worte.' *Musiktherapeutische Umschau 11*, 120–126.

Gutterman, L. (1990) 'A day treatment program for persons with AIDS.' *American Journal of Occupational Therapy 44*, 3, 234–237.

Guyatt, G., Satchett, D., Taylor, D., Chong, J., Roberts, R. and Pugsley, S. (1986) 'Determining optimal therapy randomized trials in individual patients.' *New England Journal of Medicine 314*, 889–892.

Guyatt, G., Sackett, D., Taylor, D., Chong, J., Rosenbloom, D. and Keller, J. (1988) 'A clinician's guide for conducting randomized trials in individual patients.' *Canadian Medical Association Journal 139*, 6, 497–503.

Guzzetta, C. (1989) 'Effects of relaxation and music therapy on patients in a coronary care unit with presumptive acute myocardial infarction.' *Heart and Lung 18*, 6, 609–616.

Haag, G. (1985) 'Psychosoziale rehabilitation im alter.' *Rehabilitation Stuttgart 24*, 1, 6–8.

Haag, G. and Lucius, G. (1984) 'Psychologie in der rehabilitation.' *Rehabilitation Stuttgart 23*, 1, 1–9.

Haas, F., Distenfeld, S. and Axen, K. (1986) 'Effects of perceived musical rhythm on respiratory pattern.' *Journal of Applied Physiology 61*, 3, 1185–1191.

Hagopian, L.P., Fisher, W., Piazza, C.C. and Wierzbicki, J.J. (1993) 'A water-prompting procedure for the treatment of urinary incontinence.' *Journal of Applied Behavior Analysis 26*, 4, 473–474.

Hall, D. (1977) *Klee*. London: Phaidon.

Hammeke, T., McQuillen, M. and Cohen, B. (1983) 'Musical hallucinations associated with acquired deafness.' *Journal of Neurology, Neurosurgery and Psychiatry 46*, 6, 570–572.

Hannich, H. (1988) 'Überlegen zum handlungsprimat in der intensivmedizin.' *Medizin Mensch und Gesellschaft 13*, 238–244.

Hanser, S. (1995) 'Applied behavior analysis.' In B. Wheeler (ed) *Music Therapy Research: Quantitative and Qualitative Perspectives*. Phoenixville, PA: Barcelona.

Harré, R. and Secord, P. (1971) *The Explanation of Social Behaviour*. London: Basil Blackwell.

Hart, J. (1984) 'Where is general practice going?' *New Doctor 33*, 8–10.

Harvey, S. and Kelly, E. (1993) 'Evaluation of the quality of parent–child relationships: a longitudinal case study.' *The Arts in Psychotherapy 20*, 387–395.

Hayes, S., Hussian, R., Turner, A., Anderson, N. and Grubb, T. (1983) 'The effect of coping statements on progress through a desensitization hierarchy.' *Journal of Behavioral Therapy and Experimental Psychiatry 14*, 2, 117–129.

Hays, R., Catania, J., McKusick, L. and Coates, T. (1990) 'Help-seeking for AIDS-related concerns: a comparison of gay men with various HIV diagnoses.' *American Journal of Community Psychology 18*, 5, 743–755.

Heidegger, M. (1962) *Being and Time*. London: SCM Press.

Helman, C. (1985) 'Psyche, soma and society: the social construction of psychosomatic disorders.' *Culture, Medicine and Psychiatry 9*, 1–26.

Helman, C. (1987) 'Heart disease and the cultural construction of time: The type A behaviour pattern as a western culture-bound syndrome.' *Social Science and Medicine 25*, 969–979.

Henson, R. (1988) 'Maurice Ravel's illness: a tragedy of lost creativity.' *British Medical Journal of Clinical Research 296*, 6636, 1585–1588.

Heron, J. (1984) 'Critique of conventional research methodology.' *Complementary Medicinal Research 1*, 12–22.

Herrigel, E. (1988) *The Method of Zen*. London: Penguin Arkana.

Herskowitz, J., Rosman, N. and Geschwind, N. (1984) 'Seizures induced by singing and recitation: a unique form of reflex epilepsy in childhood.' *Archives of Neurology 41*, 10, 1102–1103.

Herth, K. (1990) 'Fostering hope in terminally-ill people.' *Journal of Advanced Nursing 15*, 11, 1250–1259.

Herth, K. (1991) 'Development and refinement of an instrument to measure hope.' *Scholarly Inquiry for Nursing Practice: An International Journal 5*, 1, 39–51.

Heyde, W. and von Langsdorff, P. (1983) '[Rehabilitation of cancer patients including creative therapies].' *Rehabilitation Stuttgart 22*, 1, 25–27.

Heyink, J. and Tymstra, T. (1993) 'The function of qualitative research.' *Social Indicators Research 20*, 291–305.

Hiatt, J. (1986) 'Spirituality, medicine, and healing.' *Southern Medical Journal 79*, 6, 736–743.

Hilliard, R.B. (1993) 'Single-case methodology in psychotherapy process and outcome research.' *Journal of Consulting and Clinical Psychology 61*, 3, 373–380.

Hoefkens, A. and Allen, D. (1990) 'Evaluation of a special behaviour unit for people with mental handicaps and challenging behaviour.' *Journal of Mental Deficiency Research 34*, 3, 213–228 (discussion 229–235).

Horder, J. and Horder, E. (1954) 'Illness in general practice.' *The Practitioner 173*, 177–185.

Howat, R. (1995) 'Elizabeth: a case study of an autistic child in individual music therapy.' In T. Wigram, B. Saperston and R. West (eds) *The Art and Science of Music Therapy: A Handbook.* Chur, Switzerland: Harwood Academic Publishers.

Howie, J. (1984) 'Research in general practice: pursuit of knowledge or defence of wisdom.' *British Medical Journal 289*, 1770–1772.

Huebner, E.S. and Dew, T. (1993) 'Is life satisfaction multidimensional – the factor structure of the perceived life satisfaction scale.' *Journal of Psychoeducational Assessment 11*, 4, 345–350.

Hydén, L-C. (1995) 'The rhetoric of recovery.' *Culture, Medicine and Psychiatry 19*, 73–90.

Jacob, S. (1986) 'Soothing the ragged edge of pain. Bring on the music.' *American Journal of Nursing 86*, 9, 1034.

Jacobsen, P.B., Bovbjerg, D.H. and Redd, W.H. (1993) 'Anticipatory Anxiety in Women Receiving Chemotherapy for Breast Cancer.' *Health Psychology 12*, 6, 469–475.

Jacobsen, T., Edelstein, W. and Hofmann, V. (1994) 'A longitudinal study of the relation between representations of attachment in childhood and cognitive functioning in childhood and adolescence.' *Developmental Psychology 30*, 1, 112–124.

Jacome, D. (1984) 'Aphasia with elation, hypermusia, musicophilia and compulsive whistling.' *Journal of Neurology, Neurosurgery and Psychiatry 47*, 3, 308–310.

Jairath, N. and Campbell, H. (1990) 'Two mental status assessment methods: an evaluation.' *Journal of Ophthalmic Nursing Technology 9*, 3, 102–105.

Jeannerod, M. (1994) 'The representing brain: neural correlates of motor intention and imagery.' *Behavioral and Brain Sciences 17*, 187–245.

Joachim, G.B. (1987) 'Inflammatory bowel disease: effects on lifestyle.' *Journal of Advanced Nursing 12*, 483–487.

Jochims, S. (1990) 'Krankheitsverarbeitung in der fruhphase schwerer neurologischer erkrankungen: ein beitrag der musiktherapie zur psychischen betreuung bei ausgewahlten neurologischen krankheitsbildern.' *Psychotherapie, Psychosomatik, Medizin und Psychologie 40*, 3–4, 115–122.

Johnson, C. and Woodland-Hastings, J. (1986) 'The elusive mechanism of the circadian clock.' *American Scientist 74*, 29–36.

Johnston, M. (1988) 'AIDS related psychosocial issues for the patient and physician.' *Journal of the American Osteopathy Association 88*, 2, 234–238.

Jonas, J.L. (1991) 'Preferences of elderly music listeners residing in nursing homes for art music, traditional jazz, popular music of today, and country music.' *Journal of Music Therapy 28*, 3, 149–160.

Jones, C. (1990) 'Spark of life.' *Geriatric Nursing in New York 11*, 4, 194–196.

Jones, E.E. (1993) 'Introduction to special section – single-case research in psychotherapy.' *Journal of Consulting and Clinical Psychology 61*, 3, 371–372.

Jones, E.E., Ghannam, J., Nigg, J.T. and Dyer, J.F.P. (1993) 'A paradigm for single-case research – the time series study of a long-term psychotherapy for depression.' *Journal of Consulting and Clinical Psychology 61*, 3, 381–394.

Jones, M., Kidd, G. and Wetzel, R. (1981) 'Evidence for rhythmic attention.' *Journal of Experimental Psychology 7*, 1059–1073.

Jusczyk, P.W., Cutler, A. and Redanz, N.J. (1993) 'Infants' preference for the predominant stress patterns of English words.' *Child Development 64*, 3, 675–687.

Kaczorowski, J. (1989) 'Spiritual weel-being and anxiety in adults diagnosed with cancer.' *Hospital Journal 5*(3–4), 105–16.

Kalayam, B. and Shamoian, C. (1990) 'Geriatric psychiatry: an update.' *Journal of Clinical Psychiatry 51*, 5, 177–183.

Kammrath, I. (1989) 'Musiktherapie wahrend der chemotherapie. Bericht uber den beginn einer studie.' *Krankenpflege Frankfurt 43*, 6, 282–283.

Karanth, P. and Rangamani, G. (1988) 'Crossed aphasia in multilinguals.' *Brain and Language 34*, 1, 169–180.

Karnofsky, D., Abelmann, W. and Craver, L. (1948) 'The use of nitrogen mustards in the palliative treatment of carcinoma.' *Cancer 1*, 634–656.

Kartman, L. (1984) 'Music hath charms....' *Journal of Gerontological Nursing 10*, 6, 20–24.'

Kartman, L. (1990) 'Fun and entertainment: One aspect of making meaningful music for the elderly.' *Activities, Adaptation and Aging 14*, 4, 39–44.

Kaufmann, G. (1983) 'Zur kombination musiktherapeutischer methoden in der dynamischen gruppenpsychotherapie.' *Psychiatrie, Neurologie, Medizin und Psychologie, Leipzig 35*, 3, 148–153.

Kaufmann, G. (1985) 'Rezeptive einzelmusiktherapie in der ambulanten psychotherapie-konzeption.' *Psychiatrie, Neurologie, Medizin und Psychologie, Leipzig 37*, 6, 347–352.

Kazdin, A. (1982) *Single Case Research Designs: Methods For Clinical and Applied Settings.* New York: Oxford University Press.

Kazdin, A. (1983) 'Single-case research designs in clinical child psychiatry.' *Journal of American Academic Child Psychiatry 22*, 5, 423–432.

Kellar, L. and Bever, T. (1980) 'Hemispheric asymmetries in the perception of musical intervals as a function of musical experience.' *Brain and Language 10*, 24–38.

Kellner, D. (1988) 'Expressionism and rebellion.' In S. Bronner and D. Kellner (eds) *Passion and Rebellion.* New York: Columbia University Press.

Kelly, G.A. (1955) *The Psychology of Personal Constructs*, Vols I and II. New York: Norton.

Kempton, W. (1980) 'The rhythmic basis of interactional microsynchrony.' In M. Key (ed) *The Relationship of Verbal and Non-verbal Communication.* The Hague: Mouton.

Keshavan, M., Kahn, E. and Brar, J. (1988) 'Musical hallucinations following removal of a right frontal meningioma [letter].' *Journal of Neurology, Neurosurgery and Psychiatry 51*, 9, 1235–1236.

Kett, K., Rognum, T.O. and Brandzaeg, P. (1987) 'Mucosal subclass distribution of immunoglobulin G-producing cells is different in ulcerative colitis and Crohn's disease of the colon.' *Gastroenterology 93*, 919–924.

Key, M. (ed) (1980) *The Relationship of Verbal and Non-verbal Communication.* The Hague: Mouton.

Khan Inayat, H. (1979) *The Bowl of Saki.* Geneva: Sufi Publishing Co. Ltd.

Khan Inayat, H. (1983) *The Music of Life.* Santa Fe: Omega Press.

Kidd, G., Boltz, M. and Jones, M. (1984) 'Some effects of rhythmic context on melody recognition.' *American Journal of Psychology 97*, 2, 153–173.

Kirshner, B. and Guyatt, G. (1985) 'A methodological framework for assessing health indices.' *Journal of Chronic Diseases 38*, 27–36.

Kleinman, A. (1973) 'Medicine's symbolic reality.' *Inquiry 16*, 206–213.

Kleinman, A. (1978) 'Culture, illness and care.' *Annals of Internal Medicine 88*, 251–258.

Kleinman, A. and Sung, L. (1979) 'Why do indigenous practitioners successfully heal?' *Social Science and Medicine 13*, 7–26.

Knill, C. (1983) 'Body awareness, communication and development: a programme employing music with the profoundly handicapped.' *International Journal of Rehabilitation Research 6*, 4, 489–492.

Koch, T. (1994) 'Establishing rigour in qualitative research: the decision trail.' *Journal of Advanced Nursing 19*, 976–986.

Kolkmeier, L. (1989) 'Clinical application of relaxation, imagery, and music in contemporary nursing.' *Journal of Advanced Medical Surgical Nursing 1*, 4, 73–80.

Krupnick, J. and Pincus, H. (1992) 'The cost effectiveness of psychotherapy.' *American Journal of Psychiatry 149*, 10, 1295–1305.

Kuhn, C. (1988) 'A spiritual inventory of the medically ill patient.' *Psychiatric Medicine 6*, 2, 87–100.

Labun, E. (1988) 'Spiritual care: an element in nursing care planning.' *Journal of Advanced Nursing 13*, 3, 314–320.

Langenberg, M., Frommer, J. and Tress, W. (1992) 'A qualitative research approach to Analytical Music Therapy.' *Musiktherapeutische Umschau 13*, 258–298.

Langer, S. (1953) *Feeling and Form: A Theory of Art*. London: Routledge and Kegan Paul.

Lankheit, K. (1989) *Der blaue Reiter*. Munich: Piper.

Lask, B. (1986) 'Psychological aspects of inflammatory bowel disease.' *Wiener klinische Wochenschrift 29*, 544–547.

Laszlo, J.I. and Sainsbury, K.M. (1993) 'Perceptual-motor development and prevention of clumsiness.' *Psychological Research – Psychologische Forschung 55*, 2, 167–174.

Lavigne, J., Schulein, M. and Hahn, Y. (1986) 'Psychological aspects of painful medical conditions in children. II. Personality factors, family characteristics and treatment.' *Pain 27*, 2, 147–169.

LeBlanc, A. (1986) 'Quantitative analysis of cardiac arrhythmias.' *Critical Review of Biomedical Engineering 14*, 1, 1–43.

Lecourt, E. (1991) 'Off-beat music therapy: A psychoanalytic approach to autism.' In K. Bruscia (ed) *Case Studies in Music Therapy*. Phoenixville, PA: Barcelona.

Lecourt, E. (1992) 'The functions of music therapy in France.' Special Issue: European perspectives on the creative arts therapies. *Arts in Psychotherapy 19*, 123–126.

Lee, C. (1991) 'Foreword: Endings.' *Journal of British Music Therapy 5*, 1, 3–4.

Lehmann, K., Horrichs, G. and Hoeckle, W. (1985) 'Zur bedeutung von Tramadol als intraoperativem analgetikum. Eine randomisierte doppelblindstudie im vergleich zu placebo.' *Anaesthetist 34*, 1, 11–19.

Lehnen, R. (1988) 'Does music during dental treatment have an influence on heart and circulation parameters?' *Zahnarztlische Praxis 39*, 8, 297–300.

Lehrer, P.M., Hochron, S.M., Mayne, T., Isenberg, S., Carlson, V., Lasoski, A.M., Gilchrist, J., Morales, D. and Rausch, L. (1994) 'Relaxation and music therapies for asthma among patients prestabilized on asthma medication.' *Journal of Behavioral Medicine 17*, 1, 1–24.

Lengdobler, H. and Kiessling, W. (1989) 'Gruppenmusiktherapie bei multipler sklerose: Ein erster erfahrungsbericht.' *Psychotherapie, Psychosomatik, Medizin und Psychologie 39*, 9–10, 369–373.

Leonidas, J. (1981) 'Healing power of chants.' *New York State Journal of Medicine 81*, 6, 966–968.

Lester, B., Hoffman, J. and Brazelton, T. (1985) 'The rhythmic structure of mother–infant interaction in term and proterm infants.' *Child Development 56*, 15–27.

Lett, W. (1993) 'Therapist creativity: the art of supervision.' *The Arts in Psychotherapy 20*, 371–386.

Lewis, J.M. (1993) 'Childhood play in normality, pathology, and therapy.' *American Journal of Orthopsychiatry 63*, 1, 6–15.

Lewis, M. and Volkmar, F. (1990) *Clinical Aspects of Child and Adolescent Development.* Philadelphia: Lea and Febiger.

Lincoln, S. and Guba, E. (1985) *Naturalistic Inquiry.* Beverly Hills: Sage.

Linden, W. (1987) 'A microanalysis of autonomic activity during human speech.' *Psychosomatic Medicine 49*, 562–578.

Lindsay, S. (1993) 'Music in hospitals.' *British Journal of Hospital Medicine 50*, 11, 660–662.

Lindsay, W. (1980) 'The training and generalization of conversation behaviours in psychiatric in-patients: a controlled study employing multiple measures across settings.' *British Journal of Social and Clinical Psychology 19*, 85–98.

Lipe, A.W. (1991) 'Using music therapy to enhance the quality of life in a client with Alzheimer's dementia: a case study.' *Music Therapy Perspectives 9*, 102–105.

Locsin, R. (1988) 'Effects of preferred music and guided imagery music on the pain of selected post-operative patients.' *ANPHI-Papers 1988 23*, 1, 2–4.

Longuet-Higgins, H. (1979) 'The perception of music.' *Proceedings of the Royal Society of London 205*, 307–322.

Longuet-Higgins, H. (1982) 'The perception of musical rhythms.' *Perception 11*, 115–128.

Louis, T., Lavori, P., Bailar, J. and Polansky, M. (1984) 'Cross-over and self-controlled trials in clinical research.' *New England Journal of Medicine 310*, 24–31.

Lucia, C.M. (1987) 'Toward developing a model of music therapy intervention in the rehabilitation of head trauma patients.' *Music Therapy Perspectives 4*, 34–39.

Lynch, J. (1977) *The Broken Heart: The Medical Consequences of Loneliness.* New York: Basic Books.

Lynch, J., Long, M., Thomas, S., Malinkow, K. and Katchor, A. (1981) 'The effects of talking on blood pressure of hypertensive and normotensive individuals.' *Psychosomatic Medicine 43*, 25–33.

Macnamara, J. (1993) 'Cognitive psychology and the rejection of Brentano.' *Journal for the Theory of Social Behavior 22*, 2, 117–138.

Maher, T. (1980) 'A rigorous test of the proposition that musical intervals have different psychological effects.' *American Journal of Psychology 93*, 2, 309–327.

Maj, M. (1991) 'Psychological problems of families and health workers dealing with people infected with human immunodeficiency virus 1.' *Acta Psychiatrica Scandinavica 83*, 3, 161–8.

Marchette, L., Main, R. and Redick, E. (1989) 'Pain reduction during neonatal circumcision.' *Pediatric Nursing 15*, 2, 207–208, 210.

Mark, A. (1986) 'Adolescents discuss themselves and drugs through music.' *Journal of Substance Abuse Treatment 3*, 4, 243–249.

Mark, A. (1988) 'Metaphoric lyrics as a bridge to the adolescent's world.' *Adolescence 23*, 90, 313–323.

Marley, L. (1984) 'The use of music with hospitalized infants and toddlers: a descriptive study.' *Journal of Music Therapy 21*, 126–132.

Marshall, J. and Newcombe, F. (1984) 'Putative problems and pure progress in neuropsychological single-case studies.' *Journal of Clinical Neuropsychology 6*, 1, 65–70.

Martin, J. (1993) 'The problem with therapeutic science.' *The Journal of Psychology 127*, 4, 365–374.

Mash, E.J. (1993) 'Rochester symposium on developmental psychopathology, Vol. 3 – models and integrations, by D. Cicchetti, S.L. Toth (book review).' *Canadian Journal of Behavioral Science 25*, 4, 628–632.

May, C. (1992) 'Individual care? Power and subjectivity in therapeutic relationships.' *Sociology 26*, 4, 589–602.

McCaffery, M. (1990) 'Nursing approaches to nonpharmacological pain control.' *International Journal of Nursing Studies 27*, 1, 1–5.

McClellan, R. (1988) *The Healing Forces of Music: History, Theory and Practice.* New York: Amity House.

McCloskey, L.J. (1985) 'Music and the frail elderly.' *Activities, Adaptation and Aging 7*, 2, 73–75.

McCloskey, L.J. (1990) 'The silent heart sings. Special issue: Counselling and therapy for elders.' *Generations 14*, 1, 63–65.

McCloskey, M., Sokol, S. and Goodman, R. (1986) 'Cognitive processes in verbal-number production: inferences from the performance of brain-damaged subjects.' *Journal of Experimental and Psychological Genetics 115*, 4, 307–330.

McCormick, W., Inui, T., Deyo, R. and Wood, R. (1991) 'Long-term care needs of hospitalized persons with AIDS: a prospective cohort study.' *Journal of General Internal Medicine 6*, 1, 27–34.

McLean, A., Stanton, K., Cardenas, D. and Bergerud, D. (1987) 'Memory training combined with the use of oral physosstigmine.' *Brain Injury 1*, 2, 145–159.

McLellan, R. (1988) *The Healing Forces of Music.* New York: Amity House.

McLeod, R., Taylor, D., Cohen, Z. and Cullen, J. (1986) 'Single patient randomised clinical trials.' *Lancet 29*, 726–728.

McLoughlin, I. (1990) 'Musical hallucinations [letter].' *British Journal of Psychiatry 156*, 452.

McNiff, S. (1987) 'Research and scholarship in the creative arts therapies.' *The Arts in Psychotherapy 14*, 285–292.

Mechanic, D. (1986) 'The concept of illness behaviour: culture, situation and personal disposition.' *Psychological Medicine 16*, 1–7.

Meehan, J. (1986) 'Cardiovascular adjustments are part of behavior.' *Behavioral and Brain Sciences 9*, 2, 299.

Melzack, R. (1975) 'The McGill Pain Questionnaire: major properties and scoring methods.' *Pain 1*, 3, 227–299.

Menninger, K. (1959) 'Hope.' *The American Journal of Psychiatry 116*, 12, 481–491.

Merleau-Ponty, M. (1968) *The Visible and the Invisible.* Evanston, IL: Northwestern University Press.

Merlin, D. (1993) 'Human cognitive evolution: what we were, what we are becoming.' *Social Research 60*, 1, 143–170.

Meschede, H., Bender, W. and Pfeiffer, H. (1983) '[Music therapy with psychiatric problem patients] Musiktherapie mit psychiatrischen problempatienten.' *Psychotherapie, Psychosomatik, Medizin und Psychologie 33*, 3, 101–106.

Millard, T., Wacker, D.P., Cooper, L.J., Harding, J., Drew, J., Plagmann, L.A., Asmus, J., McComas, J. and Jensenkovalan, P. (1993) 'A brief component analysis of potential treatment packages in an outpatient clinic setting with young children.' *Journal of Applied Behavior Analysis 26*, 4, 475–476.

Milne, B., Joachim, G. and Niehardt, J. (1986) 'A stress management programme for inflammatory bowel disease patients.' *Journal of Advanced Nursing 11*, 561–567.

Milne, D. (1984) 'The development and evaluation of a structured learning format introduction to behaviour therapy for psychiatric nurses.' *British Journal of Clinical Psychology 23*, Pt 3, 175–185.

Mindell, A. (1989) *Coma: Key to Awakening.* Boston, MA: Shambala.

Moore-Ede, M., Czeisler, C. and Richardson, G. (1983) 'Circadian timekeeping in health and disease.' *New England Journal of Medicine 309*, 469–479.

Moran, G. and Fonagy, P. (1987) 'Psychoanalysis and diabetic control: a single-case study.' *British Journal of Medical Psychology 60*, Pt 4, 357–372.

Moras, K., Telfer, L. and Barlow, D. (1993) 'Efficacy and specific effects data on new treatments: A case study strategy with mixed anxiety-depression.' *Journal of Consulting and Clinical psychology 61*, 412–420.

Moreno, J. (1946) *Psychodrama.* New York: Beacon House.

Moreno, J. (1988) 'The music therapist: creative arts therapist and contemporary shaman.' *Journal of the Arts in Psychotherapy 15*, 271–280.

Morgan, O. and Tilluckdharry, R. (1982) 'Presentation of singing function in severe aphasia.' *West Indian Medical Journal 31*, 159–161.

Morley, J. (1981) 'Music and neurology.' *Clinical and Experimental Neurology 17*, 15–25.

Morris, M. (1986) 'Music and movement for the elderly.' *Nursing Times 82*, 8, 44–45.

Morrongiello, B., Trehub, S., Thorpe, L. and Capodilupo, S. (1985) 'Children's perception of melodies: the role of contour, frequency, and rate of presentation.' *Journal of Experimental Child Psychology 40*, 2, 279–292.

Morss, J. (1992) 'Making waves: deconstruction and developmental psychology.' *Theory and Psychology 2*, 4, 445–465.

Moss, R., Wedding, D. and Sanders, S. (1983) 'The comparative efficacy of relaxation training and masseter EMG feedback in the treatment of TMJ dysfunction.' *Journal of Oral Rehabilitation 10*, 1, 9–17.

Moss, V. (1987) 'The effect of music on anxiety in the surgical patient.' *Perioperative Nursing Quarterly 3*, 1, 9–16.

Moustakas, C. (1990) *Heuristic Research.* London: Sage.

Muenzenmaier, K., Meyer, I. and Ferber, J. (1993) 'Childhood abuse and neglect – reply.' *Hospital and Community Psychiatry 44*, 12, 1193–1194.

Mullooly, V., Levin, R. and Feldman, H. (1988) 'Music for postoperative pain and anxiety.' *Journal of New York State Nurses Association 19*, 3, 4–7.

Murphy, R., Doughty, N. and Nunes, D. (1979) 'Multi-element designs: an alternative to reversal and multi-element evaluative strategies.' *Mental Retardation 17*, 23–27.

Murray, J. (1985) 'The use of health care diaries in the field of psychiatric illness in general practice.' *Psychological Medicine 15*, 827–840.

Murray, L. and Trevarthen, C. (1986) 'The infant's role in mother–infant communications.' *Journal of Child Language 13*, 15–29.

Naeser, M. and Helm-Estabrooks, N. (1985) 'CT scan lesion localization and response to melodic intonation therapy with nonfluent aphasia cases.' *Cortex 21*, 2, 203–223.

Nagai Jacobson, M. and Burkhardt, M. (1989) 'Spirituality: cornerstone of holistic nursing practice.' *Holistic Nursing Practice 3*, 3, 18–26.

Nattiez, J.-J. (1990) *Music and Discourse: Towards a Semiology of Music*. Princeton, NJ: Princeton University Press.

Needleman, J. (1988) *A Sense of the Cosmos*. New York: Arkana.

Neef, N.A. (1993) 'Introduction.' *Journal of Applied Behavior Analysis 26*, 4, 419.

Nelson, H. (1992) 'USA: new AIDS definition.' *The Lancet 340*, 1151.

Neufeldt, J. (1987) 'Helping the IBD patient cope with the unpredictable.' *Nursing 17*, 47–49.

Neugebauer, L. (1992) Therapy as dialogue. Unpublished doctoral dissertation. University Witten Herdecke.

Niederreiter, L. (1990) 'Kreatives gestalten: Kunsttherapie mit HIV-infizierten.' *Münchener Medizinische Wochenschrift 41*, supplement without page numbers.

Norberg, A., Melin, E. and Asplund, K. (1986) 'Reactions to music, touch and object presentation in the final stage of dementia: an exploratory study.' *International Journal of Nursing Studies 23*, 4, 315–323.

Nordoff, P. and Robbins, C. (1971) *Therapy in Music for Handicapped Children*. London: Victor Gollancz.

Nordoff, P. and Robbins, C. (1975) *Music Therapy in Special Education*. London: Macdonald and Evans.

Nordoff, P. and Robbins, C. (1977) *Creative Music Therapy*. New York: John Day.

O'Boyle, M. and Sanford, M. (1988) 'Hemispheric asymmetry in the matching of melodies to rhythm sequences tapped in the right and left palms.' *Cortex 24*, 2, 211–221.

Odenheimer, G. (1989) 'Acquired cognitive disorders of the elderly.' *Medical Clinics of North America 73*, 6, 1383–1411.

Olderog Millard, K.A. and Smith, J.M. (1989) 'The influence of group singing therapy on the behavior of Alzheimer's disease patients.' *Journal of Music Therapy 26*, 2, 58–70.

Oldfield, A. (1995) 'Communicating through music: the balance between following and imitating.' In T. Wigram, B. Saperston and R. West (eds) *The Art and Science of Music Therapy: A Handbook*. Chur, Switzerland: Harwood Academic Publishers.

Oldfield, A. and Adams, M. (1990) 'The effects of music therapy on a group of profoundly mentally handicapped adults.' *Journal of Mental Deficiency Research 34*, Pt 2, 107–125.

Oleske, D., Heinze, S. and Otte, D. (1990) 'The diary as a means of understanding the quality of life of persons with cancer receiving home nursing care.' *Cancer Nurse 13*, 3, 158–166.

Oliveri, G. (1991) 'Malen als versuch der krankheitsbewältigung. Anmerkungen zu den bildern eines HIV-infizierten.' *Psychosozial 14*, 4, 43–47.

Onghena, P. (1992) 'Randomization tests for extensions and variations of ABAB single-case experimental designs – a rejoinder.' *Behavioral Assessment 14*, 2, 153–171.

Palmer, M. (1983) 'Music therapy in a comprehensive program of treatment and rehabilitation for the geriatric resident.' *Activities, Adaptation and Aging 3*, 3, 53–59.

Palmer, M. (1989) 'Music therapy in gerontology: a review and a projection. National Association for Music Therapy California Symposium on Clinical Practices (1987, Costa Mesa, California).' *Music Therapy Perspectives 6*, 52–56.

Parncutt, R. (1987) 'The perception of pulse in musical rhythm.' In A. Gabrielsson (ed) *Action and Perception in Rhythm and Music.* Stockholm: The Royal Swedish Academy of Music.

Parncutt, R. (1994) 'A perceptual model of pulse salience and metrical accent in musical rhythms.' *Music Perception 11*, 4, 409–464.

Parsons, T. (1951) *The Social System.* New York: Free Press.

Patel, H., Keshavan, M. and Martin, S. (1987) 'A case of Charles Bonnet syndrome with musical hallucinations.' *Canadian Journal of Psychiatry 32*, 4, 303–304.

Patterson, J.M. (1988) 'Families experiencing stress.' *Family Systems Medicine 6*, 202–237.

Pavlicevic, M. and Trevarthen, C. (1989) 'A musical assessment of psychiatric states in adults.' *Psychopathology 22*, 6, 325–334.

Pearce, W.B. and Cronen, V.E. (1980) *Communication, Action and Meaning. The Creation of Social Realities.* New York: Praeger Scientific.

Pearce, W.B., Cronen, V.E. and Conklin, F. (1979) 'On what to look for when analyzing communication: an hierarchical model of actors' meanings.' *Communication 4*, 195–220.

Penn, P. (1983) 'Coalitions and binding interactions in families with chronic illness.' *Family Systems Medicine 1*, 16–26.

Persson, P.-G. and Hellers, G. (1987) 'Crohn's disease and ulcerative colitis: a review of dietary studies.' *Scandinavian Journal of Gastroenterology 22*, 385–389.

Peterson, L. and Schick, B. (1993) 'Empirically derived injury prevention rules.' *Journal of Applied Behavior Analysis 26*, 4, 451–460.

Pfeiffer, H., Wunderlich, S., Bender, W., Elz, U. and Horn, B. (1987) 'Music improvisation with schizophrenic patients – a controlled study in the assessment of therapeutic effects.' *Rehabilitation Stuttgart 26*, 184–92.

Philip, Y. (1989) 'Effects of music on patient anxiety in coronary care units [letter].' *Heart and Lung 18*, 3, 322.

Phillips, R. (1988) 'The creative moment: improvising in jazz and psychotherapy.' *Adolescent Psychiatry 15*, 182–193.

Pollack, N.J. and Namazi, K.H. (1992) 'The effect of music participation on the social behavior of Alzheimer's disease patients.' *Journal of Music Therapy 29*, 1, 54–67.

Porchet-Munro, S. (1988) 'Music therapy in support of cancer patients.' *Recent Results in Cancer Research 108*, 289–294.

Porter, R. (1986) 'Psychotherapy research: physiological measures and intrapsychic events.' *Journal of the Royal Society of Medicine 76*, 257–261.

Povel, D. (1984) 'A theoretical framework for rhythm perception.' *Psychological Research 45*, 315–337.

Prange, P. (1990) 'Categories of music therapy at Judson Retirement Community.' *Music Therapy Perspectives 8*, 88–89.

Preza, B., Baboci, H., Ashta, A. and Lleshi, L. (1990) 'The Rett syndrome – clinical presentation of the first 9 Albanian cases.' *Brain Development 12*, 1, 40–43.

Prickett, C.A. and Moore, R.S. (1991) 'The use of music to aid memory of Alzheimer's patients.' *Journal of Music Therapy 28*, 2, 101–110.

Pringle, M. (1984) 'A minority interest: why?' *British Medical Journal 289*, 163–164.

Prinsley, D. (1986) 'Music therapy in geriatric care.' *Australian Nurses Journal 15*, 9, 48–9.

Probst, W. (1976) *Musik in der Sonderschule für Lernbehinderte.* Berlin: Marhold.

Quail, J. and Peavy, V. (1994) 'A phenomenological research study of a client's experience in art therapy.' *The Arts in Psychotherapy 21*, 1, 45–57.

Rabinow, P. (1986) *The Foucault Reader.* London: Penguin.

Rawlinson, M. (1987) 'Foucault's strategy: knowledge, power, and the specificity of truth.' *The Journal of Philosophy and Medicine 12*, 371–395.

Reason, P. and Rowan, J. (1981) *Human Inquiry.* Chichester: John Wiley.

Reed, P. (1987) 'Spirituality and well-being in terminally ill hospitalized adults.' *Research Nursing and Health 10*, 5, 335–344.

Reed, S. (1995) 'The ecological approach to language development: a radical solution to Chomsky's and Quine's problems.' *Language and Communication 15*, 1, 1–29.

Reidy, M., Taggart, M.E. and Asselin, L. (1991) 'Psychosocial needs expressed by the natural caregivers of HIV infected children.' *Aids Care 3*, 3, 331–343.

Reinberg, A. and Halberg, F. (1971) 'Circadian chronopharmacology.' *Annual Review of Pharmacology 11*, 455–492.

Reinhardt, A. and Ficker, F. (1983) 'Erste erfahrungen mit regulativer musiktherapie bei psychiatrischen patienten.' *Psychiatrie, Neurologie, Medizin und Psychologie Leipzig 35*, 10, 604–610.

Reinhardt, A., Rohrborn, H. and Schwabe, C. (1986) 'Regulative musiktherapie (rmt) bei depressiven erkrankungen – ein beitrag zur psychotherapie-entwicklung in der psychiatrie.' *Psychiatrie, Neurologie, Medizin und Psychologie, Leipzig 38*, 9, 547–553.

Ribble, D. (1989) 'Psychosocial support groups for people with HIV infection and AIDS.' *Holistic Nursing Practice 3*, 4, 52–62.

Richter, P. and Benzenhofer, U. (1985) 'Time estimation and chronopathology in endogenous depression.' *Acta Psychiatra Scandanavia 72*, 3, 246–253.

Richter, R. and Kayser, M. (1991) 'Rhythmic abilities in patients with functional cardiac arrythmias.' 7th Meeting of the European Society for Chronobiology, Marburg, 30 May – 2 June.

Rider, M.S. (1985) 'The effects of music imagery and relaxation on adrenal corticosteroids and the re-entrainment of circadian rhythms.' *Journal of Music Therapy 22*, 1, 46–56.

Rider, M.S. (1985a) 'Entrainment mechanisms are involved in pain reduction, muscle relaxation, and music-mediated imagery.' *Journal of Music Therapy 22*, 4, 183–192.

Robbins, A. (1992) 'The play of psychotherapeutic artistry and psychoaesthetics.' *The Arts in Psychotherapy 19*, 177–186.

Robertson, D., Ray, J., Diamond, I. and Edwards, J. (1989) 'Personality profile and mood state of patients with inflammatory bowel disease.' *Gut 30*, 5, 623–626.

Robinson, D. (1971) *The Process of Becoming Ill.* London: Routledge and Kegan Paul.

Robinson, E.J. and Mitchell, P. (1994) 'Young children's false-belief reasoning – interpretation of messages is no easier than the classic task.' *Developmental Psychology 30*, 1, 67–72.

Roche, J. (1989) 'Spirituality and the ALS patient.' *Rehabilitation Nursing 14*, 3, 139–141.

Rose, A. (1984) 'Chronic illness in general practice.' *Family Practice 1*, 162–167.

Rose, T. (1978) 'The functional relationship between artificial food colors and hyperactivity.' *Journal of Applied Behavior Analysis 11*, 439–446.

Rosling, L.K. and Kitchen, J. (1992) 'Music and drawing with institutionalized elderly. Miniconference in Music and Geriatrics (1990, Coquitlam, Canada).' *Activities, Adaptation and Aging 17*, 2, 27–38.

Ross, L. (1994) 'Spiritual aspects of nursing.' *Journal of Advanced Nursing 19*, 439–447.

Ross, L.V., Friman, P.C. and Christophersen, E.R. (1993) 'An appointment-keeping improvement package for outpatient pediatrics – systematic replication and component analysis.' *Journal of Applied Behavior Analysis 26*, 4, 461–467.

Ross, M. (1990) 'The relationship between life events and mental health in homosexual men.' *Journal of Clinical Psychology 46*, 4, 402–411.

Rossi, E. (1987) 'From mind to molecule: a state-dependent memory, learning and behavior theory of mind–body healing.' *Advances 4*, 46–60.

Ruud, E. (1995) 'Music in the media: the soundtrack behind the construction of identity.' *Young* (in press).

Saari, C. (1986) 'The use of metaphor in therapeutic communication with young adolescents.' *Child and Adolescent Social Work 3*, 1, 16–17.

Sacks, O. (1986) *The Man who Mistook his Wife for a Hat.* London: Pan.

Sadler, J. and Hulgus, Y. (1990) 'Knowing, valuing, casting: clues to revising the biopsychosocial model.' *Comprehensive Psychiatry 31*, (3), 185–195.

Safranek, M., Koshland, G. and Raymond, G. (1982) 'Effect of auditory rhythm on muscle activity.' *Physical Therapy 62*, 161–168.

Salkovskis, P. (1983) 'Treatment of an obsessional patient using habituation to audiotaped ruminations.' *British Journal of Clinical Psychology 22*, Pt 4, 311–313.

Salkovskis, P. and Westbrook, D. (1989) 'Behaviour therapy and obsessional ruminations: can failure be turned into success?' *Behavioral Research and Therapy 27*, 2, 149–60.

Salmon, D., Thal, L., Butters, N. and Heindel, W. (1990) 'Longitudinal evaluation of dementia of the Alzheimer type: a comparison of 3 standardized mental status examinations.' *Neurology 40*, 8, 1225–1230.

Sammons, L. (1984) 'The use of music by women during childbirth.' *Journal of Nursing and Midwifery 29*, 4, 266–270.

Sanderson, I.R. (1986) 'Chronic inflammatory bowel disease.' *Clinical Gastroenterology 15*, 71–87.

Sandman, C. (1984) 'Afferent influences on the cortical evoked response.' In M. Coles, L. Jennings and J. Stern (eds) *Psychological Perspectives (Festschrift for Beatrice and John Lacey).* Stroudberg, PA: Hutchinson and Ross.

Sandman, C. (1984a) 'Augmentation of the auditory event related to potentials of the brain during diastole.' *International Journal of Physiology 2*, 111–119.

Saudia, T.L., Kinney, M.R., Brown, K.C. and Young, W.L. (1991) 'Health locus of control and helpfulness of prayer.' *Heart Lung 20*, 1, 60–65.

Scambler, A., Scambler, G. and Craig, D. (1981) 'Kinship and friendship networks and women's demand for primary care.' *Journal of the Royal College of General Practitioners 31*, 746–750.

Schlottmann, A. and Anderson, N.H. (1994) 'Children's judgements of expected value.' *Developmental Psychology 30*, 1, 56–66.

Schmais, C. (1988) 'Creative arts therapies and shamanism: a comparison.' *Journal of the Arts in Psychotherapy 15*, 281–291.

Schmuttermayer, R. (1983) 'Möglichkeiten der einbeziehung gruppenmusiktherapeutischer methoden in die Behandlung von Psychotikern.' *Psychiatrie, Neurologie, Medizin und Psychologie, Leipzig 35*, 1, 49–53.

Schneider, S., Taylor, S., Hammen, C., Kemeny, M. and Dudley, J. (1991) 'Factor influencing suicide intent in gay and bisexual suicide ideators: differing models for men with and without human immunodeficiency virus.' *Journal of Personal and Social Psychology 61*, 5, 776–788.

Schorr, J. (1993) 'Music and pattern change in chronic pain.' *Advanced Nursing Science 15*, 4, 27–36.

Scrambler, A., Scrambler, G. and Craig, D. (1981) 'Kinship and friendship networks and women's demand for primary care.' *Journal of the Royal College of General Practitioners 31*, 746–750.

Schroeder-Sheker, T. (1993) 'Music for the dying: the new field of music thanatology.' *Advances 9*, 1, 36–48.

Schullian, D. and Schoen, M. (1948) *Music and Medicine.* New York: Henry Schuman.

Schwabe, C. (1978) *Methodik der Musiktherapie und deren theoretische Grundlagen.* Leipzig: Joh. Ambrosius Barth.

Schwalbe, M. (1993) 'Goffman against postmodernism: emotion and the reality of the self.' *Symbolic Interaction 16*, 4, 333–350.

Seed, A. (1995) 'Conducting a longitudinal study: an unsanitized account.' *Journal of Advanced Nursing 21*, 845–852.

Segal, R. (1990) 'Helping older mentally retarded persons expand their socialization skills through the use of expressive therapies. (Special Issue: Activities with developmentally disabled elderly and older adults.)' *Activities, Adaptation and Aging 15*, 1–2, 99–109.

Shadish, W. and Fuller, S. (1994) *The Social Psychology of Science.* London: Guilford Press.

Shah, I. (1964) *The Sufis.* London: Octagon Press.

Sharon, J. (1985) 'Healing and the arts.' *Child-Today 14*, 3, 29–31.

Shibles, A. (1995) 'Hanslick on hearing beauty.' *Iyyun, The Jerusalem Philosophical Quarterly 44*, 73–89.

Shivananda, S., Pena, A.S., Nap, M., Weterman, I.T., Mayberry, J.F., Ruitenberg, E.J. and Hoedemaeker, P.J. (1987) 'Epidemiology of Crohn's disease in Regio Lieden, the Netherlands.' *Gastroenterology 93*, 966–974.

Shuren, J., Geldmacher, D. and Heilman, K. (1993) 'Nonoptic aphasia: Aphasia with preserved confrontation naming in Alzheimer's disease.' *Neurology 43*, 1900–1907.

Siegel, L.S. (1993) 'Amazing new discovery – Piaget was wrong.' *Canadian Psychology-Psychologie Canadienne 34*, 3, 239–245.

Siegman, A. *et al.* (1987) 'Expressive vocal behavior and the severity of coronary disease.' *Psychosomatic Medicine 49*, 545–561.

Sipiora, M. (1993) 'Repression in the child's conception of the world: a phenomenological reading of Piaget.' *Philosophical Psychology 6*, 2, 167–179.

Slifer, K.J., Penn Jones, K., Cataldo, M., Conner, R. and Zerhouni, E. (1993) 'Behavior analysis of motion control for pediatric neuroimaging.' *Journal of Applied Behavior Analysis 26*, 4, 469–470.

Smith, B.B. (1992) 'Treatment of dementia: healing through cultural arts.' *Pride Institute Journal of Long Term Home Health Care 11*, 3, 37–45.

Smith, D.S. (1990) 'Therapeutic treatment effectiveness as documented in the gerontology literature: implications for music therapy.' *Music Therapy Perspectives 8*, 36–40.

Smith, D.S. (1991) 'A comparison of group performance and song familiarity on cued recall tasks with older adults.' *Journal of Music Therapy 28*, 1, 2–13.

Smith, G.H. (1986) 'A comparison of the effects of three treatment interventions on cognitive functioning of Alzheimer patients.' *Music Therapy 6a*, 1, 41–56.

Smith, S. (1990) 'The unique power of music therapy benefits Alzheimer's patients.' *Activities, Adaptation and Aging 14*, 4, 59–63.

Smith, T. and Rhodewalt, F. (1986) 'States, traits and processes: a transactional alternative to the individual difference assumptions in Type A behavior and physiological reactivity.' *Journal of Research in Personality 20*, 717–729.

Smyth, P. and Bellemare, D. (1988) 'Spirituality, pastoral care, and religion: the need for clear distinctions.' *Journal of Palliative Care 4*, 86–88.

Soeken, K. and Carson, V. (1987) 'Responding to the spiritual needs of the chronically ill.' *Nursing Clinics of North America 22*, 3, 603–611.

Solomon, G. (1987) 'Psychoneuroimmunology: interactions between central nervous system and immune system.' *Journal of Neuroscience Research 18*, 1–9.

Solomon, G., Fiatarone, M., Benton, D., Morlet, J., Bloom, E. and Makinodan, T. (1988) 'Psychoimmunologic and endorphin function in the aged.' *Annals New York Academy of Sciences 521*, 43–58.

Sontag, S. (1990) *Illness as Metaphor.* New York: Anchor Books, Doubleday.

Spickard, J. (1994) 'Body, nature and culture in spiritual healing.' In H. Johannessen, S. Gosvig Olesen and J.O. Andersen (eds) *Studies in Alternative Therapy 2*, 65–81. Odense: Denamrk: International Research in Alternative Therapies (INRAT) Odense University Press.

Spiegel, D. (1991) 'A psychosocial intervention and survival time of patients with metastatic breast cancer.' *Advances 7*, 3, 10–19.

Spieker, S.J. and Bensley, L. (1994) 'Roles of living arrangements and grandmother social support in adolescent mothering and infant attachment.' *Developmental Psychology 30*, 1, 102–111.

Spielberger, C. (1983) *Manual for State Trait Anxiety Inventory.* Palo Alto, CA: Consulting Psychologists' Press, Inc.

Spitzer, W. (1987) 'State of the science 1986: quality of life and functional status as target variables for research.' *Journal of Chronic Diseases 6*, 465–471.

Standley, J.M. (1986) 'Music research in medical/dental treatment: meta analysis and clinical applications.' *Journal of Music Therapy 23*, 2, 56–122.

Stanley, P. and Miller, M. (1993) 'Short-term art therapy with an adolescent male.' *The Arts in Psychotherapy 20*, 397–402.

Stanwyck, D. and Arnson, C. (1986) 'Is personality related to illness?' *Advances 3*, 4–15.

Stark, L.J., Knapp, L.G., Bowen, A.M., Powers, S.W., Jelalian, E., Evans, S., Passero, M.A., Mulvihill, M.M. and Hovell, M. (1993) 'Increasing calorie consumption in children with cystic fibrosis – replication with 2-year follow-up.' *Journal of Applied Behavior Analysis 26*, 4, 435–450.

Steedman, M. (1977) 'The perception of musical rhythm and metre.' *Perception 6*, 555–569.

Steg, R. (1990) 'Determining the cause of dementia.' *Nebraska Medical Journal 75*, 4, 59–63.

Stein, M., Keller, S. and Schleifer, S. (1985) 'Stress and neuro-immodulation: the role of depression and neuroendocrine function.' *The Journal of Immunology 135*, 827s–833s.

Steinberg, R. and Raith, L. (1985) 'Music psychopathology. I. Musical tempo and psychiatric disease.' *Psychopathology 18*, 5–6, 254–264.

Steinberg, R. and Raith, L. (1985a) 'Music psychopathology. II. Assessment of musical expression.' *Psychopathology 18*, 5–6, 265–273.

Steinberg, R., Raith, L., Rossnagl, G. and Eben, E. (1985) 'Music psychopathology. III. Musical expression and psychiatric disease.' *Psychopathology 18*, 5–6, 274–285.

Steiner, R. (1970) *Theosophy*. New York: Anthroposophic Press.

Stern, D. (1985) *The Interpersonal World of the Infant*. New York: Basic Books.

Stern, D., Jaffe, J., Bebbe, B. and Bennett, S. (1975) 'Vocalizing in unison and in alternation: two modes of communication within the mother infant dyad.' *Annals of the New York Academy of Science 263*, 89–100.

Stierlin, H. (1989) 'The psychosomatic dimension: relational aspects.' *Family Systems Medicine 7*, 3, 254–263.

Street, R.J. and Cappella, J. (1989) 'Social and linguistic factors influencing adaptation in children's speech.' *Journal of Psycholinguistic Research 18*, 5, 497–519.

Strober, W. and James, S.P. (1986) 'The immunologic basis of inflammatory bowel disease.' *Journal of Clinical Immunology 6*, 415–432.

Stuart, E., Deckro, J. and Mandle, C. (1989) 'Spirituality in health and healing: a clinical program.' *Holistic Nursing Practice 3*, 3, 35–46.

Summer, L. (1981) 'Guided imagery and music with the elderly.' *Music Therapy 1*, 1, 39–42.

Summers, W., DeBoynton, V., Marsh, G. and Majovski, L. (1990) 'Comparison of seven psychometric instruments used for evaluation of treatment effect in Alzheimer's dementia.' *Neuroepidemiology 9*, 4, 193–207.

Svedlund, J., Sjödin, I., Ottosson, J.-O. and Dotevall, G. (1983) 'Controlled study of psychotherapy in irritable bowel syndrome.' *Lancet 2*, 589–591.

Swartz, K., Hantz, E., Crummer, G., Walton, J. and Frisina, R. (1989) 'Does the melody linger on? Music cognition in Alzheimer's disease.' *Seminars in Neurology 9*, 152–158.

Tang, W., Yao, X. and Zheng, Z. (1994) 'Rehabilitative effect of music therapy for residual schizophrenia.' *British Journal of Psychiatry 165*, (Supplement 24), 38–44.

Tarter, R.E., Switala, J., Carra, J. and Edwards, K. (1987) 'Inflammatory bowel disease: psychiatric status of patients before and after disease onset.' *International Journal of Psychiatry 17*, 173–181.

Tauber, A. (1994) 'A typology of Nietzsche's biology.' *Biology and Philosophy 9*, 25–44.

Tee, D. (1987) 'Another look at the interaction of psyche and soma.' *Complementary Medical Research 2*, 1–2.

Thaut, M. (1985) 'The use of auditory rhythm and rhythmic speech to aid temporal muscular control in children with gross motor dysfunction.' *The Journal of Music Therapy 22*, 129–145.

Thaut, M. (1987) 'Visual versus auditory (musical) stimulus preferences in autistic children: a pilot study.' *Journal of Autism and Developmental Disorders 17*, 3, 425–432.

Thaut, M. (1988) 'Measuring musical responsiveness in autistic children: a comparative analysis of improvised musical tone sequences of autistic, normal, and mentally retarded individuals.' *Journal of Autism and Developmental Disorders 18*, 4, 561–571.

Thomas, K. (1995) 'Biorhythms in infants and role of the care environment.' *Journal of Perinatal and Neonatal Nursing 9*, 2, 61–75.

Thomas, L. and Harri-Augstein, E. (1985) *Self-organised Learning: Foundations of a Conversational Science for Psychology*. London: Routledge and Kegan Paul.

Tiep, B., Burns, M., Kao, D., Madison, R. and Herrera, J. (1986) 'Pursed lips breathing training using ear oximetry.' *Chest 90*, 2, 218–221.

Tournier, P. (1981) *Creative Suffering*. London: SCM Press.

Touw-Otten, F. and Spreeuwenberg, C. (1985) 'Multi-disciplinary research between natural and social sciences in general medical practice.' *Family Practice 2*, 42–45.

Trabucchi, E., Mukenge, S., Barrati, C., Colombo, R. and Fregoni, F.W. (1986) 'Differential diagnosis of Crohn's disease of the colon from ulcerative colitis: ultrastructure study with the scanning electron microscope.' *International Journal of Tissue Reactions 8*, 79–84.

Trevarthen, C. (1985) 'Facial expressions of emotion in mother infant interaction.' *Human Neurobiology 4*, 4–21.

Tröhler, U. (1988) 'The history of therapeutic evaluation.' In J. Watt (ed) *Talking Health*. London: Royal Society of Medicine.

Tsouyopoulos, N. (1984) 'German philosophy and the rise of modern clinical medicine.' *Theoretical Medicine 5*, 345–347.

Tsouyopoulos, N. (1994) 'Postmodernist theory and the physician–patient relationship.' *Theoretical Medicine 15*, 267–275.

Tsunoda, T. (1983) 'The difference in the cerebral processing mechanism for musical sounds between Japanese and non-Japanese and its relation to mother tongue.' In R. Spintge and R. Droh (eds) *Musik in der Medizin*. Berlin: Springer Verlag.

Tüpker, R. (1990) 'Auf der suche nach angemessenen formen wissenschaftlichen vorgehens in kunsttherapeutischer forschung.' In P. Petersen (ed) *Ansätze kunsttherapeutischer Forschung*. Berlin: Springer-Verlag.

Tyson, J. (1989) 'Meeting the needs of dementia.' *Nursing the Elderly 1*, 5, 18–19.

Ulrich, R. (1984) 'View through a window may influence recovery from surgery.' *Science 224*, 420–421.

Underwood, P., Gray, D. and Winkler, R. (1985) 'Cutting open Newton's apple to find the cause of gravity: a reply to Julian Tudor Hart on the future of general practice.' *British Medical Journal 291*, 1322–1324.

Updike, P. (1990) 'Music therapy results for ICU patients.' *Dimensions of Critical Care Nursing 9*, 1, 39–45.

van der Geest, S. (1994) 'Christ as a pharmacist: medical symbols in German devotion.' *Social Science and Medicine 39*, 5, 727–732.

Van Spreuuwel, J.P., Lindeman, J. and Meijer, C.J. (1986) 'Quantitative analysis of immunoglobulin-containing cells in gastrointestinal pathology.' *The International Academy of Analytical and Quantitative Cytology and Histology 8*, 314–320.

Vandenberg, B. (1991) 'Is epistemology enough? An existential consideration of development.' *American Psychologist 46*, 12, 1278–1286.

VanderArk, S., Newman, I. and Bell, S. (1983) 'The effects of music participation on quality of life of the elderly.' *Music Therapy 3*, 1, 71–81.

Vedeler, D. (1994) 'Infant intentionality as object directedness: a method for observation.' *Scandinavian Journal of Psychology 35*, 343–366.

Velanovitch, V. (1992) 'The function of the case report in medical epistemology.' *Theoretical Surgery 7*, 91–94.

Vergo, P. (1977) *The Blue Rider*. London: Phaidon.

Vincent, S. and Thompson, J. (1929) 'The effects of music on the human blood pressure.' *Lancet 1*, 9 March, 534–537.

von Hofsten, C. (1993) 'Prospective control: a basic aspect of action development.' *Human Development 36*, 253–270.

Vygotsky, L. (1978) *Mind in Society*. Cambridge, MA: Harvard University Press.

Wagner, M. and Hannon, R. (1981) 'Hemispheric asymmetries in faculty and student musicians and nonmusicians during melody recognition tasks.' *Brain and Language 13*, 379–388.

Wagner, R.K., Torgesen, J.K. and Rashotte, C.A. (1994) 'Development of reading-related phonological processing abilities – new evidence of bidirectional causality from a latent variable longitudinal study.' *Developmental Psychology 30*, 1, 73–87.

Walker, A. (1979) 'Music and the unconscious.' *British Medical Journal 2*, 1641–1643.

Walker, B. and Sandman, C. (1979) 'Human visual evoked responses are related to heart rate.' *Journal of Comparative and Physiological Psychology 93*, 717–729.

Walker, B. and Sandman, C. (1982) 'Visual evoked potentials change as heart rate and carotid pressure change.' *Psychophysiology 19*, 520–527.

Walsh, J., Welch, H. and Larson, E. (1990) 'Survival of outpatients with Alzheimer-type dementia.' *Annals of Internal Medicine 113*, 6, 429–434.

Walter, B. (1983) 'A little music: why the dying aren't allowed to die.' *Nursing Life 3*, 5, 52–7.

Warde, A. (1994) 'Consumption, identity-formation and uncertainty.' *Sociology 28*, 4, 877–898.

Warwick, A. (1995) 'Music therapy in the education service: research with autistic children and their mothers.' In T. Wigram, B. Saperston and R. West (eds) *The Art and Science of Music Therapy: A Handbook*. Chur, Switzerland: Harwood Academic Publishers.

Waterhouse, R. (1993) 'The inverted gaze.' In D. Morgan and S. Scott (eds) *Body Matters*. Brighton: The Falmer Press.

Watzlawick, P. (1984) *The Invented Reality*. New York: W.W. Norton and Co.

Watzlawick, P., Beavin, J. and Jackson, D. (1967) *Pragmatics of Human Communication*. New York: W.W. Norton and Co.

Wear, D. (1993) 'Your breasts/sliced off: literary images of breast cancer.' *Woman and Health 20*, 4, 81–100.

Weaver, T.L. and Clum, G.A. (1993) 'Early family environments and traumatic experiences associated with borderline personality disorder.' *Journal of Consulting and Clinical Psychology 61*, 6, 1068–1075.

Wein, B. (1987) 'Body and soul music.' *American Health 6*, 3, 66–75.

Weinert, S. (1992) 'Deficits in Acquiring Language Structure – The Importance of Using Prosodic Cues.' *Applied Cognitive Psychology 6*, 6, 545–571.

Wengel, S., Burke, W. and Holemon, D. (1989) 'Musical hallucinations: the sounds of silence?' *Journal of the American Geriatric Society 37*, 2, 163–166.

Wenglert, L. and Rosén, A.-S. (1995) 'Optimism, self-esteem, mood and subjective health.' *Personal and Individual Difference 18*, 5, 653–661.

Werle, M.A., Murphy, T.B. and Budd, K.S. (1993) 'Treating chronic food refusal in young children – home-based parent training.' *Journal of Applied Behavior Analysis 26*, 4, 421–433.

Wesecky, A. (1986) 'Music therapy for children with Rett syndrome.' *American Journal of Medical Genetics-Supplement 1*, 253–257.

Wheeler, B. (ed) (1995) *Music Therapy Research: Quantitative and Qualitative Perspectives.* Phoenixville: Barcelona.

Wiedermann, C. and Wiedermann, M. (1988) 'Psychoimmunology: systems medicine at the molecular level.' *Family Systems Medicine 6,* 94–106.

Wienties, C. and Grossman, P. (1994) 'Overreactivity of the psyche or the soma? Interindividual associations between psychosomatic symptoms, anxiety, heart rate, and end-tidal partial carbon dioxide pressure.' *Psychosomatic Medicine 56,* 533–540.

Wigram, T. (1995) 'A model of assessment and differential diagnosis of handicap in children through the medium of music therapy.' In T. Wigram, B. Saperston and R. West (eds) *The Art and Science of Music Therapy: A Handbook.* Chur, Switzerland: Harwood Academic Publishers.

Wilkin, D. (1986) 'Outcomes research in general practice.' *Journal of the Royal College of General Practitioners,* January, 4–5.

Wilkinson, S. and Kitzinger, C. (1993) 'Whose breast is it anyway? A feminist consideration of advice and treatment for breast cancer.' *Women's Studies International Forum 16,* 3, 229–238.

Willoughby, C. and Polatajko, H. (1995) 'Motor problems in children with developmental coordination disorder: review of the literature.' *The American Journal of Occupational Therapy 49,* 8, 787–794.

Wilson, B. (1987) 'Single-case experimental designs in neuropsychological rehabilitation.' *Journal of Clinical and Experimental Neuropsychology 9,* 5, 527–544.

Wilson, F. and Roehmann, F. (1987) *Music and Child Development.* St Louis, MO: MMB.

Winnicott, D. (1971) 'Transitional objects and transitional phenomena.' In *Playing with Reality.* New York: Basic Books.

Wittig, R. (1989) 'Adjustment, stress and coping with stress in breast cancer. Results of single case studies.' *Zeitschrift für Klinische Psychologie Psychopathologie Psychotherapie 37,* 3, 303–316.

Wolf, T., Dralle, P., Morse, E., Simon, P., Balson, P., Gaumer, R. and Williams, M. (1991) 'A biopsychosocial examination of symptomatic and asymptomatic HIV-infected patients.' *International Journal of Psychiatry in Medicine 21,* 3, 263–279.

Wolfe, D. (1978) 'Pain rehabilitation and music therapy.' *Journal of Music Therapy 15,* 162–178.

Wong, C.A. and Bramwell, L. (1992) 'Uncertainty and anxiety after mastectomy for breast cancer.' *Cancer Nursing 15,* 5, 363–371.

Yates, P. (1993) 'Towards a reconceptualization of hope for patients with a diagnosis of cancer.' *Journal of Advanced Nursing 18,* 701–706.

Yin, R. (1989) *Case Study Research: Design and Methods.* Newbury Park, CA: Sage.

You, H. (1994) 'Defining rhythm: aspects of an anthropology of rhythm.' *Culture, Medicine and Psychiatry 18,* 361–384.

Zappella, M. (1986) 'Motivational conflicts in Rett syndrome.' *American Journal of Medical Genetics Supplement 1,* 143–51.

Zigmond, A.S. and Snaith, R.P. (1983) 'The hospital anxiety and depression scale.' *Acta Psychiatrica Scandinavica 67,* 361–370.

Zillmer, E., Fowler, P., Gutnick, H. and Becker, E. (1990) 'Comparison of two cognitive bedside screening instruments in nursing home residents: a factor analytic study.' *Journal of Gerontology 45,* 2, 69–74.

Zimmerman, L. (1989) 'Reply to a letter asking what "white noise" was.' *Heart and Lung* *18*, 3, 322.

Zimmerman, L., Pierson, M. and Marker, J. (1988) 'Effects of music on patient anxiety in coronary care units.' *Heart and Lung 17*, 5, 560–566.

Zimmerman, L., Pozehl, B., Duncan, K. and Schmitz, R. (1989) 'Effects of music in patients who had chronic cancer pain.' *Western Journal of Nursing Research 11*, 3, 298–309.

Subject
Index

References in italic indicate figures or tables.

Author Index

Lightning Source UK Ltd.
Milton Keynes UK
10 December 2010

164175UK00001B/14/A

9 781853 022968